To David Bull,

who made this book possible

Contents

THIRD EDITION

Self-management of Long-term Health Conditions

A Handbook for People with Chronic Disease

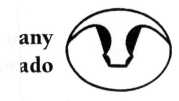

...any
...ado

Published by Bull Publishing Company

P.O. Box 1377

Boulder, CO, USA 80306

www.bullpub.com

Supported by AHCPR Grant HSO 6680 and California State Tobacco-Related Disease Research Program Award 1RT 156.

Library of Congress Cataloging-in-Publication Data

Lorig, Kate.
Self-management of long-term health conditions : a handbook for people with chronic disease / Kate Lorig, DrPH [and five others]. -- Third edition.
    pages cm
Includes bibliographical references and index.

ISBN 978-1-936693-62-7 (alk. paper)

1. Chronic diseases--Psychological aspects. 2. Chronically ill--Care. 3. Long-term care of the sick. 4. Self-care, Health. I. Title.

RC108.L56512 2014
616'.044--dc23

                                                                2013046195

Printed and bound by CPI Group (UK) Ltd, Croydon, CR0 4YY

Third Edition

19 18 17 16 15 14 13 12 11 10 9 8 7 6 5 4

Interior design and project management: Dovetail Publishing Services
Cover design and production: Shannon Bodie, Lightbourne, Inc.

Acknowledgments to the UK Third Edition

Acknowledgments to the UK original and second editions

Thank you to the many people who have helped compile the original and second editions of this helpbook. In particular, Jim Bull, Kate Lorig, Dr. Peter Collins, Jane Cooper, Ayesha Dost, Roy Jones, Anne Kennedy, Dave McHattie, Pete Moore, Brendan O'Rourke, Alison Pollard, Jim Phillips, Dr. Vivienne Press, Jean Thompson and Carolyn Townsend. We would also like to thank the many participants and tutors that have given their feedback after attending a self-management course and using the helpbook.

Acknowledgments to the original US Edition

Many people have helped us write this book. Among the most important are the first 1,000 participants of the Stanford University Chronic Disease Self-Management study. These have been followed by thousands of other course partici-pants in the United States, Australia, New Zealand, Canada, and Great Britain. All of the people, along with our wonderful course leaders, have told us what information they needed and helped us make adjustments as we went along.

There are also many professionals who have assisted us: Susan Kayman, Suephy Chen, Sandra Wilson, Margo Harris, Nancy Branni-gan, Jim Phillips, Jean Thompson, Lynne New-combe, John Lynch, Mary Hobbs, Marty Klein, Nazanin Dashtara, Vivian Vestal, María Hernán-dez-Marin, Richard Rubio, and Laurie Doyle. To all of you, your help has been greatly received. A special thanks to Gloria Samuel, who kept us all on track and put this book together.

Finally, thanks to David Bull to whom this book is dedicated. David was our first publisher and had faith in this project that allowed us to proceed. Without him, there may never have been a book. His son Jim has continued the fam-ily tradition with support and encouragement for this third edition.

Acknowledgments to the UK third edition

The Reference Group

Kathy Hawley, M.A., PhD, Post Grad Diploma (Research Theory and Methodology).

Jean Thompson (MBE), Director *Talking Health, Taking Action* and Lead T-Trainer for the UK

Cheryl Berry, *Self-management UK* (Formerly EPPCIC)

Sharon Hudswell, EPP/Self-care Lead, Guys and St Thomas' Community Health Services

Clare Evans, Self-Management Programme Manager, Office of Public Health, Dudley Metropolitan Borough Council

Jacqui Pollock, *Self-Management* UK (Formerly EPPCIC)

James Locke, Independent Self-Management Practitioner.

Special Thanks to:

Dr. Daniele Bryden, for her detailed knowledge on critical and end of life care and also for her knowledge of medical ethics and the legal system (Chapter 19); The Clinical Advisory Team at *Diabetes UK* for answering all our questions on diabetes management (Chapters 18 and 11); Dr. Chris Green (Oxford), for his detailed knowledge of diabetes and his suggestions (Chapter 18); Angela Hawley, the Long-Term Conditions Team, Department of Health, for her help and advice, for reading through the book and for being instrumental in obtaining a small grant from the DH to assist with the rewriting of the UK edition; Jean, a patient, for her comments on heart disease (Chapter 16); Rachy, a patient, for her comments and suggestions on COPD (Chapter 15); Susan Summers, Head of Long,Term Conditions, Nursing Directorate, NHS England, who read 15 Chapters of the book in detail, and for her suggestions to add additional information; Professor David Taylor, University College London, for pointing us in the direction of *Healthy Living Pharmacies* (Chapter 13).

Origins of lay-led self-management in the UK

"What lies behind us and what lies before us are tiny matters compared to what lies within us."

—Emerson

A lay-led structured training programme was pioneered by Professor Kate Lorig of Stanford University, California in the 1970s. Her initial practical approach to self-management was enhanced with reference to her colleague Albert Bandura's work on social learning theory. Their first courses were based on the experiences of people living with arthritis. In the UK Arthritis Care built upon this work and led the way for other organisations to make use of Stanford self-management programmes.

In the late 1990s the Department of Health (England) supported the Long-term Medical Conditions Alliance (LMCA) to work with other national voluntary organisations to increase knowledge about, and use of, lay led self-management programmes among people living with long-term conditions. At the same time, the Chief Medical Officer for England pioneered the establishment of the NHS Expert Patients Programme (NHS EPP), which was launched in 2002. Over the next five years NHS EPP delivered programmes and built capacity among third sector agencies and Primary Care Trusts (PCTs) in England, while the development of self-management within the rest of the UK was taken forward by initiatives within each of the Nations. On 1 April, 2007 the Expert Patients Programme Community Interest Company (EPP CIC) was created and delivery of Stanford programmes is now carried out by a wide range of organisations.

There are two capacity building bodies dedicated to supporting the growing number of organisations delivering Stanford University and other self-management interventions. *Talking Health, Taking Action* is the only UK organisation exclusively dedicated to providing self-management capacity building training and support; and QISMET (Quality Institute for Self-management Education and Training) provides independent verification of programmes through their Certification Schemes.

There is now widespread recognition of the potential for partnerships between patients and health care professionals – working together to make decisions about an individual's care – to transform the way in which people living with long term conditions make use of health care resources. However, in order to make such shared decision making an everyday reality there is a need for approaches that support patients to develop the ability to participate in their healthcare. Stanford University programmes provide this by supporting people living with long term conditions to acquire the knowledge, information, confidence and skills needed to ensure that there are "no decisions about me without me". The Stanford approach is therefore as relevant now as it has ever been; providing part of the future solution to the economic and demographic challenges that growing numbers of people living with long term conditions will bring to the UK over the next 25 years.

February 2014
Jean Thompson, MBE
Talking Health, Taking Action

Disclaimer

This book is not intended to replace common sense, professional medical or psychological advice. You should seek and get appropriate professional evaluation and treatment for problems – especially unusual, unexplained, severe, or persistent symptoms. Many symptoms and diseases require and benefit from specific medical or psychological evaluation and treatment. Don't deny yourself proper professional care.

- If your symptoms or problems persist beyond a reasonable period despite using self-care recommendations, you should consult a health professional. What is a reasonable period will vary; if you're not sure and you're feeling anxious, consult a health care professional.

- If you receive professional advice in conflict with this book, you should rely upon the guidance provided by your health care professional. He or she is likely to be able to take your specific situation, history, and needs into consideration.

- If you are having thoughts of harming yourself in any way, please seek professional care immediately.

This book is as accurate as its publisher and authors can make it, but we cannot guarantee that it will work for you in every case. The authors and publisher disclaim any and all liability for any claims or injuries that you may believe arose from following the recommendations set forth in this book. This book is only a guide; your common sense, good judgment, and partnership with health professionals are also needed.

Editor's Notes

This handbook draws on the material in the US fourth edition of *Living a Healthy Life with Chronic Conditions*, by Kate Lorig, Halsted Holman, David Sobel, Diana Laurent, Virginia González, Marian Minor and Peg Harrison.

While keeping to the integrity of the US edition, some text has been revised for UK users of the handbook taking into account feedback received.

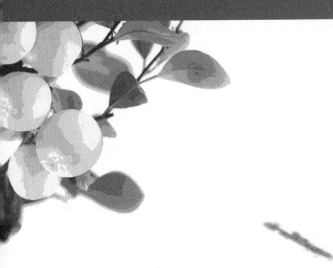

Overview of Self-Management

NOBODY WANTS TO HAVE A CHRONIC LONG-TERM CONDITION. Unfortunately, most of us will experience two or more of these conditions during our lives. This book has been written to help people with a chronic illness explore healthy ways to live with a physical or mental condition. This may seem like a strange concept. How can you have a medical condition and yet live a healthy life? To answer this, we need to look at what happens with most long-term health problems. These conditions, such as heart disease, diabetes, depression, liver disease, bipolar disorder, emphysema, or any one of a host of others, cause most people to experience fatigue and to lose physical strength and endurance. In addition, they may cause emotional distress, such as frustration, anger, anxiety, or a sense of help-lessness. Health is *soundness of body and mind*, and a healthy life is one that seeks that soundness. Therefore, a healthy way to live with a long term condition is to work at overcoming the physical, mental, and emotional problems caused by the condition. The challenge is to learn how to function at your best, regardless of the difficulties life

1

presents. The goal is to achieve the things you want to do and to get pleasure from life. That is what this book is all about.

Before we go any further, let's talk about how to use this book. In it you will find information to help you learn and practise self-management skills. This is not a textbook; you might think of it as a workbook. You do not need to read every word in every chapter. The best approach is to read the first two chapters and then use the table of contents to find the information you need. Feel free to skip around and to make notes in the book. This will help you learn the skills you need in order to follow your individual path.

You will not find any miracles or cures in these pages. Rather, you will find hundreds of tips and ideas to make your life easier. This advice comes from doctors and other health professionals, as well as people like you who have learned to manage their health problems in a positive way. Please note that we said *manage in a positive way*. There is no way to avoid managing a

long-term condition. If you choose to do nothing, that is one way of managing. If you only take medication, that is another. If, on the other hand, you choose to be a positive self-manager and undergo all the best treatments that health care professionals have to offer, and to be proactive in your own day-to-day management, then you will live a healthier life.

In this chapter we discuss long-term health conditions in general as well as pointing out the most common problems. In addition, we give some guidance on the self-management skills that are unique to particular conditions. You will soon see that the problems and skills have much more in common than you think, no matter what the health problem may be. This is good news because most people have more than one condition. Therefore, learning common life skills allows you to successfully manage your life, not just a single condition. This book gives you the tools you need to become a great manager of both your long-term conditions and all the other aspects of your life.

What Exactly Is a Long-term Health Condition?

Very simply, a long term condition is a health condition that cannot be cured but can be managed through medication or therapy.

Health problems can be characterised as either *acute* or *chronic*. Acute health problems usually begin suddenly, have a single cause, are often easily diagnosed, last a short time, and get better with medication, and/or surgery, rest, and time. Most people with acute illnesses are cured and return to normal health. There is relatively little uncertainty for the patient or the doctor; both

usually know what to expect. The illness typically follows a cycle of becoming worse for a while, followed by carefully treating or observing the symptoms, and then getting better. Finally, the care of acute illness depends on the body's ability to heal itself and sometimes on a health professional's knowledge and experience in finding and administering the correct treatment.

Table 1.1 **Differences Between Acute and Chronic Disease**

	Acute Disease	Chronic Disease (long-term)
Beginning	Usually rapid	Slow
Cause	Usually one, identifiable	Often uncertain, especially early on
Duration	Short	Usually for life
Diagnosis	Commonly accurate	Sometimes difficult
Tests	Give good answers	Often of limited value
Role of professional	Select and conduct treatment	Become teacher and partner
Role of patient	To follow orders	To partner health professionals, responsible for daily management

Appendicitis is an example of an acute illness. It typically begins rapidly, signalled by nausea and pain in the abdomen. The diagnosis of appendicitis, once established by examination, leads to surgery for removal of the inflamed appendix. There follows a period of recovery and then a return to normal health.

Long-term conditions are different and some details are indicated in Table 1.1. They usually begin slowly and proceed slowly. For example, a person may slowly develop blockage of the arteries over decades and then might have a heart attack or a stroke. Arthritis generally starts with brief annoying twinges that gradually increase. Unlike acute disease, long-term conditions usually have multiple causes that vary over time. These causes may include heredity, lifestyle, exposure to environmental factors such as second-hand smoke or air pollution and to physiological factors such as low levels of thyroid hormone or changes in brain chemistry that may cause depression. Lifestyle encompasses matters like smoking, lack of exercise, poor diet, and stress.

The combination of many causes and unknown factors can be frustrating for those of us who want quick answers. It is difficult for both the doctor and the patient when clear answers are not available. In some cases, even when the diagnosis is rapid, as in the case of a stroke or heart attack, the long-term effects may be hard to predict. The lack of a regular or predictable pattern is a major characteristic of most long-term conditions.

Unlike acute disease, where full recovery is expected, a long-term condition usually leads to more symptoms and a loss of physical or mental functioning. With chronic conditions many people assume that the symptoms they are experiencing are due to the disease itself. Although the disease can cause pain, shortness of breath, fatigue, and the like, it is not the only cause. Each of these symptoms can contribute to the other symptoms and all these can feed on each other. For example, depression causes fatigue, pain causes physical limitations, and these can lead to poor sleep and more fatigue. The interactions of these symptoms make the condition

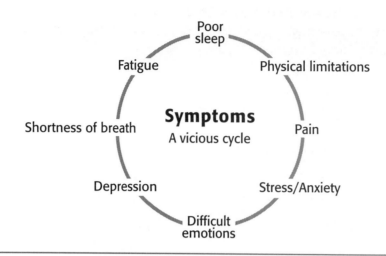

Figure 1.1 **The Symptoms Cycle**

worse. These interactions can create a *vicious cycle* that will get worse unless we find a way to break into it. Take a look at Figure 1.1.

To break the cycle, we need to understand how the body operates. As you know, cells are the building blocks of tissues and organs: the heart, lungs, brain, blood, blood vessels, bones, muscles, and in fact, everything in the body. For a cell to remain alive and function normally, three things must happen: it must be nourished, receive oxygen, and get rid of waste products. If anything goes wrong with any of these three functions, the cell becomes diseased. If cells are diseased, the organ or tissue suffers. If this happens you may experience limitations in your ability to be active in daily life. The differences between long-term conditions depend on which cells and organs are affected and the processes by which the disruption occurs, for example:

■ *When you are having a stroke,* a blood vessel in the brain becomes blocked or bursts. Oxygen and nutrition are cut off for the part of the brain supplied by that artery. As a result, the part of your body controlled by the damaged brain cells, such as an arm, a leg, or a portion of your face, loses function.

■ *If you have heart disease,* heart attacks occur when the vessels supplying blood to the heart muscle become blocked. This is called a coronary thrombosis. When this happens, oxygen is cut off, the heart muscle is injured, and pain results. Afterwards, the heart may be less effective in supplying the rest of your body with oxygen-carrying blood. Because the heart is pumping blood less efficiently through your body, fluid accumulates in tissues, and you may experience shortness of breath and fatigue.

■ *With diseases of the lungs,* there is either a problem getting oxygen to the lungs, as with bronchitis or asthma, or the lungs cannot effectively transfer oxygen to the blood, as with emphysema. In both cases the body is deprived of oxygen.

■ *In diabetes,* the pancreas does not produce enough insulin or produces insulin that cannot be used efficiently by the body. Without this insulin the body's cells are not able to use the glucose or sugar, in the blood for energy.

■ *In liver and kidney disease*, the cells of these organs do not work properly, making it difficult for the body to get rid of waste products.

The basic consequences of these diseases are similar: loss of function due to a reduction in oxygen, accumulation of waste products, or the inability of the body to use glucose for energy. You should also note that:

■ *Loss of function also occurs in arthritis*. In osteoarthritis, as the cartilage which is the cushioning material found on the ends of bones, and the *discs* between the vertebrae of the back become worn, frayed, or dis-

placed, ends by causing pain. We often do not know exactly why the cartilage cells begin to weaken or die. But the results are pain and disability.

■ *Most mental illnesses are caused by imbalances in chemicals and structural changes in the brain*. Too much or too little of these chemical neurotransmitters can affect our moods, thoughts, and behaviours. Treatment of such conditions as depression, bipolar disorder, and schizophrenia often includes restoring chemical balance with medications, and making changes in the environment or self-care practices designed to support effective coping.

Different Diseases, Similar Symptoms

Because a long-term disease starts with a malfunction at the cellular level, we may not notice the disease either until it intrudes in our life by causing symptoms, or as it declares itself through an abnormal test result. Although the biological causes of chronic illnesses differ, the problems they cause for people are similar. For example, most people with a long-term condition suffer fatigue and loss of energy. Sleeping problems are common. In one case there is pain, but in another case there is trouble breathing. Disability is, to some extent, a part of having a long-term condition. It may be the inability to use your hands well because of arthritis or stroke, or difficulty in walking due to shortness of breath, stroke, arthritis, or diabetes. Indeed, sometimes disability is caused by a lack of energy, extreme

fatigue, or change in mood. Depression can be a reflection of a chronic or recurrent imbalance in your brain chemicals. It is also a consequence of the negative feelings, *feeling down* or *feeling blue*, that result from having other long-term conditions. It is hard to maintain a cheerful disposition when your condition causes annoying problems that are unlikely to go away. Along with the depression come fear and concern for the future. *Will I be able to remain independent? If I can't care for myself, who will care for me? Will I get worse? How bad will it get?* Both disability and depression can also contribute to a loss of self-esteem.

Because there are similarities among long-term conditions, the essential management tasks and skills you need to learn in order to

What are Self-Management Skills?

- Solving problems and responding to your disease as it gets better or worse.
- Maintaining a healthy lifestyle with regular exercise, healthy eating, sound sleep habits, and stress management.
- Managing common symptoms.
- Making decisions about when to seek medical help and what treatments to try.

- Working effectively with your health care team.
- Using medications safely and effectively while minimising side-effects.
- Finding and using community resources.
- Talking about your illness with family and friends.
- Adapting your social activities.

Table 1.2 **Problems for the Self-Management of Common Long-term Conditions**

Chronic Condition	Possible Problems Caused by Chronic Conditions				
	Pain	Fatigue	Shortness of Breath	Physical Function	Difficult Emotions
Anxiety/Panic Disorder		✔	✔	✔	✔
Arthritis	✔	✔		✔	✔
Asthma and Lung Disease		✔	✔	✔	✔
Cancer	✔	✔	✔	✔	✔
Chronic Heartburn and Acid Reflux	✔				✔
Chronic Pain	✔	✔		✔	✔
Congestive Heart Failure		✔	✔		✔
Depression		✔		✔	✔
Diabetes	✔	✔		✔	✔
Heart Disease	✔	✔	✔	✔	✔
Hepatitis	✔	✔			✔
High Blood Pressure					✔
HIV Disease or AIDS	✔	✔	✔	✔	✔
Inflammatory Bowel Disease	✔				✔
Irritable Bowel Syndrome	✔				✔
Kidney Stones	✔				
Multiple Sclerosis	✔	✔		✔	✔
Parkinson's Disease	✔	✔		✔	✔
Peptic Ulcer Disease	✔				✔
Renal Failure		✔			✔
Stroke		✔		✔	✔

live with different conditions are also similar. Perhaps the most important skill of all is learning to respond to your condition on an ongoing basis to solve day-to-day problems. After all, you live with your condition 24 hours a day whereas your health care professional sees you for only a tiny portion of this time. This means that *you* must manage your condition. Table 1.2 on page 6 illustrates some of the self-management problems caused by long-term conditions. From this brief introduction you can see that long-term conditions have more in common than first meets the eye. In this book we talk about *managing* these conditions. For most of the book, however, we will talk more about the management tasks common across many conditions. If you have more than one health problem, you need not be confused about how to start. The approaches that work for heart disease will also help with lung disease, arthritis, depression, or a stroke. Start with the problem or condition that bothers you most. Table 1.3 on pages 8 and 9 outlines some

of the management skills that you may need to deal with disease-specific problems. Some of these skills are also discussed later in the book in the chapters dealing with specific diseases.

A Note about NHS Care Plans

The NHS *Guide to Long-term Conditions and Self-care*, says that everyone with a long-term condition can have a *Care Plan* if they want one. This Care Plan is an agreement between you and your healthcare professional, together with social services, to help you manage your health on a daily basis. It can be a formal document or notes inserted into your medical records. The plan can be amended at any time and it can be an annual process. The most important thing about the plan is that *you are involved* in working it out with the help of the health care professional. In fact, it is primarily for *your benefit* rather than the benefit of your GP or other healthcare professional. It helps you to set your own goals and at the heart of achieving these goals are self-management skills.

Same Disease, Different Response

Arthur suffers from severe arthritis. He is in pain most of the time and can't sleep. He took early retirement because of his arthritis and now, at age 55, he spends his days sitting at home bored. He avoids most physical activity because of the pain, weakness, and shortness of breath. He has become very irritable. Most people, including his family, don't enjoy his company. It even seems too much trouble when the grandchildren he adores come to visit.

Isabel, age 66, also suffers from severe arthritis. Every day she manages to walk several blocks to the local library or the park. When the pain is severe, she practises relaxation techniques and tries to distract herself. She works several hours a week as a volunteer at a local hospital. She also loves going to see her young grandchildren and even manages to take care of them for a time when her daughter has to go shopping. Her husband is amazed at how much zest she has for life.

Table 1.3 **Management Skills for Dealing with Chronic Conditions**

Chronic Condition	Management Skills							Other Management Tools
	Pain Management	Fatigue Management	Breathing Techniques	Relaxation and Managing Emotions	Nutrition	Exercise	Medications	
Anxiety/Panic Disorder		✓	✓	✓	✓	✓	✓	• Behavioral techniques to decondition triggers
Arthritis	✓	✓		✓	✓	✓	✓	• Use of assistive devices • Appropriate use of joints • Use of cold/heat • Pacing of activities
Asthma and Lung Disease		✓	✓	✓		✓	✓	• Use of inhalers and peak flow meters • Avoid triggers
Cancer	✓	✓		✓	✓	✓	✓	• Varies with site of the cancer • Managing effects of surgery, radiation, and chemotherapy
Chronic Pain	✓	✓		✓		✓	✓	• Pacing of activities • Specific exercises • Use of pain management techniques
Congestive Heart Failure		✓	✓	✓	✓	✓	✓	• Monitoring of daily weight • Sodium/salt restriction
Depression		✓		✓	✓	✓	✓	• Engaging in pleasant activities • Exposure to light (phototherapy)
Diabetes	✓	✓		✓	✓	✓	✓	• Home blood glucose monitoring • Insulin injection • Foot care • Regular eye (retinal) exams
Heartburn and Acid Reflux					✓		✓	• Avoid stomach irritants (e.g., coffee, alcohol, aspirin, nonsteroidal anti-inflammatory medications) • Elevation of bed

Management Skills

Chronic Condition	Pain Management	Fatigue Management	Breathing Techniques	Relaxation and Managing Emotions	Nutrition	Exercise	Medications	Other Management Tools
Heart Disease	✓	✓	✓	✓	✓	✓	✓	• Know and watch for warning signs of heart attack
Hepatitis	✓	✓		✓	✓		✓	• Avoid use of alcohol, IV drugs, medications toxic to liver • Preventing spread of infection (e.g, for hepatitis B and C, safer sex practices, hygiene)
High Blood Pressure				✓	✓	✓	✓	• Home blood pressure monitoring • Sodium/salt restriction
HIV Disease or AIDS	✓	✓	✓	✓	✓	✓	✓	• Preventing spread of infection (e.g., safer sex practices, hygiene) • Watch for signs of early infection • Avoid IV drugs
Inflammatory Bowel Disease	✓			✓	✓		✓	
Irritable Bowel Syndrome	✓			✓	✓		✓	
Kidney Stones	✓			✓	✓		✓	• Maintain fluid intake • Avoid calcium or oxalates, depending on type of stones
Multiple Sclerosis	✓	✓		✓	✓	✓	✓	• Management of incontinence • Management of mobility
Parkinson's Disease		✓		✓	✓	✓	✓	• Mobility
Peptic Ulcer Disease	✓			✓	✓	✓	✓	• Avoid stomach irritants (e.g., coffee, alcohol, aspirin, nonsteroidal anti-inflammatory medications) and early infection
Renal Failure		✓		✓	✓		✓	• Dialysis
Stroke		✓		✓		✓	✓	• Use of assistive devices

Arthur and Isabel both live with the same condition with similar physical problems. Yet their ability to function and enjoy life is very different. *Why?* The difference lies largely in their attitude toward the disease and their lives. Arthur has allowed his life and physical capacities to wither. Isabel has learned to take an active role in managing her long-term condition. Even though she has limitations, she controls her life instead of letting the condition control her.

Attitude cannot cure a long-term condition, but positive attitudes and certain self-management skills can make it much easier to live with. Much research now shows that the experience of pain, discomfort, and disability can be modified by circumstances, beliefs, mood, and the attention we pay to symptoms. For example, with arthritis of the knee, a person's degree of depression is a better predictor of how disabled, limited, and uncomfortable the person is than the evidence of physical damage to the knee on X-rays. What goes on in a person's mind is at least as important as what is going on in the person's body.

In other words, why is it that two people with similar long-term conditions can function so differently? One person may be able to minimise the effect of the symptoms, although they are both extremely disabled. One person is focused on healthy living, but the other is concentrated on the disease. One of the keys to shaping the impact of any disease is how effective and engaged the person is in self-management.

Understanding the Chronic Condition Path

The first responsibility of any *long-term condition self-manager* is to understand the condition. This means more than learning about what causes the illness, the symptoms it may cause, and what you can do about it. It also means observing how the condition and its treatment affect you. An illness is different for each person, and with experience you and your family will become experts at determining the effects of the illness and its treatment. In fact, you are the only person who lives with your health problem for every minute of every day. Therefore, observing how it affects you and making accurate reports to your health care providers are essential parts of being a good self-manager. Most long-term conditions go up and down in intensity. They do not follow a steady path. Let's look at an example.

John, Sandra, and *Mary* all have a blood pressure of 160/100, which is too high.

- *Mary tells her doctor that she sometimes forgets to take her medications and is not getting much exercise.* She is also overweight. Her doctor talks with her and together they work out a plan, to help her remember her medications, start an exercise programme, and cut down on the amount of food she eats.

- *John says he is taking his medications, exercising, and eating well.* The doctor decides to change his medications, because what he is currently taking is probably not working.

■ *Sandra does not want to take medication.* She is doing everything she can to lower her blood pressure: eating well, losing weight, and exercising. Unfortunately, although her blood pressure has improved a bit, it is not good enough. The doctor talks to her about the dangers of high blood pressure and advises starting a medication. In the end Sandra decides that this might be best.

The successful management of high blood pressure varied for each of these patients but it depended on each one communicating their unique situation, experiences, and preferences to their doctor. In other words, effective control of the condition involved an observant patient, communicating openly with their health care provider.

When you develop a chronic condition you become more aware of your body. Minor symptoms, previously ignored may now cause concerns. For example, *Is my chest pain a sign of a heart attack?* or *Is this pain in my knee a sign that the arthritis is getting worse?* There are no simple reassuring answers. Nor is there a fail-safe way of sorting out serious signals from minor temporary symptoms that can be ignored. It is helpful to know and understand the natural rhythms of your chronic condition. In general, if your symptoms are unusual, severe, or persistent or occur after starting a new medication or treatment plan they should be checked out with your doctor.

Throughout this book we give some specific examples of what actions to take if you experience certain symptoms. But this is where your partnership with your health care provider becomes critical. Self-management does not mean going it alone. Always get help or advice when you are concerned or uncertain. From what we have said, self-management may seem like a simple enough concept. Both at home and in the business world, managers direct the show. But they don't do everything themselves; they work with others, including consultants, to get the job done. What makes them managers is that they are responsible for making decisions and making sure that their decisions are carried out.

Managing a chronic condition, like managing a family or a business, is a complex undertaking. There are many twists, turns, and mid-course corrections. By learning self-management skills, you can ease the problems of living with your condition. The key to success in any undertaking is, *first*, deciding what you want to do; *second*, deciding how you are going to do it; and, *finally*, learning a set of skills and practising them until they have been mastered. Success in self-management of long-term conditions is just the same. In fact, mastering self-management skills is one of the most important tasks of life.

We will describe hundreds of skills and tools to help you relieve the problems caused by your long-term condition. We do not expect you to use them all. You have to pick and choose and experiment. Set your own goals. *What you actually do may not be as important as the sense of confidence and control that comes from successfully doing it.* However, knowing the skills is not enough. We need a way of incorporating these skills into our daily lives. Whenever we try out a new skill, the first attempts may be clumsy, slow, and show few results. It is easier to return to old ways than to continue trying to master new and sometimes difficult tasks. The best way to master new skills is through practice and the evaluation of results.

More about Self-Management Skills

What you do about something is largely determined by how you think about it. For example, if you think that having a long-term condition is like falling into a deep pit, you may have a hard time motivating yourself to escape! You may even think the task is impossible. The thoughts you have can influence what happens to you and how you handle your health problems.

Some of the most successful self-managers are people who think of their illness as a path. This path, like any other path, goes up and down. Sometimes it is flat and smooth. At other times it is rough. To negotiate the path one has to use many strategies. Sometimes you can go fast; other times you must slow down. There are obstacles to negotiate.

Good self-managers are people who have learned some key skills that will help to negotiate the path:

- *Skills needed to deal with the illness:* Any illness requires that you do new things. These may include taking medicine, using an inhaler, or using oxygen. It means more frequent interactions with your doctor and the health care system. Sometimes there are new exercises or a new diet. Even diseases such as cancer require self-management. Chemotherapy, radiation, and surgery can all be made easier through good day-to-day self-management. All of these skills constitute the work you must do to manage your condition.

- *Skills needed to continue your normal life:* Just because you have a long-term condition does not mean that life does not go on. There are still chores to do, friendships to maintain, jobs to perform, and family relationships to continue. Things that you once took for granted can become much more complicated in the face of a long-term condition. You may need to learn new skills or adapt the way you do things in order to maintain the things you want to do.

- *Skills needed to deal with emotion:* Diagnosis of a long-term condition means your future changes and with this come changes in plans and in your emotions. Many of the new emotions are negative. They may include anger, *It's not fair*, or fear *I am afraid of becoming dependent on others*, or depression *I can't do anything anymore, and I'm no use any more*, or frustration *No matter what I do, it doesn't make any difference, I just can't do what I want to do*, or isolation *No-one understands, no one wants to be around someone who is sick*. Negotiating the path of a long-term condition means learning skills to work with these negative emotions. We will teach you some skills which will help.

With this as background, you can think of self-management as the use of skills to manage the practicalities of living with your condition, continuing your daily activities, and dealing with emotions brought about by your condition.

Final Points to Ponder

■ *You are not to blame:* Long-term conditions are caused by a combination of genetic, biological, environmental, and psychological factors. For example, stress alone does not cause most long-term conditions. The mind matters, but your mind cannot always triumph over matter. If you fail to recover, it is not because you lack the right mental attitude. There are many things you can control that will help you to cope with a long-term condition. Remember, you are not responsible for causing the disease or failing to cure it. You are responsible for taking action to manage your condition.

■ *Don't do it alone:* One of the side-effects of a long-term condition is a feeling of isolation. Supportive as friends and family members may be, they often cannot understand what you are experiencing as you struggle to cope with your condition. The chances are, however, that there are other people who know first-hand what it is like to live with a condition just like yours. Connecting to those with similar conditions can reduce your sense of isolation and help you understand what to expect based on a fellow patient's perspective. These people can offer practical tips about managing symptoms and feelings on a day-to-day basis, give you the opportunity to help others to cope with your condition, help you appreciate your strengths and realise that things

could be worse, and inspire you to take a more active role in managing your own condition by seeing others doing it successfully. Support can sometimes come from reading a book or a newsletter about how someone lives with a long-term condition. Or, it can come from talking with others on the telephone, in face-to-face support groups, or linking online through computer support groups.

■ *You're more than your disease:* When you have a chronic disease, too often the centre of attention becomes your disease. But you are *more* than your disease, *more* than just a *heart patient* or *lung patient*. And life is more than trips to the doctor and managing symptoms. It is essential to cultivate areas of your life that you enjoy. Small daily pleasures can help balance the other parts in which you have to manage uncomfortable symptoms or emotions. For example, find ways to enjoy nature by growing a plant or watching a sunset, or indulge in the pleasure of human touch, or a tasty meal, or celebrate companionship with family or friends. Finding ways to introduce moments of pleasure is vital to the self-management of long-term conditions. Focus on your abilities and strengths rather than disabilities and problems. Helping others is one way to increase your own sense of what you can do instead of focusing on what you can't. Celebrate small improvements. If a long-term condition teaches anything, it is the importance of living each moment more fully. Within the true limits of whatever disease you have, there are always ways to enhance your function, your sense of control, and your enjoyment of life.

■ *You can treat your illness as an opportunity.* Illness, even with its pain and disability, can enrich your life. It can make us re-evaluate what is really important to us, it can shift priorities and move us in exciting new directions that we may never have considered before.

Consider these cases:

Jill has breast cancer. Since her diagnosis, she lives more fully than ever:

> *I was a housewife, lost and aimless after my children grew up and left home. One of the first things I did after the diagnosis was to teach myself to swim with my head in the water. I had always kept it above, too scared to put my whole self in. That had been the story of my life. Now I do whatever I want. I don't think about how much time there is, just what I want to do with it. Surprisingly, I feel less afraid of living.*

Sometimes a heart attack makes people decide to slow down. They would rather use their time to deepen their relationships with family and friends. A chronic condition that restricts movement may lead some to think again about unused intellectual talents:

> *Meg* learned a new language and found an overseas pen pal. *Fred* dared to write the novel he always thought he was too stupid to write.

Though chronic illness may close some doors, you can choose to use it to open new ones.

Suggested Further Reading

Baker, B. *Coping with Long-term Illness.* London: Sheldon Press, 2001. This book helps with overcoming common problems.

Butler, G. and Hope, T. *Manage Your Mind.* Oxford: Oxford University Press, 1995.

Campling, F. and Sharpe, M. *Living with a Long-term Illness.* Oxford: Oxford University Press, 2006. This book provides considerable factual information.

Jones, F. R. (Editor), et al. *Working with Self-management Courses: The Thoughts of Participants, Planners and Policy Makers.* Oxford: Oxford University Press, 2010.

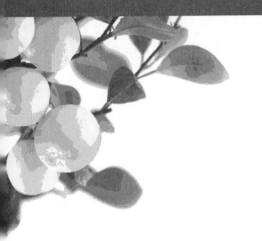

CHAPTER 2

Becoming an Active Self-Manager

*I*T IS IMPOSSIBLE TO HAVE A LONG-TERM CONDITION without being a self-manager of some kind. Some people manage by withdrawing from life. They stay in bed or socialise less. The disease becomes the centre of their existence. Other people, with the same condition and symptoms, somehow manage to get on with life. They may have to change some of the things they do or the way that things get done. Nevertheless, life continues to be full and active. The difference between these two extremes is not the condition but rather how the person with the condition decides to manage it. Please note the word *decides*. Self-management is always a *decision*: a decision to be active or a decision to do nothing, a decision to seek help or a decision to suffer in silence. This book will help you deal with these decisions.

Like any skill, active self-management must be learned and practised. This chapter will help you to start by presenting the three most important self-management tools: problem solving, decision making, and action planning. Remember: *you* are the

15

manager. So, like any manager of an organisation or a household, you must do all of the following things:

1. Decide what you want to accomplish.

2. Look for various ways to accomplish your goals.

3. Make a short-term action plan.

4. Carry out your action plan.

5. Check the results.

6. Make any changes needed.

7. Reward yourself for your success.

Problem Solving

Problems sometimes start with a general uneasiness. Let's say you are unhappy but not sure why. On closer examination, you find that you miss having contact with some close relatives who live far away. With the problem identified, you decide to take a trip to visit these relatives. You know what you want to accomplish, but now you need to make a list of ways in which you can solve the problem.

In the past you have always driven, but you now find driving too tiring, so you think about other ways of travelling. You consider leaving at noon instead of early in the morning and making the trip in two days instead of one. You consider asking a friend along to share the driving. There is also a train that stops within 20 miles of your destination, or you might fly. Eventually, you decide to take the train.

The trip still seems overwhelming, as there is so much to do to prepare. You decide to write down all the steps necessary to make the trip a reality. These include:

■ Finding a good time to go.

■ Buying a ticket.

■ Working out how to handle luggage.

■ Wondering if you can walk about on a moving train to get food or go to the toilet.

■ Working out how you will get to the station.

Each of these steps can be an action plan. To start making your action plan, you promise yourself that this week you will phone to find out just how much the rail services can help. You also decide to start taking a short walk each day, including walking up and down a few steps so that you will be steadier on your feet. You then carry out your action plan by calling train enquiries and starting your walking programme.

A week later you check the results. Looking back at all the steps to be accomplished, you see that a single phone call answered many of your questions. The rail services can help people who have mobility problems and have ways of dealing with many of your concerns. However, you are still worried about walking. Even though you are walking better, you are still unsteady. You make a change in your plan by asking a physiotherapist about this. He suggests using a cane or walking stick. Although you don't like using it, you realise that a walking stick will give you the extra security needed on a moving train. You have just been engaged in problem solving to achieve your goal to take a trip. Now let's review the specific steps in problem solving.

Steps in Problem Solving

1. *Identify the problem:* This is the first and most important step in problem solving. It is usually the most difficult step, as well. You may know, for example, that stairs are a problem, but it will take a little more effort to determine that the real problem is a fear of falling.

2. *List ideas to solve the problem:* You may be able to come up with a good list yourself, but you may sometimes want to call on other people for support. These can be friends, family, members of your health care team, or community resources. One thing to note about using supporters: these people cannot help you if you do not describe the problem well. For example, there is a big difference between saying that you can't walk because your feet hurt and saying that your feet hurt because you cannot find walking shoes that fit properly.

3. *Pick an idea to try:* As you try something new, remember that new activities can sometimes be difficult. Be certain to give your potential solution a fair chance before deciding it won't work.

4. *Once you've given your idea a fair trial, check the results:* If all goes well, your problem will be solved.

5. *Try again, if necessary:* If you still have the problem, pick another idea from your list and try again.

6. *Use other resources:* For example, you could involve a person from your support circle to seek for more ideas if you still do not have a solution.

7. *If the problem is still unresolved:* if you have gone through all of the steps until your ideas have been exhausted and the problem is still there, you may need to accept that your problem maybe insoluble. This is sometimes hard to admit. The fact that a problem can't be solved immediately doesn't mean that it won't be later on, nor does it mean that other problems cannot be solved. Even if your path is blocked, there are probably alternative paths. Don't give up. Keep going.

Living with Uncertainty

Living with uncertainty is one of the hardest of all self-management tasks. It is something that most of us cannot avoid. Uncertainty is also one of the causes of emotional *ups and downs*. The diagnosis of a chronic condition takes away some of our sense of security and control. It can be frightening. We are following our life path, and suddenly we are forced to detour to a different, unwanted path. Even as we work with health professionals and start new treatments, this uncertainty continues. Of course, we all have an uncertain future, but most people do not think about this. However, when we have a long-term health condition this becomes an important part of our lives. We are uncertain about our future health, and perhaps about our ability to continue to do the things we want, need, and like to do. Many people find it very challenging to make decisions when things are uncertain.

Making Decisions: Weighing the Pros and Cons

Making decisions is an important tool in our self-management toolbox. It is part of problem solving and we present here a useful process which can help:

1. *Identify the options:* For example, you may have to make a decision about getting help in the house or continuing to do all the work yourself. Sometimes the options are either to change your behaviour or not change at all.

2. *Identify what you want:* It may be important for you to continue your life as normally as possible, to have more time for your family, cut the grass, or clean the house. Sometimes identifying your deepest, most important values, like spending time with family, helps you to set priorities and increase your motivation to change.

3. *Write down the pros and cons for each option:* List as many items as you can for both pros and cons. And don't forget about the emotional and social effects.

4. *Rate each item on your list on a five-point scale:* with 0 indicating *not at all important* and five indicating *extremely important.*

5. *Add up the ratings for the Pro and Con columns and compare them:* The column with the higher total should guide your decision. If the totals are close or you are still not sure, skip to the next step.

6. *Apply the gut test:* An example is, whether *going back to work part-time feels right to you.* If it does, then you have probably reached a decision. If the decision is on a knife edge, then the way you feel should probably win out over the maths.

Decision-Making Example: Should I get help in the house?

Pro	Rating	Con	Rating
I'll have more time	4	It's expensive	3
I'll be less tired	4	It's hard to find good help	1
I'll have a clean house	3	They won't do things my way	2
		I don't want a stranger in the house	1
Total	11		7

Add up the points for the pro and con lists. The decision in this example would be to get help because the *Pro Score* (11) is significantly higher than the *Con Score* (7). If this feels right in your gut, then you have a clear answer.

Now it's your turn! Think of a decision you need to make. Now, try coming to a decision by using the following chart. It's perfectly OK to write in this book.

The decision to be made: _____

Pro	Rating	Con	Rating
Total			

The key to successful problem solving and decision making is taking action. We will talk about this next.

Taking Action

You have looked at a problem or made a difficult decision. Knowing what to do is not enough. It is time to do something, to take action. We suggest that you start by doing one thing at a time.

Setting Your Goal

Before you can take action, you must decide what you want to do. You must be realistic and specific when stating this *goal*. Think of all the things you would like to do. For example, one self-manager wanted to climb 20 steps to her daughter's home so that she could join her family for a holiday meal. Another individual wanted to overcome anxiety and attend social events. And yet another wanted to continue to ride his motorcycle even though he could no longer lift his heavy bike when it was lying on the ground.

One of the problems with such goals is that they often seem like dreams. They are so far off, so big, or so difficult that we are overwhelmed and don't even try to accomplish them. We'll tackle this problem next. For now, take a few minutes to write down some of your goals. Add extra lines if you need to:

Choose some personal goals

_____

_____

_____

_____

Put a star (★) next to the goal that you would like to work on first. Don't reject a goal until you have thought about alternatives. Sometimes we can reject the alternatives without knowing much about them. In the earlier example, our traveller was able to make a list of alternative travel arrangements before finally choosing the train as her best option.

Work out how to reach your goal

There are many ways to reach any specific goal. For example, our self-manager who wanted to climb 20 steps, might decide to start off with a slow walking programme and could start to climb a few steps each day. Alternatively she could look into having the family gathering at a different place. The man who wanted to attend social events could start with going on very short outings, asking a friend to go along to help, using distraction techniques when he's feeling anxious, or talking to his health care team about therapy or medication. Our motorcycle rider could buy a lighter motorcycle, use a sidecar, put *training wheels* on his bike, buy a three-wheeled motorcycle, or give up riding.

As you can see, there are many options for reaching our goals. The job here is to list the options and then choose one or two to try out.

Sometimes it is hard to think of all the options yourself. If you are having problems deciding, then it is time to use a mentor or someone who provides you with support. Share your goal with your family, friends, and health professionals. You can call community organisations such as *The British Heart Foundation* or *The Multiple Sclerosis Society*. You can use the Internet. Don't ask what you should do. Instead, ask for suggestions. It is always good to have a list of options.

In doing all this be cautious: Many of your options are never seriously considered because you assume that solutions do not exist or are simply impractical. Never make this assumption until you have thoroughly investigated each option. In one case, a woman who had lived in the same town all her life, felt that she knew all about the full range of community resources. When she was having problems with welfare benefits, a friend from another town suggested contacting a local financial advice centre. However, the woman dismissed this suggestion because she was certain that this service did not exist in her town. It was only when, months later, the friend came to visit and called the local *Age UK* Offices that the woman learned that *Age UK* and three other local organisations nearby all offered advice on benefits. Our motorcycle rider thought that training wheels on a Harley motorbike was a crazy idea but nevertheless he investigated. He added 15 years to his riding life using training wheels. In short, never assume anything. Assumptions are major enemies of self-management.

Now write down your list of options for your *Main Goal* here. Then put a star (★) next to the two or three options on which you would like to work:

Select your options

_____

_____

_____

_____

Making Short-Term Plans: Action Planning

You now need to devise your Action Plans: Once you've made some decisions about Goals and Options, you will have a pretty good idea of where you are going. However, the *Goal* you have set may still feel overwhelming. You ask yourself, *How will I ever move*; or *How will I ever be able to paint again*; and now it's your turn:

How will I ever be able to

_____
(You fill in this blank)

The secret is to not try to do everything at once. Instead, look at what you can realistically expect to accomplish within *the next week*. We call this an *Action Plan*: something that is short-term, is do-able, and sets you on the road toward your Goal. The Action Plan should be about something you want to do. It is a tool to help you do what you wish. Do not make Action Plans simply to please your friends, your family, or doctor.

Action Plans are probably your most important self-management tool. Most of us can do things to make us healthier but fail to do them. For example, most people with a long-term condition can walk, some just across the room, others for a hundred yards. Most can walk several hundred yards, and some can walk a mile or more. However, few people have a systematic exercise programme to help them.

Spelling out the steps in your action plan

An action plan helps you do the things you know you should do. However, you should start with what you *want* to do. Let's go through all the steps for making a realistic action plan.

1. Decide what you will do this week. For a step climber, this might be climbing three steps on four consecutive days. The man who wants to continue riding his motorcycle might spend half an hour on two days researching lighter motorcycles and motorcycle training wheels. Make very sure that your plans are *action-specific*. For example, rather than just deciding "to lose weight" (which is *not* an action but the result of an action); you will "replace a fizzy drink with tea."

2. Make a specific plan. Deciding what you want to do is worthless without a plan to do it. The plan should answer all of the following questions:

   ■ *Exactly* **what** *are you going to do?* Are you going to walk? Will you eat less? What distraction techniques will you practise?

   ■ **How much** *will you do?* This question is answered in terms of time, distance, portions, or repetitions. Will you walk a hundred yards, walk for 15 minutes, eat half portions at lunch and dinner or practise relaxation exercises for 15 minutes?

■ **When** *will you do this?* Again, this must be specific: will you do this before lunch, in the shower, on coming home from work? Connecting a new activity with an old habit is a good way to make sure it gets done. Consider what comes right before the action plan that could be used to trigger the new behaviour. For example, brushing your teeth might remind you to take your medication. Another trick is to do your new activity before one of your favourite activities, such as reading the paper or watching a favourite TV programme.

■ **How often** *will you do the activity?* This can be a bit tricky. We would all like to do things every day, but that is not always possible. It is usually best to decide to do an activity three or four times a week to give yourself some *wriggle room* because something might come up. If you do more, that's a bonus. If you are like most people, you will feel less pressure if you can do your activity three or four times a week and still feel successful. Note that taking medications is an exception to this. This must be done exactly as directed by your doctor.

Deciding on Some Guidelines

Here are some general guidelines for writing your Action Plan which may help you:

1. *Start where you are and start slowly*: If you can walk for only one minute, start your walking programme by walking one minute

every hour or two, rather than setting off to walk a hundred yards. If you have never done any exercise before, start with a few minutes of warm-up. A total of five or ten minutes is enough. If you want to lose weight, set a goal based on your existing eating behaviours, for example by eating half portions. *Losing a pound this week* is *not* an action plan because it does not involve a specific action; by contrast, *not eating after your main meal for four days this week* would be a good action plan.

2. *Give yourself some time off*: All people have days when they don't feel like doing anything. This is a very good reason for saying that you will do something three times a week rather than every day.

3. *Once you've made your action plan, ask yourself the following question:* On a scale of zero to ten, with zero being totally unsure and ten being totally certain, *how sure are you that you can complete this entire plan?"* If your answer is seven or above, then this is probably realistic. If your answer is below seven, you should think again. Ask yourself *why* you are unsure. What problems do you foresee? At this point, see if you can either solve the problems or change your plan to make yourself more confident of success.

4. *When you are happy with your plan, write it down and place it where you will see it every day*: Thinking through an action plan is one thing; writing it down makes it more likely you will take action. It also helps you to keep track of how you are doing and the problems you encounter. A blank action plan form is provided at the end of this

chapter. You may wish to make photocopies of it to use on a weekly basis.

Carrying Out Your Action Plan

If the action plan is well written and realistic, completing it is generally pretty easy. Ask your family or friends to check with you on how you are doing. Having to report your progress also provides good motivation. Keep track of your daily activities while carrying out your plan. Many good managers have lists of what they want to accomplish. Check things off as they are completed. This will give you guidance on how realistic your planning is—and will also be useful in making better plans in future. Make daily notes, even of those things you don't understand at the time. Later, these notes may be useful in helping you to establish a pattern for problem solving.

For example, our stair-climbing friend never did her climbing. Each day she had a different problem: not enough time, being too tired, the weather being too cold, and so on. When she looked back at her notes, she began to realise that the real problem was her fear of falling when there was no one around to help her. She then decided to use a stick when climbing stairs and to do it when a friend or neighbour was around.

The Basics of a Successful Action Plan

- It is something *you* want to do.
- It is achievable and something you expect to be able to accomplish.
- It is action-specific.
- It answers the questions *What? How much? When?* and *How often?*
- You are sure that you will complete your entire plan at a level of seven or higher on a scale from zero *not at all sure* to ten *absolutely sure.*

Checking the Results

At the end of each week, see if you completed your action plan and if you are any nearer to accomplishing your goal. Are you able to walk further? Have you lost weight? Are you less anxious? Taking stock is important. You may not see progress day by day, but you should see a little progress each week. At the end of each week, check on how well you have fulfilled your action plan. If you are having problems, this is the time to use your problem-solving skills.

Making Mid-Course Corrections

Mid-course corrections may send you back to problem solving. When you are trying to overcome obstacles, the first plan is not always the most workable one. If something doesn't work, don't give up. Try something else; modify your short-term plans so that the steps are easier,

give yourself more time to accomplish difficult tasks, choose some new steps towards your goal, or check with your supporters and mentors for advice and assistance. If you are not sure how to go about this, go back and read about problem solving on pages 16 and 17.

How People Change

Thousands of studies have been done to learn how people change themselves—or why they don't change. Here's what we have learned:

Most people change by themselves, when they are ready. Even though doctors, counsellors, spouses, and self-help groups can coax, persuade, nag, and try to assist people to change their lifestyle and habits, most people do so without much help from others.

Change is not an all-or-nothing process. It happens in stages. Most of us think of change as occurring one step at a time: each step is an improvement over the one before. Although a few people do make changes like this, it is rare. For example, more than 95% of people who successfully quit smoking do so only after a series of setbacks and relapses.

In most cases, change resembles a spiral more than a straight line, with people reverting to previous stages before proceeding further, taking *two steps forward and one step back.* So, relapses are not failures but setbacks, which are an integral part of change. In fact, dealing with a relapse is frequently a helpful way for people to learn how to maintain change. Relapsing provides feedback about what doesn't work.

Efficient self-change depends on doing the right things at the right time. There's evidence that people who are given strategies which are inappropriate to their particular stage are less successful in changing themselves than people who receive no assistance at all. For example, making an elaborate written plan of action when you really haven't decided that you *want* to change is a prescription for failure. You're likely to get bored, discouraged, or frustrated before you even start.

Confidence in your ability to change is a key ingredient for success. Your belief in your own ability to succeed will determine whether you will attempt to change in the first place, whether you will persist, if you relapse, and whether you will ultimately be successful in making the desired change.

Rewarding Yourself

The best part of being a good self-manager is the reward that comes from accomplishing your goals and then living a fuller and more comfortable life. However, don't wait for rewards until your goal is reached; it's better to reward yourself frequently for your *short-term successes.* For example, decide that you won't read the paper until after you exercise. In this way reading the paper becomes your reward. One self-manager buys only one or two pieces of fruit at a time and walks the half-mile to the supermarket every day or two to get more fruit. Another, who stopped smoking, used the money

Your Success Improves Your Health

The benefits of change go beyond the pay-offs of adopting healthier habits. Obviously, you will feel better when you exercise, eat well, keep regular sleeping hours, stop smoking, and take time to relax. But regardless of the behavior that's altered, there's evidence that the feelings of self-confidence and control over your life that come from making any successful change does improve your health.

As we age, or develop a chronic health condition, physical abilities and self-image may decline. For many people, it is discouraging to find that they can't do what they used to do or want to do. By changing and improving even one area of your life, whether it is boosting your physical fitness or learning a new skill, you will regain a sense of optimism and vitality. By *focusing on what you can do* rather than what you can't do, you're likely to lead a more positive and happier life.

he would have spent on cigarettes to have his house professionally cleaned, and there was even enough left over to go to a football match with a friend. Rewards don't have to be fancy, expensive, or fattening. There are many healthy pleasures that can add enjoyment to your life.

One last note: not all goals are achievable. Chronic (long-term) conditions may mean having to give up some options. If this is true for you, don't dwell too much on what you can't do. Instead, start working on another goal you would like to accomplish. One self-manager we know, who uses a wheelchair, talks about the 90% of things he *can* do. He devotes his life to developing this 90% to the fullest possible extent.

Tools for Becoming a Self-Manager

Now that you understand the meaning of self-management, you are ready to begin using the tools that will make you a successful one. Most self-management skills are similar for all conditions. Chapters 15 to 18 contain information about some of the more common long-term conditions. If your condition is not covered, we apologise. If we had included everything, then you would

not even be able to carry this book! In Chapter 13 we talk about medications and their uses. The rest of the book is devoted to the *tools of the trade*. These include exercise, nutrition, symptom management, preventing falls, communication, making decisions about the future, finding resources, information about advance decisions for health care, and the delicate matter of sex and intimacy.

My Action Plan

In writing your action plan, be sure it includes all of the following:

1.   *What* you are going to do (a specific action)

2.   *How much* you are going to do (time, distance, portions, repetitions, etc.)

3.   *When* you are going to do it (time of the day, day of the week)

4.   *How often* or *how many days a week* you are going to do it

Example: This week, I will walk (what) to the park and back (how much) before lunch (when) three times (how many).

This week I will _____ (what)

_____ (how much)

_____ (when)

_____ (how often)

How sure are you? (0 = not at all sure; 10 = absolutely sure) _____

Comments

Monday _____

Tuesday _____

Wednesday _____

Thursday _____

Friday _____

Saturday _____

Sunday _____

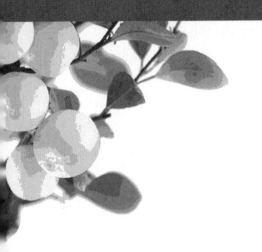

CHAPTER 3

Finding Resources

A MAJOR PART OF BECOMING A SELF-MANAGER is knowing about when you need help and how to find support. When you seek help, you are not just a victim of your condition. You are becoming a good self-manager. Start by evaluating your condition; consider what you can do and what you want to do. You may find that there is a difference between what you can and what you want to do. If so, it may be time to seek help so that you can do those things that are most important to you.

When you begin to look for help you will probably start by asking family or friends. Sometimes this can be difficult. We are often afraid that others will see us as weak. Sometimes our pride gets in the way. Most people we ask want to be helpful but do not know how. Your job is to tell them what you need. Finding the right words when you are seeking help is discussed in Chapter 9. Unfortunately, some people do not have family or close friends, and others cannot bring themselves to ask. It is often true that your family and friends cannot offer all the help that you need. Thankfully, we have another wonderful resource available; our community.

Finding resources can be a little like a treasure hunt. Just as in a treasure hunt, creative thinking often wins the game. Finding what you need may be as simple as looking in the telephone book, or making a couple of phone calls or using the Internet. Other times it may take careful sleuthing. All good *community resource detectives* must find clues and follow them. Sometimes this will mean starting again when a clue leads you to a dead end.

First, you need to define the problem and then decide what It is that you want. For example, suppose you find it is increasingly difficult to get in and out of the bath, either because you now lack confidence or you don't have enough strength in your arms. After some thought, you decide that you want to continue being responsible for your own baths and wish to avoid relying on someone else. You work out you could do this if you had some hand grips fitted on the side of your bath. Your task is working out how to get this done.

You look at some hand grips in a local DIY shop but suspect that they are not substantial enough for what you need. So you decide to get some professional advice. The hunt is on. Where can you find a professional who will know about the needs of people like you? You need a *starting point* for your treasure hunt. The phone book has pages of adverts and listings for bath installers. Some advertisers say they specialise in adaptations for people with physical disabilities. However, because you don't want any *major* alterations done, you decide to talk to a friend who also had this problem some months earlier. She makes various useful suggestions.

Her suggestions then lead to a long list of possibilities: these include occupational therapists, medical supply shops, centres for independent living, and voluntary organisations such as *Arthritis Care* or *Age UK*. There is a local branch of *Age UK* close to where you live so you pay a visit. This soon provides you with all the information you need about the best way to get the hand grips installed and also how to get help with the cost of doing the job.

There are also people in every community who are natural resources. These *networkers* seem to know everyone and everything about their community. They tend to be people who have lived in your community for a long time and have been closely involved in it. They are also natural problem solvers. These *naturals* are individuals that other people turn to for advice. They always seems to be helpful. A *natural* could be: a friend, a business associate, the postman, your doctor, the lady at the local newsagents, the pharmacist, the taxi driver, or the librarian. All *you* need to do is to think of this person as an information resource. Let's review the lessons we have learned from this example. The most important steps in finding the resources you need are these:

1. Identify the problem.

2. Identify what you want or need.

3. Look for resources in the phone book or on the Internet.

4. Ask friends, family, and neighbours for ideas.

5. Contact organisations that might deal with similar issues.

6. Identify and ask the *naturals*.

One last note: the best detectives usually follow several clues at the same time. Doing this will save you lots of time and shorten the treasure hunt. Watch out, though. once you get good at thinking about community resources creatively, you will become a *natural* in your own right!

Resources for Resources

When we need to find goods or services, there are helpful resources we can call on. The telephone directory, including the *Business* or *Yellow Pages*, and internet search engines are the most frequently used tools. These are particularly helpful if you are looking for someone to employ for jobs such as plumbing or gardening. For most searches this is where to start. One resource often leads to another . . . and another. When we are looking for a resource specifically relating to general health or for our specific medical condition, our *community resource detective kit* must offer a variety of other useful tools. The next section will clarify what these are and how to use them.

Organisations and Referral Services

Your local library is a vital starting point

Despite financial cuts local libraries remain a good resource for information likely to be useful to you. Librarians are very ready to help you to use the variety of options available and to suggest which of these will be most appropriate for your needs. The available options include:

■ *Hard Copies of Books*: These are important for people who do not, or cannot, use computers. In addition, many health-related books will contain details of further reading and resource lists, either at the end of each chapter or at the back of the book.

Books on health tend to be specialised and therefore can sometimes be expensive to buy. So, if the library does not have a copy of the book you need, it is worth asking if it can be ordered for you from another library. Make sure that any book you decide to use is as up-to-date as possible. Information on health matters can change very quickly. We know, from reading newspapers and listening to the radio or television, that hardly a week goes by without a report highlighting new research and new guidance on medical conditions which may be relevant to you personally.

■ *Electronic Books and Electronic Audio titles*: Many libraries can offer you free downloads of e-books and e-Audio titles to use on your computer. They will also help you to set up the software you need to use this service.

■ *Computers*: If you do not own a computer you can often have free access to one in the library. However, there is often a queue to use them, so it is worth reserving one in advance. The use of the computers is usually free but there will be a small charge if you need to print out any material. If you are completely new to using computers and worried about how to set about learning this new skill, you may find your local library also runs training sessions for beginners.

Newspapers and Magazines

Most national newspapers have a weekly section on health issues covering new research and guidance on daily living issues. The content is usually gleaned from new reports and press releases issued by researchers and their organisations. These sources may be drug companies or academic institutions. If you are doubtful about the advice offered in a newspaper article, you can check this out with your GP or get hold of the original report to verify what was actually said.

Local newspapers are often a good resource for finding exercise classes, lectures and meetings that you can attend. An example of this is a list of *Healthy Walks Schemes* which are organised by your local NHS. This is usually advertised in the newspapers under the heading of *Local Activities*.

Disabled Living Foundation

The *Disabled Living Foundation* is a national charity which provides impartial advice, information and training on aids for daily living. They work in partnership with other organisations, such as *Assist UK*. Assist UK mounts permanent exhibitions of equipment that provide people with the opportunity to see and try out a range of products. You can also get professional advice from the staff about what might suit you best.

Voluntary patient support groups

These organisations are often concerned with specific long-term conditions. So, they provide one of your best resources when looking for help relating to your particular medical condition. They may provide:

- *Help-lines* for advice on daily living.

- *Simple information* about the facts of your condition.

- *Research and development* relating to your medical condition.

- *Newsletters and information leaflets* which can be sent to you on request.

- *On-line Forums* are sometimes offered where you can hear about other people's experiences of living with the condition that you suffer from.

- *News from a huge range of other organisations* representing well-known conditions such as diabetes, but also rarer conditions like *Hughes Syndrome* which is sometimes known as *Sticky Blood Syndrome*

At the end of this chapter you will find a list of contact details for useful organizations.

Financial matters

There are several agencies that specialise in giving free, confidential independent advice on financial and legal matters. The *Citizens Advice Bureau* is one such organisation, providing help on a wide range of subjects such as debt, welfare benefits, housing, discrimination, employment and immigration. Locally based *Law Centres* are not-for-profit legal practices which give free advice and representation to disadvantaged people in the UK. Although local government benefit agencies will provide you with accurate information, it is the independent agencies that may have the time and knowledge to work out the best options for *you* as an individual. *Age UK* can also offer help and advice on welfare benefits and a whole range of other relevant topics ranging from exercise classes to computer courses.

Please be aware that the legislation related to welfare benefits is complicated and often subject to major changes. Because of this, professional advice can be very helpful, informative and sometimes essential on welfare benefits.

Ex-military organisations

If you, or a close relative have been involved in the military there are several agencies that are useful resources. These include the *Royal British Legion*, the *Soldiers, Sailors and Airmen's Families Association (SSAFA)* and *Help for Heroes*. The last of these is a comparatively new charity offering financial assistance and long-term support to those who have suffered a life changing injury or illness whilst in service.

Religious organisations

Many religious organisations have advisory services. You do not have to be a member of a religious organisation to receive their help. Local parishes, the Salvation Army, Mosques, Temples and Gurdwaras for example, have information about help services in your neighbourhood.

Housing

Local Authority *Housing Advice Centres*, social service departments and voluntary organisations such as *Shelter* can advise you about homelessness, bad housing and your statutory rights. Local Authority social services have a duty to provide advice for disabled people. The provision of adaptations or special equipment which will help you live in your own home may be mandatory, other things may be discretionary. Shelter produces a booklet called *Housing: Key Facts* which can help to guide you through the maze of legislation.

Domestic violence organisations

Sometimes people with long-term conditions or disabilities can experience domestic violence. Local refuges for such people will treat all enquiries seriously and in confidence. Their addresses are not made public but they can be contacted through the police or social services.

Disability Employment Advisors

If your health or disability is affecting your chances of getting or keeping a job then you can access *Disability Employment Advisors* (DEA's) at your local Jobcentre. They can offer specialist advice and support to disabled job seekers and to those already in work. Two important aspects of their service are:

1. *They can do an employment assessment:* This will help to identify what work or training is most suitable for you.

2. *They can help you with the Access to Work Scheme:* This scheme can for example, pay for specialist equipment or travel expenses to work when you can't use public transport. You will not have to pay the money back and it will not affect your benefits.

NHS Direct

In 2013 *NHS Direct* underwent a major reform and the old service was replaced in some parts of the country by the simple three digit number 111. This new service has been introduced to make it easier to access local NHS healthcare services. The service is not yet available throughout England and has yet to be introduced in Scotland, Wales and Northern Ireland. You are advised to dial 111 when:

- *You need medical help fast* but it is not a 999 emergency.

- *You think you may need to go to A&E* or you need another NHS urgent care service.

- *You do not know who to call* – for example, when you do not have a GP to call.

- *You need health information, reassurance or advice* to deal with a situation where you need to know what to do.

The service will then refer you to the most appropriate support. This could be A&E, an out-of-hours doctor, an urgent care centre, a walk-in centre, a community nurse, an emergency dentist or a late-opening chemist. If the advisor feels you need an ambulance they will call one for you. For your less urgent health needs you should contact your GP or pharmacist in the usual way.

The Internet

Today many people have access to the *Internet*. Even if you are not an Internet user, you will know someone who is. Some people who do not have computers can use them in their local library. Alternatively, ask a friend who *does* have a computer for help. The Internet is the fastest-growing source of information today. Information is being added every second of every day. It offers information about health and anything else you can imagine. It also provides several ways in which you can interact with people all over the world. For example, someone who has *Gaucher disease*, which is a rare health condition, might find it difficult to locate others with the same disease near to home. The Internet can put them in touch with a whole group of such people; with the Internet it doesn't matter whether they are across the street or on the other side of the world.

Another good thing about the Internet is that anyone can take an active part by maintaining a *website*, joining *Facebook* or another social network, writing a blog, or establishing a group. This *openness* can also be a bad thing. There are virtually no controls over who is posting information, or any guarantee that the information is accurate or even safe. This can mean that although there is a mass of information out there that might be very useful, it also means that you may encounter incorrect or even dangerous misinformation. Therefore, you should never assume that information found on the Internet is always entirely trustworthy. Approach information obtained online with scepticism and caution. Ask yourself:

- Is the author or sponsor of the website clearly identified?

- Is the author or the source reputable?

- Is the information contrary to what everyone else seems to be saying about the subject?

- Does common sense support the information?

- What is the purpose of the website?

- Is someone trying to sell you something or win you over to a particular point of view?

One way to start analysing the purpose of the website is to look at the web address: so for example the web address of the *National Osteoporosis Society* is:

www.nos.org.uk

At the end of the main part of a UK-based website, you will most commonly see *.edu, .ac, .org, .gov,* or *.com.* This will give you a clue about the nature of the organisation that owns the website:

- A college or university will have *.edu* or *.ac.*

- A non-profit organisation will have *.org.*

- A government agency will have *.gov.*

- A commercial organisation will have *.com.*

As a general rule of thumb, *.edu, .org, .ac* and *.gov* are fairly trustworthy sites, although a non-profit organisation can sometimes be formed to promote just about anything. A website with *.com* is trying to sell you a product or service, or it is selling advertising space on its site to others trying to sell you something. This doesn't mean that a commercial website can't be a good one. On the contrary, there are many outstanding commercial sites dedicated to providing high-quality, trustworthy information. The *BMJ,* signalled by bmj.com is one such example, which was formerly known as the *British Medical Journal.* These sites are often only able to cover the costs of providing their service by selling advertising or by accepting grants from commercial firms. The addresses for some of our most useful and reliable websites are listed at the end of this chapter.

In the case of the example we used earlier, *www.nos.org.uk,* we know that *www* stands for World Wide Web; *.nos* stands for National

Osteoporosis Society; *.org* tells us it is a non-profit making organisation and *.uk* tells us it is a United Kingdom website. When you search for Government websites in the UK it is advisable to add *.uk* at the end of the address. Without this you may be referred to US sites. Although these are likely to be reliable they do not have information relating specifically to the UK situation. A note of caution should be added about the use of the website *Wikipedia.* This is a free Internet encyclopaedia that is created by general users. These users are able to change or edit anything on the site and although most of the information is accurate it is not always so. There are some editorial controls in place, but you need to be careful in how you use it.

The Internet and social networking

Social networking sites and blogs are exploding on the Internet. Sites such as *Facebook* and *Twitter* are currently very popular. These sites enable ordinary people to communicate easily with others. Some sites, like *Facebook,* require users to decide who will be allowed to read what they post on their page by using the privacy settings.

Many of these sites have been started by people living with particular health conditions who are eager to share their experiences. Some have discussion forums attached to them. The information and support offered can be valuable. However, you should be cautious as some sites may be proposing unproven and dangerous ideas.

Discussion groups on the Internet

Yahoo, Google, and other websites offer discussion groups for just about anything you can imagine. In fact, anyone can start a discussion group about any subject. These groups are run by the people who start them. For any one health problem, you will probably find dozens of discussion groups. You can join in the discussion if you wish, or just read things without interacting. For example in the case of a person with *Gaucher* disease, a discussion group may provide a connection to people who share similar experiences. This may provide the only opportunity to talk with someone else with this rare disease. The other person involved can live in any part of the world. Also, for someone with bipolar disorder, it can sometimes be difficult to talk with someone face-to-face about problems. To find discussion groups, you can go to *Google* or *Yahoo* or another home page and search for a link to *groups*.

Keep in mind that the Internet changes by the second. Indeed things will have changed while you have been reading this.

Technology: Apps and Telehealth

Increasingly we use technology in managing our health. We live in a society where new science and technology arrives almost daily and at the speed of light. Some people are exhilarated by this progress and what it can mean for them. However, some have a natural apprehension and anxiety about how to use new gadgets. Recently something called the *4G Network,* or the *Fourth Generation Network* was introduced. This means more information will be available to people using certain types of mobile phones, such as *smart-phones*, and at a much faster rate. These phones operate like mini-computers with many of the facilities normally found on laptop and desk-top computers. For example, they can receive e-mails and solve problems such as

finding bus timetables. One of the ways these phones can assist people living with a long term condition is that they enable us to use *Apps*. These *Applications* are available to download onto advanced phones. The NHS provides many *Apps* which you can download, ranging from calculating your Body Mass Index (BMI) to dealing with allergies. Sometimes there are even video demonstrations.

Something which is very important to people living with a long-term condition who are often spending lots of time attending hospital and doctor appointments or having blood tests, is the use of *Telehealth*. This *Telehealth* equipment can monitor your health in your own home; for example monitoring your blood pressure or blood glucose levels and many other procedures that people living with a long-term condition need to undertake.

This means you do not have to make so many visits to your GP or Hospital; for example, spending time attending routine appointments for blood tests at the surgery. You are taught how to do the test yourself and the equipment will automatically send your results to the healthcare professional. In this way they can monitor your condition and contact you if they are worried about the readings they receive. The technology to do this is very simple to use. There is a patient information leaflet available entitled "Supporting your independence and well being with Telehealth and Telecare."

You can order a hard copy by calling 0300 123 1002 and *quoting 2900546/telehealthtelecare*. This will give you helpful explanations about Telehealth. At the time of writing this, the Telehealth service is not available to all patients in the UK.

Conclusion

Becoming an effective resource detective is one of the most important jobs of a good self-manager. We hope that this chapter has given you some ideas about the process of finding resources in your community. Knowing *how* to search for resources *yourself* will serve you better than being handed a list of resource agencies. If you find resources that you think we should add to future editions of this book, kindly send them to *self-management@stanford. edu* or to *jean@talkinghealthtakingaction.org* for the UK version of this book.

Resources

The Mayo Clinic

The Mayo Clinic is a well-respected US institution offering information and advice on all medical conditions. www.mayoclinic.org.

The NHS

This offers a comprehensive website with good up-to-date information about most health conditions and NHS organisations. www.nhs.uk.

NHS Direct

NHS Direct will provide information on using the new 111 phone service. Website www.nhs.direct.uk.

Health Talk Online

This site lets you share more than 2000 people's experiences of over 80 health-related conditions and illnesses ranging from breast cancer to epilepsy. The site was formerly known as *DIPEx*. Much of the information gathering was conducted by Oxford University Department of Primary Health Care. Tel: 01865 201330, E-mail info@healthtalkonline.org.uk. www.healthtalkonline.org.

Disabled Living Foundation

Tel: 0845 130 9177, E-mail info@dlf.org.uk.

Patient UK

This is UK medical resource supplying evidence-based information on a wide range of health and medical topics to patients and health professionals. www.patient.co.uk.

Age UK

This is the charity formed by the amalgamation of *Age Concern* and *Help the Aged*. Tel: 0800 169 6565, www.ageuk.org.uk

Arthritis Care

This is an organisation supporting people with arthritis and offering a range of services. Tel: 0808 0800 4050, E-mail info@arthritiscare.org.uk, www.arthritiscare.org.uk.

British Heart Foundation

The organisation offers help and advice in managing heart conditions. The helpline is staffed by cardiac nurses and health advisors, Tel: 0300 330 3311, www.bhf.org.uk.

Diabetes UK

Diabetes UK offers a wide range of support services including information, publications, events and a patient forum. They also support research into various aspects of diabetes Tel: 0845 120 2960, E-mail info@diabetes.org.uk, www.diabetes.org.uk.

Multiple Sclerosis Society

This organisation offers help through information, support campaigning and research. Tel: 0808 800 8000, E-mail Helpline@mssociety.org.uk.

Parkinson's Society

They offer help and support through their trained advisors who include specialist nurses dealing with all aspects of living with the condition. Tel: 0808 800 0303, E-mail hello@parkinson.org.uk, www.parkinsons.org.uk.

Macmillan Cancer Support

This organisation offers advice on how to deal with the practical and emotional effects that a cancer diagnosis may have. Tel: 0808 808 0000, www.macmillan@org.uk.

British Liver Trust

The Trust provides information for those who have a diagnosis of Liver Disease or for relatives or friends who want more information about the condition. The Trust information line is 0800 652 7330, www.britishlivertrust.org.uk.

Terence Higgins Trust

This is a British charity that campaigns on behalf people diagnosed with HIV or Aids. www.tht.org.uk.

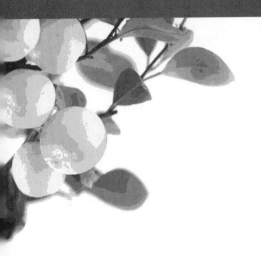

CHAPTER 4

Understanding and Managing Common Symptoms

CHRONIC CONDITIONS COME WITH SYMPTOMS. These are signals from the body that something unusual is happening. These symptoms may include fatigue, stress, shortness of breath, pain, itching, anger, depression, and sleep problems. Sometimes they cannot be seen by others, some are very difficult to describe, and we often don't know when they will occur. Although some symptoms are common, the *times* when they occur and the *ways* in which they affect us are very personal. What's more, these symptoms can interact, which may worsen existing symptoms and may lead to new symptoms or problems.

Regardless of the causes of these symptoms, the ways in which we manage them are often similar. The way we do this comprises our set of *self-management tools*. This chapter discusses several common symptoms, their causes, and some of the *tools* you can use to manage them. Other ways in which you can use your *mind* to help you deal with these symptoms are discussed in Chapter 5. We call these *cognitive tools*.

Dealing with Common Symptoms

Learning to manage symptoms is very similar to problem solving, which we discussed in Chapter 2. It is important to identify the symptom you are experiencing and then to determine why you might be having this symptom *now*. This may sound like a simple process, but it is not always easy.

For example, you can experience many different symptoms with each symptom having various causes and interacting with other symptoms. In addition, the ways in which these symptoms affect your life can be very different. All of these factors can become tangled, like the frayed threads of a cloth. To manage these symptoms, it is helpful to work out how to untangle the threads. One way to do this is to keep a *daily diary* or *journal*. This can be done simply by writing your symptoms on the calendar. You can add some notes about what you were doing before the symptom started or before it got worse. Check the example of this in Figure 4.1. After a week or two, you may begin to see a pattern. For Instance, you go out to for a meal on Saturday evening and wake up later in the night with stomach pain. Once you realise that when you go out, you over eat, you know to adjust the food you order in future. Or every time you go dancing, your feet hurt, but this does not occur when you walk. Could the shoes you wear for dancing account for the difference? Seeing patterns is for many people the first step in symptom self-management.

As you read through this chapter, you will note that many symptoms have the same causes. Also, one symptom may actually cause other symptoms. For example, pain may change the way you walk. In turn, this new way of walking may alter your balance and cause a new pain, or cause you to fall. As you gain more understanding of the possible causes of your symptoms,

Figure 4.1 **A Sample Calendar Journal**

Sample Calendar Journal

Mon.	Tue.	Wed.	Thur.	Fri.	Sat.	Sun.
Grocery shop	Babysit grandkids Pain p.m.	Tired	Water exercise Feel great	Little stiff Clean house	Dinner out Poor sleep	Tired
Mon.	**Tue.**	**Wed.**	**Thur.**	**Fri.**	**Sat.**	**Sun.**
Grocery shop	Babysit grandkids Pain p.m.	Tired	Water exercise Feel great	Clean house	Feel great	Feel great Dinner out Poor sleep

you will be able to identify better ways to deal with them. You may also find ways to prevent or reduce certain symptoms.

Let's look at what you can do to lessen some of the common symptoms experienced because of particular long-term conditions:

Common Symptoms

These common symptoms are discussed in this chapter on the pages shown:

Choosing and Using Different Symptom-Management Tools

- *Choose a tool to try:* Be sure to give this method a fair trial. We recommend that you practise it for at least two weeks before deciding whether or not the tool is going to be helpful.

- *Try some other tools, giving each a trial period:* It is important to try more than one tool because some tools may be more useful for certain symptoms or you may find that you prefer some techniques to others.

- *Think about how and when you will use each tool:* For example, some of these tools may require more lifestyle change than others. The best symptom-managers learn to use a variety of techniques. These will depend on your condition and what you want and need to do each day.

- *Place some cues in your environment to remind you to practise these techniques:* Both practice and consistency are important for mastering new skills. For example, place notes in visible places such as on your mirror, near the phone, in your office, on your computer, or on the car dashboard. Change the notes from time to time so that you'll continue to see them.

- *Try linking the practice of each new tool with some other established daily behaviour:* For example, practise relaxation as part of your cool-down from exercise. Also, you could ask a friend or family member to remind you to practise each day; these individuals may even wish to participate.

Fatigue

A long-term condition can drain your energy. So, fatigue is a very real problem for many people. It is not to be dismissed as, *all in the mind*. Fatigue can keep you from doing things you'd like to do. It is often misunderstood by people who do not have a long-term condition. This is because other people cannot usually see your fatigue. Unfortunately, spouses, family members and friends sometimes fail to understand the unpredictable way in which the fatigue associated with your condition can affect you. They may conclude, incorrectly, that you are just not interested in certain activities or that you want to be alone. Sometimes even *you* may not know why you feel this way.

To be able to manage fatigue, it is important to understand that your fatigue may be related to several factors, such as these:

- *The disease itself:* No matter what illness or illnesses you have, what you do demands the use of more energy. When a chronic condition is present, the body uses energy less efficiently. This is because the energy that would normally be supporting everyday activities, is instead being used to help to heal your body. In response, your body may release chemical signals to conserve energy and make you rest more. Some long-term conditions are also associated with anaemia. This *low blood haemoglobin*, can then contribute to your fatigue.

- *Inactivity:* Muscles that are not used regularly become de-conditioned and less efficient at doing what they are supposed to do. The heart, which is made of muscle

tissue, can also become de-conditioned. When this happens, the ability of the heart to pump blood, which carries necessary nutrients and oxygen to other parts of the body decreases. When muscles do not receive these necessary nutrients and oxygen, they cannot function properly. De-conditioned muscles tire more easily than muscles in good condition.

- *Poor nutrition:* Food is our basic source of energy. If the fuel we take in is of inferior quality, or not consumed in the appropriate quantities, or is improperly digested, fatigue can result. However, vitamin deficiencies are rarely a cause of fatigue. For some people, body weight is the problem. Extra weight causes an increase in the amount of energy needed to perform daily activities. Conversely, being under-weight can also cause problems associated with fatigue. This is especially true for individuals with Chronic Obstructive Pulmonary Disease (COPD). Many people with COPD experience weight loss because of a change in their eating habits and increased fatigue as a consequence.

- *Not enough rest:* For a variety of reasons, there are times when we do not get enough sleep or do not sleep well. This can result in fatigue. We will discuss how to manage sleep problems in more detail later in this chapter.

- *Emotions:* Stress, anxiety, fear, and depression can cause fatigue. Most people are aware of the connection between stress and feeling tired, but fewer are aware of the fact that fatigue is a *major symptom of depression.*

- *Medications:* Some medications can cause fatigue. If you think your experience is medication-related, talk to your doctor. Sometimes the medications or the dose can be changed.

If fatigue is a problem for you, start by trying to determine the cause. Again, a diary may be helpful. Begin with the easiest things that are under your control. Are you eating healthy foods? Are you exercising? Are you getting enough good-quality sleep? Are you effectively managing your stress? If you answer *no* to any of these questions, you may be well on your way to finding one or more of the reasons for your fatigue.

The important thing to remember is that your fatigue *may be caused by things other than your illness.* To prevent fatigue, you must address the real causes. This may mean trying out a variety of self-management tools.

If your fatigue is the result of not eating well, such as consuming too much junk food or drinking too much alcohol, then the solution in each case is to eat better quality foods, in the proper quantities, or to drink less alcohol. For others, the problem may be a decreased interest in food, leading to a lack of calories and subsequent weight loss. Chapter 11 discusses some eating problems and provides tips for healthy eating.

People often say they can't exercise because they feel fatigued. If *you* believe this, then you are creating a vicious cycle. So, people are fatigued because of a lack of exercise, and they don't exercise because they fear the fatigue! Believe it or not, motivating yourself to do a little exercise might be the right answer. You don't have to run a marathon. One important example is to get outdoors and take a short walk. If this is not possible, walk around your house or try some gentle chair exercises. Chapter 6 provides more information on getting started with an exercise programme.

If it is your emotions that are causing your fatigue, rest will probably not help. In fact, it may make you feel worse, especially if your fatigue is also associated with depression. We will talk about how to deal with depression a little later in this chapter. If, on the other hand, you feel that your fatigue may be related to stress, read the section dealing with *Managing Stress* on page 65.

Pain or Physical Discomfort

Pain or physical discomfort is a problem shared by many people with a long-term condition. As with most symptoms, such pain or discomfort can have many causes. The following are some of the most common:

- *The disease itself:* Pain can come from inflammation, damage in or around joints

and tissues, insufficient blood supply to muscles or organs, or irritated nerves, and from other sources.

- *Tense muscles:* When something hurts, the muscles in that area become tense. This is your body's natural reaction to pain when trying to protect the damaged area. In addition, stress can also cause you to tense your muscles. These tense muscles can cause soreness or pain.

- *Muscle de-conditioning:* With chronic conditions, it is common to become less active, leading to a weakening of the muscles, or muscle de-conditioning. When a muscle becomes weak, it tends to complain whenever it is used. This is why even the slightest activity can sometimes lead to pain and stiffness.

- *Lack of sleep or poor-quality sleep:* Pain often interferes with the ability to get enough good quality sleep. But poor sleep by itself can also make pain worse and lessen your ability to cope.

- *Stress, anxiety, and emotions such as depression, anger, fear, and frustration:* These are all normal responses to living with a long-term condition and they can increase your pain or discomfort. When you are stressed, angry, afraid, or depressed, everything, including your pain, seems worse.

- *Medications:* The medicine you are taking can sometimes cause abdominal or other discomfort, pain, weakness and changes in the way you think. If you suspect that medications are the cause, talk to your doctor.

Controlling the 'Pain Gates'

Research suggests that we are not helpless in the face of pain. Your brain can regulate the flow of pain messages by sending electrical and chemical signals that open and close *pain gates* along your nerve pathways.

For example, the brain can release powerful opiate-like chemicals, such as *endorphins* that can effectively block pain. When people are very seriously injured, they sometimes experience little pain in the period when they are focused on survival. It follows that the way you focus your attention, your mood, and the way you view your situation can open or close the *pain gates*. The techniques recorded in Chapter 5 can be helpful.

Thinking about Chronic Pain

Chronic pain is pain that extends over months or years and is often difficult to explain. Most experts now believe that almost all unexplained chronic pain is caused by some sort of physical problem: damaged or inflamed nerves, blood vessels, muscles, or other tissues. These underlying physical problems can't always be pinpointed. This means that the pain is not *all in your head*.

Your day-to-day pain level is based on how your mind and body respond to pain. For example, your body quickly attempts to limit movement in the damaged area. This causes muscle tension, which can increase your pain. Chronic pain often leads to inactivity. As a consequence, muscles may become weakened and hurt with even the slightest use.

Feelings of anxiety, anger, frustration, and loss of control also amplify the experience of pain. This doesn't mean that the pain is not real; it simply means that your emotions can make a painful situation worse.

Here are four examples of how pain relates to the way your mind and body interact:

Keep a Pain Diary

To get a clear understanding of how your moods, activities, and conditions affect your pain, keep a pain diary. You can begin by recording your activities and pain levels three times a day, at regular intervals.

1. **Record** the date and time.

2. **Describe** the situation or activity, for example, you might be watching TV, doing housework, or simply arguing.

3. **Rate** the physical sensation of your pain on a scale from 0 (no pain), to 10 (excruciating pain).

4. **Describe** your pain sensation, for example, (it's a deep aching pain in my left lower back).

5. **Rate** your emotional distress from this pain on a scale from 0 (no distress), to 10 (severely distressed).

6. **Describe** the type of emotional distress, for example, "I felt very angry or I needed to cry."

7. **Describe** what you did, if anything, to alleviate the discomfort, for example, you took medication, had a massage, did a relaxation exercise or went for a walk. At the same time, note its effect.

Look for patterns. For example, is the pain worse after sitting for a long time? Is it less when you are engaged in a favourite hobby?

How much you notice pain can vary according to your mood, fatigue and muscle tension. It's important to distinguish between *physical* pain sensations, such as *stabbing, burning,* and *aching* and *emotional* pain distress, which includes the accompanying *anger, anxiety, frustration,* or *sadness.* This is useful because even if your physical pain may not be reduced, you can *feel* better about the pain and consequently experience less distress, anxiety, helplessness, and despair.

■ *Inactivity:* Because of the pain, you can avoid physical activity and this, in turn, causes you to lose strength and flexibility. The weaker and more out of condition you become, the more frustrated and depressed you will feel. These negative emotions can open the pain gates and cause pain levels to rise.

■ *Overdoing things:* You may be determined to prove that you can still be active, so you over-exert yourself. This increases the pain

and leads to more inactivity, more depression, and yet more pain.

■ *Misunderstanding:* Your friends, family, boss, and co-workers may not understand that you are suffering and may dismiss your pain as *not real.* This evokes yet more anger or depression.

■ *Overprotection:* Friends, family, and co-workers can sometimes coddle you and make excuses for you. This can make you feel dependent and disabled and can alter how you react.

Fortunately, this downward spiral of mind-body interaction can be interrupted. Being told you have to *learn to live with pain* doesn't have to be the end of the road. It can be a new beginning. You can learn techniques such as these:

- *Redirect* your attention to control pain.
- *Challenge* negative thoughts that support pain.
- *Cultivate* more positive emotions.
- *Increase* your activity slowly and recondition yourself.

Tools for Managing Pain

There are many tools available to help you to manage your pain. But, just as you cannot build a house with one tool, you often need several tools to accomplish this task.

Try exercise

exercise and physical activity can be excellent pain relievers. The benefits of exercise and tips for starting an exercise programme are discussed in Chapters 6, 7 and 8. If you aren't able to do the things you want and need to do because of physical limitations, a physiotherapist may also be helpful.

Try mind-made medicine

you can also use your mind to manage pain through relaxation, imagery, visualisation, distraction, and through positive thinking. This is discussed In Chapter 5. Positive thinking is a very powerful way to challenge pain. You can learn how to monitor and defeat negative thinking by using *self-talk*. If you find yourself waking up in pain and saying, *"I'm going to be miserable all day and I won't get anything done"*, instead, tell yourself *"I've got some pain this morning, so I'll start with some relaxation and stretching exercises, and then I'll do some of the less demanding things I want to get done."*

Try ice, heat, and massage

for pain in a local area such as the back or knee, the application of heat, cold, and massage are helpful. These three tools work by stimulating the skin and other tissues surrounding the painful area, which increases the blood flow and blocks the transmission of pain in nerve fibres.

Applying heat by using a heating pad or by taking a warm bath or shower, with the water flow directed at the painful area will help. You can make your own substitute heating pad by placing rice or dry beans in a sock, knotting the top, and heating it in a microwave oven for three to four minutes. Be sure to test the heat before you use it, so that you don't burn yourself.

Some people prefer *applying cold* for soothing pain, especially if there is inflammation. A bag of frozen peas makes an inexpensive and reusable *cold pack*. Whether using heat or cold, always place a towel between the source and your skin. Also, limit the application to 15 or 20 minutes at a time. Longer exposure can burn or freeze the skin.

Using Massage is one of the oldest forms of pain management. Hippocrates (460–380 BC) said that, *"Physicians must be experienced in many things, but assuredly also in the rubbing that can bind a joint that is loose and loosen a joint that is too hard."* Self-massage is a simple procedure that can be performed with little practice or preparation. It stimulates the skin, the underlying tissues, and muscles simply by rubbing with a little applied pressure. Some people like to use a mentholated cream with self-massage because this also provides a cooling effect.

Massage, although relatively simple, is not appropriate for all cases of pain. Do *not* use self-massage for a *hot joint* which is red, swollen, and hot to touch. Also avoid it for an infected area or, if you are suffering from *cellulitis*, *phlebitis*, *thrombophlebitis*, or skin eruptions.

Try medications

Acute pain usually responds to pain-killing drugs. These can range from mild over-the-counter analgesics for headaches to powerful narcotic medications for post-operative and cancer pain. Some medications can open up blood vessels in the heart or in muscles and this can relieve pain. Some types of chronic pain and arthritis respond well to anti-inflammatory medications. Surprisingly, some medications which were originally used to treat depression have been found to relieve pain in lower doses without the problem of addiction. Narcotic medications are rarely suitable for chronic pain, as they can become less effective over time and require increasing doses. They can also interfere with breathing, balance and sleep. They can also cause disturbances in mood and in the ability to think clearly. Sometimes injections of a local anaesthetic or a surgical procedure can block pain signals from a painful area and this can provide temporary, and sometimes lasting, relief from chronic pain.

Two final notes

1. If you have pain medication in the house, keep it in a place that will not be accessible to young people or visitors. The potential for *adolescent prescription drug abuse* is a real and concerning one. This is because some youngsters use these drugs to get high. It is preferable to keep the medicine locked in a cabinet.

2. If you or someone you care for is nearing the end of life, which means that they are estimated to have six months or less to live, and pain is a problem, you might consider asking for palliative or hospice care. Hospice units are staffed by specialist teams of health professionals who are experts in relieving end-of-life pain whilst allowing the patient to remain alert. At this point in life, addiction is not a concern: comfort is.

If pain continues to be a major factor in your life, discuss with your doctor the options available, including referral to a pain management clinic.

Shortness of Breath

Shortness of breath, like many other symptoms, can have several causes, all of which prevent your body from getting the oxygen it needs. Before continuing with this section, you may wish to read Chapter 15, which discusses normal lung functioning and also considers the changes that take place in the lungs with chronic lung disease. Chapter 16 goes on to discuss heart disease, which is also associated with shortness of breath.

Excess weight can cause shortness of breath because it increases the amount of energy you use and therefore the quantity of oxygen you need. Weight also increases the workload for your heart. As a result, when excess weight is coupled with chronic lung or heart disease, there is an added difficulty in supplying the body with the oxygen it needs.

The *de-conditioning of muscles* can also lead to shortness of breath. This de-conditioning can affect the breathing muscles as well as other muscles in your body. When muscles become de-conditioned, they are less efficient. They require more energy and oxygen to perform activities. In the case of de-conditioned breathing muscles, the problem is complicated. If the breathing muscles are weak, it becomes harder to cough and clear mucus from the lungs. When there is mucus in the lungs, there is less space for fresh air.

Just as there are many causes of shortness of breath, there are many things you can do to manage this problem.

- *When you feel short of breath, don't stop what you are doing or hurry up to finish:* Instead, slow down. If shortness of breath continues, stop for a few minutes. If you are still short of breath, take any medication prescribed by your doctor. Shortness of breath can be frightening, and this fear can cause two additional problems. *First,* when you are afraid, you release hormones such as adrenaline. This will increase your shortness of breath. *Second,* you may stop activity for fear that it will hurt you. If this happens, you will

never build up the endurance necessary to help your breathing. The basic rule is to take things slowly and in steps.

- *Increase your activity gradually, generally by not more than 25% each week:* So, if you are now able to garden comfortably for 20 minutes, next week increase it by up to five minutes. Once you can garden comfortably for 25 minutes, you can again add *a few more minutes.* Don't smoke, and, equally important, avoid smokers. This may sometimes be difficult because smoking friends may not realise how they are complicating your life. Your job is to tell them. Explain that their smoke is causing breathing problems for you, and that you would appreciate it if they would not smoke when you are around. Also, make your house and especially your car *no smoking zones.* Ask people to smoke *outside.*

- *Drink plenty of fluids if mucus and secretions are a problem:* Don't do this if your doctor has told you to limit what you drink. However, in normal circumstances fluid consumption will help thin the mucus and make it easier to cough up. Using a humidifier may also be helpful.

- *Use your medications and oxygen as prescribed:* We often hear that drugs are harmful and should not be used. In many cases this is correct. However, when you have a long-term condition, drugs are often very helpful and sometimes even life savers. Don't skimp, cut down, or go without. On the other hand, more is not better, so don't take more than the prescribed amount. If adjustments need to be made, let your doctor make that decision.

Breathing Self-Management Tools

Here are several tools that can help you with better breathing; you will also find more tools described in Chapter 15.

Diaphragmatic breathing – sometimes called "belly breathing"

Diaphragmatic breathing is also called *belly breathing* because when you do it properly, the diaphragm descends into the abdomen. One of the problems that causes shortness of breath, especially for people with emphysema, chronic bronchitis, or asthma, is de-conditioning of the diaphragm and chest breathing muscles. When this de-conditioning occurs, the lungs are not able to function properly. That is, they do not fill properly, nor do they get rid of the stale air.

Most of us use our upper lungs and chest mainly for breathing. As a result, because diaphragmatic or belly breathing goes deeper, it requires some practice to learn to fully expand your lungs. This *deep breathing* strengthens the breathing muscles and makes them more efficient, so breathing is easier. These are the steps to achieving effective diaphragmatic breathing:

1. *Lie on your back* with pillows under your head and knees.

2. *Place one hand on your stomach*, at the base of your breastbone, and the other hand on your upper chest.

3. *Breathe in slowly through your nose*, allowing your stomach to expand outward. Imagine that your lungs are filling with fresh air. The hand on your stomach should move upward. The hand on your chest should not move or should move only slightly.

4. *Breathe out slowly, through pursed lips.* At the same time, use your hand to gently push inward and upward on your abdomen.

5. *Practise this technique* for ten to 15 minutes, three or four times a day, until it becomes automatic. If you begin to feel a little dizzy, either rest or breathe out more slowly.

You can also practise diaphragmatic breathing whilst sitting in a chair:

1. *Relax your shoulders, arms, hands, and chest.* Do *not* grip the arms of the chair or your knees.

2. *Put one hand on your abdomen and the other on your chest.*

3. *Breathe in through your nose*, filling the area around your waist with air. Your chest hand should remain still and the hand on your abdomen should move.

4. *Breathe out* without force or effort.

Once you are comfortable with this technique, you can practise it almost anytime, when lying down, sitting, standing, or walking. Diaphragmatic breathing can help strengthen and improve the coordination and efficiency of the breathing muscles, as well as decreasing the amount of energy you need to breathe. In addition, it can be used in conjunction with any of the relaxation techniques that use the power of your mind to manage your symptoms. Again, take a look at Chapter 5.

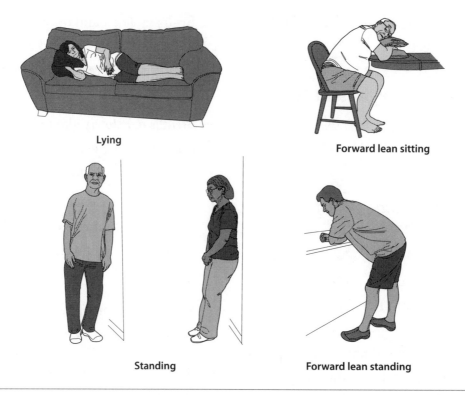

Figure 4.2 **Positions that will help if you are breathless or short of breath**

Pursed-lip breathing

The *pursed-lip breathing* technique, usually happens naturally for people who have problems emptying their lungs. It can also be used if you are breathless or relatively short of breath.

1. *Breathe in, and then purse your lips*; as if to blow across a flute or into a whistle.

2. *Breathe out through pursed lips using diaphragmatic breathing*, without any force.

3. *Remember to relax the upper chest, shoulders, arms, and hands while breathing out.* Check for tension. Breathing out should take longer than breathing in.

By mastering this technique while doing other activities, you will be better able to manage your shortness of breath. Take a look at Figure 4.2 which illustrates some of these suggestions.

The next two techniques may be helpful for removing mucus and phlegm secretions:

Huffing

This technique combines one or two forced *huff-puffs* of breath with diaphragmatic breathing. It is useful for removing secretions from small airways.

1. *Take in a breath* as you would for diaphragmatic breathing.

2. *Hold your breath* for a moment.

3. *Huff,* keeping your mouth open while squeezing your chest and abdominal muscles to force out the air. This is a little like panting.

4. *If possible, do another huff* before taking in another breath.

5. *Take two or three diaphragmatic breaths.*

6. *Huff once or twice.*

Controlled cough

This helps to remove phlegm secretions from your larger airways.

1. Take in a full, slow diaphragmatic breath.

2. Keep your shoulders and hands relaxed.

3. Hold the breath for a moment.

4. Cough, tightening the abdominal muscles to force the air out.

You can find out more about controlled coughing in Chapter 15.

If you have a bout of uncontrolled coughing, the following advice may help:

- *Avoid* very dry air or steam.

- *Swallow* as soon as the bout starts.

- *Sip* some water.

- *Suck* on a lozenge or a boiled sweet.

- *Try* diaphragmatic breathing, being sure to breathe in through your nose.

Sleep Problems

Sleep is a time during which the body can achieve healing. Little energy is required to maintain body functioning when you sleep. When you don't get enough sleep, you can experience a variety of other symptoms, such as fatigue, inability to concentrate, irritability, increased pain, and weight gain. Of course, this does not mean that these symptoms are always caused by lack of sleep. Remember, the symptoms associated with long-term conditions can have many causes. Nevertheless, improving the quality of your sleep can help you manage many symptoms, regardless of the cause.

How Much Sleep Do You Need?

The amount of sleep needed varies from person to person. Most people do best with about 7½ hours. Some feel refreshed with just six hours, but others need eight to ten to function well. If you are alert, feel rested, and function well during the day, the chances are you are getting enough sleep.

Sleep is a basic human need, like food and water. Getting less sleep for *one night* is not a big problem. But if you get less sleep than you require night after night, your quality of life and mood may suffer.

Getting a Good Night's Sleep

The self-management techniques we offer here are clinically proven, with a 75% to 80% success rate. They are not *quick fixes* like sleep medications, but they'll give you safer and more effective results in the long run. Allow yourself at least two to four weeks to see some positive results and ten to 12 weeks for long-term improvement.

Things you can do before you get into bed include the following:

- *Get a comfortable bed that allows for ease of movement and good body support:* This usually means a good-quality, firm mattress that supports the spine and does not force the body to stay in the middle of the bed. A bed board, made of 1 to 2 cm plywood, can be placed between the mattress and the box spring to increase the firmness. Heated waterbeds, airbeds, and foam mattresses are helpful for some people with chronic pain because they support weight evenly by conforming to the body's shape. If you are interested and it is possible, try some beds out at a friend's home or at a hotel for a few nights to decide what is right for you. An electric blanket, set on low heat, or a wool mattress pad are also effective at providing heat as you sleep, especially on cool or damp nights. If you decide to use electric bedding, make sure you follow the instructions carefully to prevent being burned.

- **Warm your hands and feet** with gloves or socks: For painful knees, it often helps to cut the toes off warm stockings and use them as *sleeves* for your knees.

- *Find a comfortable sleeping position:* The best position depends on you and your condition. Sometimes the use of small pillows put in the right places can relieve pain and discomfort. Experiment with different positions and the use of pillows. Also check with your health care professional for any specific recommendations given for your condition.

- **Elevate the head of the bed** by four to six inches on wooden blocks to make breathing easier: This is especially helpful if you have heartburn or gastric reflux.

- *Keep the room at a comfortable temperature:* This can be either warm or cool. Each of us has a different preference.

- *Use a vaporiser if you live where the air is dry:* Air which is warm and moist can often make breathing and sleeping easier.

- *Make your bedroom safe and comfortable:* Keep a lamp and telephone by your bed, in easy reach. If you use a walking stick, keep it where you will not trip over it and yet close to the bed. This means you can use it when you get up during the night.

- *Keep your spectacles by the bed when you go to sleep:* This way, if you need to get up in the night, you can easily put them on and see where you are going!

There are a number of things you should avoid before bedtime:

- *Avoid eating:* You may feel sleepy after eating a big meal, but that is not a good way to help you fall asleep and get a good night's sleep. Sleep is meant to allow your body time to rest and recover. So, when it is busy digesting food, this takes valuable time and attention away from the healing process. If you find that going to sleep feeling hungry keeps you awake, try drinking a glass of warm milk at bedtime.

- *Avoid drinking alcohol:* You may think that alcohol helps you sleep better because it makes you feel relaxed and sleepy, but in fact, alcohol disrupts your sleep cycle. Alcohol before bedtime can lead to shallow sleep and frequent awakenings throughout the night.

- *Avoid caffeine late in the day:* Caffeine is a stimulant, and it can keep you awake. Coffee, tea, colas, other fizzy drinks, and chocolate all contain caffeine, so go easy on them as evening approaches.

- *Avoid smoking:* Aside from the fact that smoking itself can cause complications and a worsening of your chronic condition, falling asleep with a lighted cigarette can pose a fire hazard. Furthermore, the nicotine contained in cigarettes is a stimulant.

- *Avoid diet pills:* Diet pills often contain stimulants, which may interfere with falling asleep and staying asleep.

- *Avoid sleeping pills:* Although the name *sleeping pills* sounds like the perfect solution for sleep problems, these remedies tend to become less effective over time. Also, many sleeping pills have a *rebound effect*. So, if you stop taking them, it is even more difficult to get to sleep. Consequently, as they become less effective, you can end up with more problems than you had when you first started. All in all, it is best to use other approaches and to avoid using sleeping pills.

- *Avoid using a computer or watching TV for about an hour before you go to bed:* The light from computer and TV screens can disrupt your natural sleep rhythms.

- *Avoid taking diuretics (water pills) before bedtime:* It's better to take them in the morning so that your sleep is not interrupted by frequent trips to the bathroom. Don't reduce the overall amount of fluids you drink, unless your doctor has recommended otherwise, as these are important for your health. However, you may want to limit the amount you drink just before you go to bed.

How to develop a routine

- *Maintain a regular rest and sleep schedule:* Try to go to bed at the same time every

night and get up at the same time every morning. If you wish to take a brief nap, take one in the afternoon, but do not take a nap after dinner. Stay awake until you are ready to go to bed.

- *Re-set your sleep clock when necessary:* If your sleep schedule gets off track, for example, you go to bed at 4:00 a.m. and sleep until mid-day you'll have to re-set your internal sleep clock. To do so, try going to bed an hour earlier or later each day until you reach the hour you would like to go to sleep. This may sound strange, but it seems to be the best way to re-set your sleep clock.

- *Exercise at regular times each day:* Not only will the exercise help you obtain better quality sleep, but it will also help set a regular pattern for your day. However, it's best to avoid exercising immediately before bedtime.

- *Get out in the sun every morning:* Do this even if it is only for 15 or 20 minutes. This helps regularise your body clock and rhythms.

- *Do the same things every night before going to bed:* This can be anything from listening to the news to reading a chapter of a book to taking a warm bath. By developing and sticking to a *get ready for bed* routine, you will be telling your body that it's time to start winding down and beginning to relax.

- *Only use your bedroom for sleeping and sex:* If you find that you get into bed and you can't fall asleep, get out of bed and go into another room until you begin to feel sleepy again. Keep the lighting low.

What to Do When You Can't Get Back to Sleep

Many people can get to sleep without a problem but then wake up with *early morning worries* and can't seem to turn off their minds. They then get more worried because they cannot get back to sleep. Keeping your mind occupied with pleasurable or interesting thoughts will ward off such worries and help you get back to sleep. For example, try distraction techniques such as quieting your mind by counting backward from 100 by threes or by naming a flower for every letter of the alphabet. The relaxation techniques described in Chapter 5 may also be helpful. If after some time you really can't to sleep, then get up and do something. Try reading a book, washing your hair, playing a game of solitaire, although it's probably best not to do this on the computer! After 15 or 20 minutes, try going back to bed.

It can also help to set a *worry time*. If a racing mind keeps you awake, designate a time well before bedtime, during which you write down your problems and concerns. Then make a to-do list which addresses them. Now you can relax and sleep well, knowing that you can worry again during tomorrow's *worry time*.

Don't worry too much about not getting enough sleep. If your body needs sleep, you will sleep. Also, remember that people tend to need less sleep as they get older.

Sleep Apnoea and Snoring

If you fall asleep *as soon as your head hits the pillow* or fall asleep regularly in front of the TV and are tired when you wake up in the morning, even after a full night's sleep, you may have a sleep disorder. People with the most common sleep disorder, *obstructive sleep apnoea*, often don't know.

Such individuals, when asked about their sleep, respond *"I sleep well"*. Sometimes the only clue to the problem is that others might complain about your loud snoring. Sleep specialists believe that obstructive sleep apnoea is very common and yet alarmingly under-diagnosed.

With sleep apnoea, the soft tissues in the throat or nose relax during sleep and block the airway. Extreme effort is now required to breathe. The sleeper will struggle against the blockage for up to a minute and then wakes just long enough to gasp air, and falls back to sleep to start the cycle all over again. The person is rarely aware that he or she has awakened dozens of times during the night and therefore lacks the deep sleep needed to restore the body's energy and help with the healing process. This cycle of events, in turn, leads to more symptoms such as fatigue and pain. You should note that there is a much rarer form of sleep apnoea called *central sleep apnoea* which is caused by the brain forgetting to breathe during sleep.

Getting Professional Help

The majority of sleep problems can be solved with the techniques we have mentioned, but there are times when you need professional assistance. So, when should you seek help?

- *If your insomnia persists for six months or is seriously affecting your daytime functioning:* Your job or social relationships may be badly affected, despite the fact that you have faithfully followed the self-help programme we have described.

- *If you have great difficulty staying awake during the day:* Daytime sleepiness can cause or come close to causing an accident.

- *If your sleep is disturbed by breathing difficulties:* This includes loud snoring with long pauses, chest pain, heartburn, leg twitching, excessive pain, or other physical conditions.

- *If your difficulty sleeping is accompanied by other issues:* This includes matters such as depression, or problems with alcohol, sleeping medications, or addictive drugs.

Don't put off asking for help. Most sleep problems can be solved. Once they're gone, you'll get a better night's sleep and will enjoy better health.

Depression

Most people with a long-term condition sometimes feel depressed. There are different degrees of depression, ranging from being occasionally sad or blue, to serious clinical depression. Sometimes, we are unaware that we are depressed. More often we may not want to admit it. How you handle depression makes a real difference.

Depression and Bad Moods

Feeling sad sometimes is natural. This *sadness* is a temporary feeling, often linked to a specific event or loss. We sometimes use the word *depressed* to describe feeling sad or disappointed: *"I'm really depressed about not being able to get a ticket for the concert"*. Under these circumstances we do feel *sad*, but we can still relate to others and find joy in other areas of our lives.

Sometimes depression lasts longer, for example when we lose a loved one or are diagnosed with a serious illness. If the sad feelings that you feel are severe, long-lasting, and recurrent, you may be experiencing *clinical depression*. It drains the pleasure out of life, leaving you feeling hopeless, helpless, and worthless. With severe depression, feelings may become numb, and even crying brings no relief. Depression affects everything: the way you think, the way you behave, the way you interact with others, and even the way your body functions.

What Causes Depression?

Depression is not caused by personal weakness, laziness, or a lack of will-power. Heredity, your long-term condition, and your medications may all play a part in depression. The way you think, especially negative thoughts, can also produce and sustain a depressed mood. Negative thoughts can sometimes be automatic, recur endlessly, and they may not be linked to any event or triggering cause. Certain feelings and emotions also contribute to depression, such as:

- *Fear, anxiety, or uncertainty about the future:* Feelings that result from worries about your financial situation, your disease or treatment, or concerns about your family can all lead to depression. By facing these issues as soon as possible, both you and your family will spend less time worrying and have more time to enjoy life. This can have a healing effect. We talk more about these issues and how to deal with them in Chapter 19.

■ *Frustration:* Frustration can have many causes. You may find yourself thinking, *"I just can't do what I want"*, or *"I feel so helpless"*, or *"I used to be able to do this for myself"*, or *"Why doesn't anyone understand me?"* The longer you accept and endure these feelings, the more alone and isolated you are likely to feel.

■ *Loss of control over your life:* Many things can make you feel as if you are losing control. These can include having to rely on medications, having to see a doctor on a regular basis, or having to count on others to help you do things such as bathing, dressing, and preparing your meals. This feeling of *loss of control* can make you lose faith in yourself and your abilities. Even though you may not be able to do everything yourself, you can still be in charge.

Not all depressive behaviour is negative. Sometimes unrealistic cheeriness will mask what a person is really feeling. Refusal to accept offers of help, even in the face of obvious need, is a frequent symptom of unrecognised depression.

Depressed feelings can lead to such behaviours as withdrawal, isolation, and lack of physical activity. These behaviours can in themselves create more depressed feelings. The paradox of depression-related behaviour is that the more you engage in the behaviour, the more likely it is that you will drive away the people who can support and comfort you. Most of our friends and family want to help us to feel better, but often they don't really know how. As their efforts to comfort and reassure us are frustrated, they may at some point throw up their hands and stop trying. Then the depressed person ends up

saying, *"See, nobody cares"*. This in turn reinforces feelings of loss and loneliness.

All these factors, and others, can contribute to an imbalance in the chemicals in your brain. This imbalance can change how you think, feel, and act. Changing the way you think and behave can be a powerful and effective way of changing your brain chemistry, lightening depression, and improving an ordinary bad mood.

Am I Depressed?

Here is a quick test for depression: Ask yourself what you do to have fun. If you don't have a quick answer to that, consider the other possible symptoms of depression we describe here.

Think about your mood over the past two weeks. Which of the following have you experienced?

■ *Having little interest or pleasure in doing things:* Not enjoying life or other people may be a sign of depression. Symptoms include not wanting to talk to anyone, or go out, or answer your phone or doorbell.

■ *Feeling down, depressed, or hopeless:* Feeling persistently blue in this way, can be a symptom of depression.

■ *Experiencing trouble in falling asleep, or in staying asleep or sleeping too much:* Waking up and being unable to go back to sleep, sleeping too much, or not wanting to get out of bed can all signal a problem.

■ *Feeling tired or having little energy:* Fatigue is that feeling of being tired all the time; it is often a clear symptom of depression.

■ *Having a poor appetite or over-eating:* This may range from a loss of interest in food to an unusually erratic or excessive eating pattern.

- *Feeling bad about yourself:* Have you begun to feel that you are a failure or have let yourself or your family down? Have you had a feeling of worthlessness, a negative image of your body, or doubts about your own self-worth? This is a clear indicator.

- *Having trouble concentrating:* Have you found it hard to do simple things such as reading the newspaper or watching television?

- *Experiencing lethargy or restlessness:* Have you been moving lethargically, or speaking so slowly that other people have noticed? Or, perhaps the opposite, have you been so fidgety or restless that you have been moving around a lot more than usual? Either of these can be a sign of depression.

- *Wishing yourself harm or worse:* Have you ever thought that you would be better off dead or thought about hurting yourself in some way? If so, this is the hallmark of severe depression.

Depressed people may also experience a weight loss or a weight gain, loss of interest in sex or intimacy, loss of interest in personal care and grooming, an inability to make decisions, and having accidents more frequently than usual. These are all telling signs.

If several of the symptoms we have indicated seem to apply to you, please get some help from your doctor, or good friends, a member of the clergy, a psychologist, or a social worker. Don't wait for these feelings to pass. If you are thinking about harming yourself or others, get help

now. Don't let a tragedy happen to you and your loved ones.

Fortunately, available treatments for depression, including anti-depressant medications, counselling, and self-help, are highly effective in decreasing the frequency, length, and severity of depression. Depression, like other symptoms, can be managed.

How to Lighten Depression and Bad Moods

The three most effective treatments for depression are medications, counselling, and self-help.

Medications

Anti-depressant medications that help to balance brain chemistry are highly effective. However, most anti-depressant medications take time to work. It may be several days to several weeks before they begin to change how you feel. Then they usually bring significant relief. So don't be discouraged if you don't feel better immediately. Stick with it. To get the maximum benefit you may need to take some medications for six months or more.

Side effects are usually most noticeable in the first few weeks and then reduce in severity or go away. If the side effects are not especially severe, you should continue to take your medication. As your body gets used to it, you will begin to feel better. It is important to remember to take your medication every day. If you stop the medication because you're feeling better, or worse, you may relapse. Anti-depressant medications are not addictive, but always talk with your doctor before stopping or changing the dose.

Counselling

Several types of psychotherapy can also be highly effective, relieving symptoms for up to 60% to 70% of the time. As with medications, counselling rarely has an immediate effect. It may be many weeks before you see improvement. This therapy can be brief, usually involving one to two sessions a week over several months. By learning new psychotherapy skills during counselling about ways to think and relate, you can reduce the risk of recurrent depression.

Self-help

Self-help can also be surprisingly effective. You can learn to apply many successful psychotherapy techniques on your own. The self-help strategies discussed here can sometimes be very productive in combating mild to moderate depression or just lifting your mood. One study showed that reading and practising self-help advice improved depression in nearly 70% of patients. The skills and strategies which follow can be used alone or to supplement medications and counselling:

- *Eliminate the negative:* First let's talk about some things that will certainly *not* help depression or bad moods. Being alone and isolating yourself, crying a lot, getting angry and yelling, blaming your failure or bad mood on others, or using alcohol or other drugs will usually leave you feeling worse. If you are taking tranquilisers or narcotic painkillers such as *Valium, Librium, codeine, Vicodin,* or sleeping medications, or other *downers,* they will intensify and may even cause depression as a side effect. However, do not stop taking the prescribed medication before talking to

your doctor. There may be important reasons for continuing their use and you may experience withdrawal reactions.

Do you sometimes drink alcohol to feel better? Alcohol is also a *downer.* There is virtually no way to escape depression unless you unload these negative alcoholic influences from your brain. For most people, one or two drinks in the evening will not be a problem. On the other hand, if your mind is not free of alcohol during most of the day, you are beginning to have trouble with this drug. Talk this over with your doctor or call *Alcoholics Anonymous.*

- *Plan for pleasure:* When you are feeling blue or depressed, the tendency is to withdraw, isolate yourself, and restrict activity. This is the wrong thing to do. Maintaining or increasing activity is one of the best antidotes for depression. Going for a walk, looking at a sunset, watching a funny film, getting a massage, learning another language, taking a cookery class, or joining a social club can all help to keep your spirits up and keep you from falling into a situation where you might get depressed.

But sometimes having fun isn't such an easy prescription. You may have to make a deliberate effort to plan pleasurable activities. Even if you don't feel like doing it, try to stick to your plan. You may find that the nature walk, cup of tea, or half hour of listening to music will improve your mood despite your initial misgivings. Don't leave good things to chance. Make a firm plan for your free time during the week and what you'd like to do with it.

If you are feeling hardly any emotion and the world seems devoid of colour, make an effort to put some sensation back into your life. Go to a bookshop and look through your favourite section. Listen to some upbeat music, or dance to it. Exercise, or ask someone to give you a massage, so that you can reconnect with your body. Treat yourself to a very hot bath, or try a cold shower. Go to a garden centre and smell all the flowers.

Make your plans and carry them out. Look to the future. Plant some young trees. Look forward to your grandchildren's graduation from university or college. If you know that one time of the year is especially difficult, such as Christmas or a birthday, make some specific plans for that period. Don't wait to see what happens. Be prepared.

■ *Take action:* Continue your daily activities. Get dressed every day, make your bed, get out of the house, go shopping, maybe walk your dog. Plan and cook meals. Force yourself to do these things even if you don't feel like it. Taking action to solve the problems immediately facing you, provides the surest relief from a bad mood. More important than *what* you change or *how much* you change are the confidence-building feelings that come from successfully changing something. It can be anything! *Taking action* is the important thing. Incorporating some simple things into your life can boost your mood. You might decide to clean or reorganise a room, or a cupboard or a desk drawer. Perhaps you can get a new magazine subscription or call an old friend.

Be careful not to set yourself difficult goals or take on a lot of responsibility. Break large tasks down into small ones. Set some priorities, and do what you can as well as you can. Learn some of the proven steps for taking successful action described In Chapter 2. It is probably wise when you are feeling depressed not to make big life decisions. For example, don't move house without a lot of thought. If you do, then spend some time in the area you are thinking of moving to. Learn about the resources available in your new community. Moving can be a sign of withdrawal. Certainly, depression can be intensified when you are in a location far away from friends and acquaintances. In any case, many troubles may move with you. At the same time, the support you need to deal with your troubles may have been left behind.

■ *Socialise:* Join a group. Get involved in a church, a book club, an adult education class, a self-help support group, a gardening club or *any type of group* which focuses on your own interests. If you can't get out, consider a group on the Internet. If you do this, be sure that the Internet group is moderated, that is, that someone is in charge to enforce the rules of the group. Don't isolate yourself. Try to seek out positive, optimistic people because they can lighten your heavy feelings.

■ *Move your mood:* Physical activity lifts depression and counters negative moods. Depressed people often complain that they feel too tired to exercise. But the feelings of fatigue associated with depression are rarely due to physical exhaustion. Try to get at least 20 to 30 minutes a day of some type of exercise, from chair dancing to walking. If you can get yourself moving, you may find that you have more energy. This is explained in Chapter 6.

- *Think positively:* Many people tend to be excessively self-critical, especially when they're depressed. You may find yourself thinking groundless, untrue things about yourself. As you challenge these negative thoughts, begin to re-script the negative stories you tell yourself, as indicated in Chapter 5. For example, one of your underlying beliefs may be *"Unless I do everything perfectly, I'm a failure"*. Perhaps this belief could be revised to *"Success is doing the best that I can in any situation"*. Also, when you are depressed, it's easy to forget about nice things that have happened. Make a list of some of the good or positive events in your life. Such as the time you decided to lose weight and succeeded, the time you organised a very successful birthday party or the time you helped your friend choose an outfit for her daughter's wedding.

- *Do something for someone else:* Lending a helping hand to someone in need is one of the most effective ways to change a bad mood. But it is also one of the least commonly used. Arrange to baby-sit for a friend, read a story to someone who is ill, or volunteer at a day centre. When you're depressed, you can sometimes react to helping others with gloomy thoughts like *"I've got enough troubles of my own. I don't need anyone else's"*. But if you *can* help someone else, even in a small way, you'll feel better about yourself. Feeling useful is good for self-esteem, and you will be temporarily distracted from your own problems. Helping others needier than yourself can help you to appreciate your own assets and capabilities. By comparison, your problems and difficulties may not appear so overwhelming. Sometimes helping others is the surest way to help yourself.

Don't be discouraged if it takes some time to feel better. If these self-help strategies are not sufficient on their own, seek help from your doctor or a mental health professional. Often some *talk therapy* or the use of antidepressant medications, or both, can go a long way toward relieving depression. Seeking professional help and taking medications are not signs of weakness. They are signs of strength.

Anger

Anger is one of the most common responses to a long-term health condition. The uncertainty and unpredictability of living with a chronic condition can threaten your independence. At times you may find yourself asking, *"Why me"?* This is a normal response to a chronic condition.

You may be angry with yourself, your family, friends, health care providers, God, and the world in general. For example, you may be angry for not taking better care of yourself. You may also be angry at your family and friends because they don't do things the way you want.

Or you might be angry at your doctor because he or she cannot solve your problems. Sometimes, your anger may be misplaced, as when you find yourself yelling at the cat!

Sometimes the health condition itself causes anger. For example, a stroke or Alzheimer's disease can affect the emotions, leading the person to cry inappropriately or have temper flare-ups. Some depressed people and those who have anxiety disorders express their depression or anxiety through anger. Aristotle (384–322 BC) observed, *"Anyone can get angry, that is easy . . . but to do this to the right person, to the right extent, at the right time, with the right motive, and in the right way, that is not for everyone, nor is it easy"*.

The first step is to recognise or admit that you are angry and then to identify why, or with whom. These are important steps in learning how to manage your anger effectively including the identification of constructive ways to express your anger.

Defusing Anger

Research now suggests that people who vent their anger actually get angrier. But suppressing anger isn't the answer either. Angry feelings often smoulder and can flare up later. There are a couple of strategies you can use to reduce hostile feelings:

1. *You can raise your anger threshold:* For example, by allowing fewer things to trigger your anger in the first place.

2. *You can choose how to react when you get angry:* You can do this without either denying your feelings, or giving in to the situation.

This sounds simple enough, but what gets in the way is our tendency to see anger as coming from outside ourselves. It can seem to be something over which we have little control. We see ourselves as helpless victims. We blame others and say, *"You make me so angry!"* We explode and then say, *"I couldn't help it"*. We see our friends as selfish and insensitive, our bosses as snobs or bullies, our friends as unappreciative. So, it seems that our only choice is an outburst of hostility. But with a little practice, even a seasoned hot-head can master a new repertoire of healthy and effective responses. There are several things you can do to help manage your anger.

Reason with yourself

How you interpret and explain a situation determines whether you will feel angry or not. You can learn to defuse anger by pausing and questioning your anger-producing thoughts. If you change your thoughts, you can change your response. You can decide whether or not to get angry and then decide whether or not to act. At the first sign of anger, count to three and ask yourself the following questions:

■ *Is this really important enough to get angry about?* Maybe this incident isn't serious enough to merit the time and energy. Consider if the issue is likely make any big difference in your life.

■ *Am I justified in getting angry?* You may also need to gather more information to understand the situation better. This will counteract jumping to conclusions or misinterpreting the intentions and actions of others.

■ *Will getting angry make any difference?*
More often than not, getting angry and losing your cool does not work and may even be punishing. Exploding or venting anger increases your angry feelings, puts a strain on your relationships, and potentially damages your health.

Cool off

Any technique that relaxes or distracts you, like meditating or taking a long walk, can help you put out the fire within. Slow, deep breathing is one of the quickest and simplest ways to cool off. For more on this, take a moment to read about cooling down in Chapter 8. So, when you notice your anger building up, take ten slow, relaxed breaths before responding. Sometimes, withdrawing and buying some time on your own can defuse the situation. Also, physical exercise can provide a good natural cooling off for stress and anger.

Verbalise without blame

One important technique is to communicate your anger out loud, preferably without blaming or offending other people. This can be done by learning to use "*I*", rather than "*You*" messages to express your feelings. You can refer to Chapter 9 for a discussion of "*I*" messages. However, if you choose to express your anger verbally, you should realise that many people will not be able to help you. Most of us are not very good at dealing with angry people. This is true even if the anger is justified. Therefore, you may also find it useful to seek counselling or join a support group. Voluntary organisations, such as the various heart, lung, liver, diabetes, MS, Parkinson's and arthritis organisations, are useful resources in this area.

Modify your expectations

You may also find that you would benefit from modifying your expectations. You have already done this throughout your life. For example, as a child you thought you could become a fireman, or a ballet dancer, or a doctor. When you grew older, you re-evaluated these expectations, as you accepted your capabilities, talents, and interests. Based on this re-evaluation, you modified your plans.

This same process can be used to deal with the effects of chronic illness on your life. For example, it may be unrealistic to expect that you will get *totally better*. However, it is realistic to expect that you can still do many pleasurable things. You have the ability to alter the progress of your health condition by slowing your decline or preventing it from becoming worse. Changing your expectations can help you change your perspective. Instead of dwelling on the 10% of things you can no longer do, think about the 90% of things you *can* still do.

In short, anger is a normal response to having a chronic condition. Part of learning to manage the condition involves acknowledging this anger and finding constructive ways to deal with it.

Stress

Stress is a common problem. But what exactly is it? In the 1950s, the physiologist Hans Selye described stress as *"the non-specific response of the body to any demand made upon it"*. Others have expanded on this definition to explain that the body adapts to demands, whether pleasant or unpleasant. For example, you may feel stress after experiencing negative events, such as the death of a loved one, or even joyful events such as the marriage of a child.

How Does Your Body Respond to Stress?

■ *What happens if you experience stressful change?* Your body is used to functioning at a certain level. When there is a need to change this level, your body must adjust to meet the new demand. It reacts by preparing to take some action: Your heart rate increases, your blood pressure rises, your neck and shoulder muscles become tense, your breathing becomes more rapid, your digestion slows, your mouth becomes dry, and you may begin sweating. These are all signals of what we call stress.

■ *Why does this happen?* To take an action, your muscles need to be supplied with oxygen and energy. Your breathing increases in order to inhale as much oxygen as possible, and at the same time to rid your body of as much carbon dioxide as possible. Your heart rate increases to deliver the oxygen and nutrients to the muscles. Furthermore, body functions that are not immediately necessary, such as the digestion of food and the body's natural immune responses, are slowed down.

■ *How long will these responses last?* In general, they are present only while the stressful event lasts. Your body then returns to its normal level of functioning. Sometimes, your body does not go back to its former comfortable level. When the stress is present for any length of time, your body begins adapting to it. This chronic stress can contribute to the onset of some chronic conditions and can make symptoms more difficult to manage.

Common Stressors

Regardless of the type of stressor, the changes in the body are the same. Different stressors, however, are not completely independent of one another. In fact, one stressor can often lead to others and also magnify the effects of existing stressors. Several stressors can occur at the same time. For instance, shortness of breath can cause anxiety, frustration, inactivity, and loss of endurance. Let's examine some of the most common sources of stress.

Physical stressors

Physical stressors can range from something as pleasant as picking up your new grandchild from the hospital, to everyday grocery shopping, or the physical symptoms of your chronic condition. What they have in common is that *all* of these stressors increase your body's demand for energy. If your body is not prepared to deal with this demand, the results may be anything from sore muscles and fatigue to a worsening of some of your disease symptoms.

Mental and emotional stressors

Mental and emotional stressors can also be either pleasant or uncomfortable. The joys you experience from seeing a child get married, or meeting new friends, may induce a stress response which is similar to that caused by feeling frustrated or worried because of your illness. Although this fact may seem surprising, the similarity comes from the way your brain perceives the stress.

Environmental stressors

Environmental stressors, too, can be both good and bad. They may be as varied as responding to a sunny day, uneven pavements that make it difficult to walk, loud noises, bad weather, a snoring spouse, or secondary smoke. Each one creates a pleasurable or apprehensive excitement that triggers the stress response.

Isn't the Idea of Good Stress a Contradiction?

As noted earlier, some types of stress can have good sources, such as a job promotion, a wedding, a holiday, a new friendship, or a new baby. These stressors make you feel happy but still cause the changes in your body that we have discussed. Another example of a *good stressor* is exercise.

When you exercise or do any kind of physical activity, there is a demand placed on your body. The heart has to work harder to deliver blood to your muscles; the lungs are working harder, and you breathe more rapidly to keep up with your muscles demands for oxygen. Meanwhile, your muscles are working hard to keep up with the signals from your brain, which are telling them to keep moving.

When you maintain an exercise programme for several weeks, you will begin to notice a change. What once seemed virtually impossible now becomes easier. Your body has adapted to this stress. There is less strain on your heart, lungs, and other muscles because they have become more efficient and you have become fitter. The same can happen with psychological stresses. Many people become more resilient and stronger emotionally after experiencing emotional challenges to which they have learned to adapt.

Recognising When You Feel Stressed

Everyone has a certain need for stress. It helps your life run more efficiently. Indeed, as long as you do not go past your body's breaking point, stress can be helpful. You can tolerate more stress on some days than on others. But sometimes, if you are not aware of the different types of stress, you can go beyond your breaking point and feel that your life is slipping out of control. Often it is difficult to recognise when you are under too much stress. The following are some of the warning signs:

- Biting your nails, pulling your hair, tapping your foot, or other repetitive habits.

- Grinding your teeth or clenching your jaw.

- Experiencing tension in your head, neck, or shoulders.

- Feeling anxious, nervous, helpless, or irritable.

- Falling foul of frequent accidents.

- Forgetting things you usually don't forget.

- Having difficulty concentrating.

- Feeling fatigue and exhaustion.

Sometimes you notice when you are behaving or feeling stressed. If you do, then take a few minutes to think about what it is that is making you feel tense. Take a few deep breaths and try to relax. Also, a quick body scan, a relaxation technique we describe in Chapter 5, can help you recognise stress in your body. You will find additional good ideas for coping with stress in that chapter.

Dealing with Stress

Dealing effectively with stress need not be complicated. In fact, it can start with a simple three-step process:

1. *Identify your stressors by making a list:* Consider every area of your life; family, relationships, health, financial security and living environment.

2. *Sort out your stressors:* For each stressor you have identified, ask yourself, is it *important* or *unimportant* and, whether you can change it or not? Then place each of your stressors in one of these four categories:

   - Category One: *Important and changeable.*
   - Category Two: *Important and unchangeable.*
   - Category Three: *Unimportant and changeable.*
   - Category Four: *Unimportant and unchangeable.*

Thus, the need to quit smoking is Category One, important and for most people it is changeable. By contrast, the loss of a loved one and the loss of a job, are both in Category Two, they are important and unchangeable. The poor performance of your favourite sports team, an inconvenient traffic jam, and bad weather are all unchangeable and may or may not be important. They could be in Category Three, or in Category Four. What really counts is how you think about each stressor.

3. *Match your strategy to each stressor:* Different strategies work for different stressors. Here are some strategies to help you in managing each type of problem more effectively:

   - *Managing important and changeable stressors.* These types of stressors are best managed by taking action to change the situation and thereby reduce the stress associated with them. Useful problem-solving skills include planning and goal setting which we considered in Chapter 2; imagery, positive and healthy thinking which you can read about in Chapter 5; effective communication which we dealt with in Chapter 9, and seeking social support.

   - *Managing important and unchangeable stressors.* These stressors are the most difficult to manage. They can make you feel helpless and hopeless. No matter what you do, you cannot make another person change, bring someone back from the dead, or delete traumatic experiences from your life. However, even though you may not be able to change the situation, you may be able to use one or more of the following strategies:

◆ *Change the way you think about the problem.* For example, think how much worse it could be, explore this in the section on gratitude Chapter 5, and focus on the positive and practise thankfulness. You can also deny or ignore the problem, or distract yourself as illustrated on page 75. Overall, you can simply accept what you can't change.

◆ *Find some part of the problem that you can reclassify as changeable.* For example, you can't stop the flooding, but you can take steps to repair the damage.

◆ *Reassess how important the problem is in light of your overall life and priorities.* Maybe your neighbour's criticism isn't so important after all.

◆ *Change your emotional reactions to the situation* and thereby, reduce the stress. You can't change what happened, but you can help yourself feel less distressed about it. Try writing things down or confiding your deepest thoughts and feelings to someone, a technique we discuss on page 89. Try seeking social support, helping others, enjoying your senses, relaxing, using imagery, enjoying humour, or exercising.

■ *Managing unimportant and changeable stressors:* If the stressor is unimportant, first try just letting it go. But if you can control it with relatively little effort, then go ahead

and deal with it. Solving small problems will help to build your skills and give you the confidence to tackle bigger ones. Use the same strategies that we suggested for important and changeable problems.

■ *Managing unimportant and unchangeable stressors:* The best solution for these problems is to ignore them. Starting now, you are given permission to let go of all unimportant concerns. These are common hassles and everybody has their share of them. Don't let them bother you. You can distract yourself with humour, relaxation or imagery, or by focusing on more pleasurable things.

Using Problem Solving

There are some situations that you recognise as stressful, such as being stuck in traffic, going on a trip, or preparing a meal. First, look at what it is that is stressful about this particular situation. Is it that you hate to be late? Are trips stressful because of uncertainty about your destination? Does meal preparation involve too many steps and demand too much energy?

Once you have identified what the problem is, begin looking for possible ways to reduce the stress. Can you leave earlier? Can you let someone else drive? Can you call someone at your destination and ask about wheelchair access, local public transport, and other concerns? Can you prepare food in the morning? Can you take a short nap in the early afternoon?

After you have identified some possible solutions, select one which you will try the next time you are in this situation. Then evaluate the results. You will remember that this problem-solving approach was also discussed in Chapter 2.

Managing the Stress

Whereas you can successfully manage some types of stress by modifying the situation, other types of stress can sneak up on you unexpectedly. The approach to dealing with these unexpected sources of ,stress also involves problem solving. Try to manage by:

■ *Being aware that certain situations will be stressful* and that you can develop ways to deal with them before they happen. Rehearse, in your mind, what you will do when the situation arises, so that you will be ready.

■ *Knowing that certain chemicals you ingest can also increase your stress.* These include nicotine, alcohol, and caffeine. Some people smoke a cigarette, drink a glass of wine or beer, eat chocolate, or drink a cup of coffee to soothe their tension, but these actions may actually increase your stress. Eliminating or cutting down on these stressors will help you.

■ *Using other tools which we have already discussed* aimed at dealing with stress. Don't forget to include issues such as getting enough sleep, exercising, and eating well.

■ *Recognising that that these tools are not always going to be effective,* and that sometimes stress can be overwhelming. These are times when good self-managers turn to expert supporters such as counselors, social workers, psychologists, and psychiatrists.

In summary, stress, like every other symptom, has many causes and consequently can be managed in many different ways. It is up to you to examine the problem and try to find solutions that meet your needs and suit your lifestyle.

Memory Problems

Many people worry about changes in their memory, particularly as they age. Although all of us are sometimes forgetful, there are serious illnesses that cause memory loss, including Alzheimer's disease and other types of dementia. These are not a normal part of aging. Although symptoms can vary widely, the first problem many people notice is forgetfulness, particularly when it is severe enough to affect their ability to function at home or at work or enjoy lifelong hobbies. Alzheimer's and similar diseases may cause a person to become confused, get lost in familiar places, misplace things, or have trouble with language. The disease gets worse over time.

If you suspect that you or someone you know is experiencing memory problems, then seek a diagnosis as soon as possible. There is currently no cure for dementia, but early detection allows you to get the maximum benefit from available treatments. Treatments may relieve some symptoms and help you maintain your independence for longer. An early diagnosis allows you to take part in decisions about care, transportation, living options, and financial and legal matters. You can also start building a helpful social network and increase your chances of participating in clinical drug trials that could help to advance research.

If you are concerned about Alzheimer's or a similar condition, contact the Alzheimer's Society. The *Helpline* is usually open from 9 a.m. to 5 p.m. Monday to Friday and Saturday and Sunday from 10 a.m. to 4 p.m. However the service may be closed occasionally during these times for operational reasons or because of staff shortages. Callers will be able to speak to trained *Helpline Advisers.* Further contact information is provided at the end of this chapter.

Itching

Itching is one of the most difficult symptoms to understand. It is any sensation that causes an urge to scratch. Like other symptoms, it can have many different causes. Some of these we understand. So, when you get an insect bite or come into contact with stinging nettles, your body releases histamines that irritate nerve endings and cause itching. Also, when the liver is damaged, it cannot remove bile products, and these are deposited in the skin, causing itching. In kidney disease, itching may be severe, although the exact cause is not clear. There are also other conditions, such as psoriasis, in which the causes of itching are not easily explained. We do know that factors such as warmth, wool clothing, and stress can make itching worse. There are some ways that may help you relieve your itching.

Controlling Moisture

- Dry skin tends to be itchy; therefore, try keeping the skin moisturised by applying moisturising creams several times a day. When you choose a moisturiser, be careful. Be sure to read the list of ingredients in the cream or lotion. *Avoid products that contain alcohol* or any other ingredient that ends in -ol, as they tend to dry the skin. *In general, the greasier the product, the better* it works as a moisturiser. Creams are better moisturisers than lotions, and products such as Vaseline, olive oil, and vegetable shortening can also be very effective.

- When taking a bath or shower, use warm water and soak for not less than ten or more than 20 minutes. You also may want to add bath oil, baking soda, or home made bath oil to the water. To make your own bath oil, stir two teaspoons of olive oil into a large glass of milk and add it to your bath. When you get out of the water, pat yourself dry immediately and apply your cream.

- If your itching is caused by the release of histamines during an allergic reaction, or from contact with an irritating substance, wash off the oils or offending agent, apply cold compresses, and take *Benadryl* or another anti-histamine to help stop the reaction. Of course, check with your pharmacist that the anti-histamine is OK for you to take.

■ During cold weather it can be especially difficult to deal with itching because indoor heating tends to dry the skin. If this is a problem for you, then using of a humidifier might help. Also, try to keep your home and office as cool as you can without being uncomfortable.

Choose Clothing with Care

The type of clothing you wear can also add to itching sensations. Obviously, the best rule of thumb is to wear what is comfortable. This is usually clothing made from material that is not scratchy. Most people find that natural fibres such as cotton allow the skin to *breathe* and are the least irritating to the skin.

Think about Your Medications

Anti-histamines will help if your itching is caused by the release of histamines. You can buy many of these products over the counter. They include products such as *Benadryl*, *Piriton* and *Claritin*. You can also buy creams that help soothe the nerve endings, such as *Vicks Vap-o-Rub*. If you want an anti-itch cream, look for one that contains *benzocaine*, *lidocaine*, or *pramoxine*. However, be careful, because some people can have allergic reactions to these creams, especially benzocaine. *Capsaicin* creams may also help itching, although they do cause a burning sensation. *Steroid creams* that contain cortisone can also help control some types of itching. It is always sensible to ask the pharmacist or your doctor about these *over-the-counter* products to ensure they will not cause problems with your prescribed medications.

With the exception of moisturising creams, no cream should be used on a long-term basis without talking to your doctor. If your itching continues with use of these *over-the-counter* products, you may want to talk to your doctor about trying stronger versions of these medications.

Reduce Stress Levels

Anything that you can do to reduce the stress in your life will also help to reduce itching. We have already discussed some of the ways to deal with stress earlier in this chapter, and some additional techniques are described in Chapter 5.

Stop Scratching

Although our natural tendency is to scratch what itches, this really does not help, especially for chronic itching. Rather, it leads to a vicious cycle whereby the more you scratch, the more you itch. Unfortunately, it is hard to resist scratching, you might try rubbing, pressing, or patting the skin instead, whenever you feel the need to scratch. If you are not able to break this cycle yourself, ask your doctor's advice or ask to be referred to a dermatologist who may help you to find alternative ways to control the itching.

Itching is a common and undoubtedly very frustrating symptom for both patients and doctors to manage. If the self-management tips described here do not seem to help, it may be time to seek the advice of a doctor. Often your doctor can prescribe medications that can help with specific types of itching.

Urinary Incontinence: Loss of Bladder Control

Urinary incontinence means you have trouble controlling your bladder and accidentally leak urine. If so, you are not alone. Many people have to cope with this problem. Although urinary incontinence can occur in both men and women, it is more common in women. In many cases, incontinence can be controlled, even if it is not cured outright.

It is common to experience incontinence during or after pregnancy or at the menopause, when you are aging, or gaining weight. Activities that put increased pressure on the bladder, such as coughing, laughing, sneezing, and physical activity can all cause urine leakage. Incontinence can be related to changes in your hormones, the weakening of muscles or ligaments in the pelvic area, or the use of certain medications. Infections in the bladder can also cause temporary incontinence.

Urinary incontinence can affect your quality of life and lead to other health problems. Feeling embarrassed by this problem causes some people to avoid social activities and sex. Some people experience loss of confidence or depression as a result of incontinence. Leaked urine may also cause skin irritation and infections. The frequent urge to urinate can also interfere with sound, restorative sleep. In addition, slipping and falling on leaked urine when rushing to the bathroom can result in injury.

The good news is that there are many treatments that can control or even cure this condition. It may be reassuring to know that many of these are small things you can do at home. If none of the following solves the problem, talk to your doctor about other treatments. Don't be embarrassed. Your doctor has heard it all before.

There are three types of persistent or chronic loss of bladder control:

1. *Stress incontinence:* This refers to small amounts of urine leaking out during exercise, coughing, laughing, sneezing, or other movements that squeeze the bladder. *Kegel exercises,* better known as *pelvic floor exercises,* which are described below under the heading *Home Treatments* can often improve stress incontinence.

2. *Urge incontinence, or an overactive bladder:* This happens when the need to urinate comes on so quickly that you don't have enough time to get to the toilet.

3. *Overflow incontinence:* This occurs when the bladder cannot empty completely.

Home Treatments

Small, effective changes to your lifestyle or behaviour are the first treatments for urinary incontinence. For many people, these treatments effectively control or cure the problem. *Kegel exercises* strengthen your pelvic floor muscles. This allows better control of your urine flow and prevents leaking. Learning Kegel exercises takes a bit of practice and patience. It may take a few weeks to feel an improvement in your symptoms.

Here is how to do Kegel exercises:

1. *Find the muscles that stop your urine.* You can do this by repeatedly stopping your

urine in midstream and starting again. Focus on the muscles that you feel squeezing around your urethra, the opening for the urine, and your anus, the opening for your bowels.

2. *Practise squeezing these muscles when you are not urinating.* If your stomach or buttocks move, you're not using the right muscles.

3. *Squeeze the muscles,* hold for three seconds, and then relax for three seconds.

4. *Repeat this exercise.* Do it ten to 15 times each session.

Complete at least 30 Kegel exercises every day. The wonderful thing about these exercises is that you can do them anywhere and anytime. No one will know what you are doing except you.

With *urge incontinence,* retraining your bladder may help:

■ *Practise double-voiding:* Empty your bladder as much as possible, relax for a minute, and try to empty it again. This helps empty your bladder completely.

■ *Practise waiting for a specified amount of time before urinating.* This sometimes helps as it gradually retrains your bladder to require emptying less often.

■ *Train yourself to urinate on a regular schedule.* Try about every two to four hours during the day, whether or not you feel the urge. If you now need to urinate every 30 minutes, perhaps you can start by waiting for 40 minutes and gradually work your way up to every two to four hours.

In general it is important to think about:

■ *Consuming fewer beverages*: Consuming fewer beverages can reduce your trips to the toilet. Beverages such as alcohol, tea, coffee, and other drinks that contain caffeine, stimulate the bladder and urine production and hence more trips to the toilet.

■ *Losing weight:* If you are carrying *extra weight,* losing it can reduce the pressure on your bladder. Studies show that a loss of just 10% of total body weight improves incontinence problems for many people.

■ *Wearing absorbent pads or briefs:* Whilst these will not cure incontinence they certainly help you to manage the condition.

Treatments and Medications

If the changes you make in your lifestyle or behaviour do not relieve your urinary incontinence, discuss other treatments with your doctor. Treatments such as the use of medication, or a *pessary,* or in some cases, surgery can help. A pessary is a thin, flexible ring that can be worn inside the vagina to support the pelvic area. The point is that you don't have to suffer in silence if you have urinary incontinence. Talk to your doctor.

In this chapter we have discussed the causes of some of the most common symptoms experienced by people with chronic conditions. In addition, we have described some tools that you can use to cope with your symptoms. Taking action to deal physically with your symptoms is necessary in coping with your condition on a day-to-day basis. But sometimes this just doesn't seem to be enough. There are times when you may wish to escape from your surroundings and just have *your time*, this means a time that allows you to clear your mind and gain a fresh perspective. The following chapter presents different ways to complement your physical-symptom management with *thinking techniques*. In effect, using the power of your mind to help to reduce and perhaps prevent some of the symptoms you may experience.

Suggested Further Reading

Bergstrom, K. and Kimbell, A. *100 Questions and Answers about Psoriasis.* Sudbury MA: Jones and Bartlett, 2011

Butler, G and Hope, T. *Manage Your Mind.* 2nd Edition: Oxford: Oxford University Press, 2007. This book has a host of ideas for personal change and improvement.

Caudill, M. *Managing Pain Before It Manages You.* 3rd Edition: New York: Guilford Press, 2008.

Donoghue, P. J., and Siegel M. E. *Sick and Tired of Feeling Sick and Tired: Living with Invisible Chronic Illness.* 2nd Edition: New York: Norton, 2000.

McKenzie, K. *Anxiety and Panic Attacks.* Poole: Family Doctor Publications, 2006.*

Johnstone, F. *Getting a Good Night's Sleep.* London: Sheldon Press, 2000

Williams, C. *Overcoming Depression and Low Moods.* London: Hodder Arnold, 2006.

Other Resources

☐   Alzheimer's Society. Central Office: Devon House, 58 St. Catherine's Way, London E1W 1LB. Helpline: 0300 222 1122, www.alzheimers.org.uk.

☐   Association of Continence Advice. Central Office: Winchester House, Kennington Park, Cranmer Road, London SW9 6EJ. Tel: 020 7820 8113, www.aca.uk.com.

☐   Depression Alliance. Central Office: Great Dover Street London, SE1 4LX. There is no helpline but they will send out information. Tel: 0845 123 2320, www.depressionalliance.org.

---

*This book is one of the Family Doctor series published in association with the BMJ. They can be found in many local bookshops such as WH Smith or Waterstone's and cost approximately £5. They are written by practising doctors recognised for their expertise in the field. Other books in the series cover Allergies, Alzheimer's disease and other forms of Dementia, Blood Pressure, Angina and Heart Attacks, Arthritis and Rheumatism, Asthma, Back Pain, COPD, Depression, Diabetes, Epilepsy, Heart Failure, Irritable Bowel Syndrome, Psoriasis, Osteoporosis, Parkinson's disease, Thyroid Disorders and many more. So they are particularly relevant to people living with long-term conditions. Be aware that any advice about medication written in these books will be correct at the time of publishing but because of the continuing flow of new research they may be subject to change. So you will need to clarify with your own doctor what is appropriate for you personally.

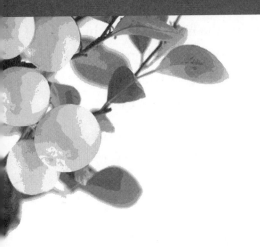

CHAPTER 5

Using Your Mind to Manage Symptoms

THERE IS A STRONG LINK BETWEEN OUR THOUGHTS, attitudes, emotions and our mental and physical health. One of our self-managers said, "It's not always mind over matter, but mind matters." Although thoughts and emotions do not directly cause our long-term health conditions, they can influence our symptoms. Research has shown that our thoughts and emotions trigger certain hormones or other chemicals that send messages throughout our body. These messages affect how our body functions; for example, thoughts and emotions can change our heart rate, blood pressure, breathing, blood sugar levels, muscle responses, immune responses, concentration, the ability to get pregnant, and even our ability to fight off other illnesses.

All of us, at one time or another, have experienced the power of the mind and its effects on the body. Both pleasant and unpleasant thoughts and emotions can cause our body to react. Our heart rate and breathing may increase or slow down; we may experience sensations such as warm or cold sweating, blushing and crying. Sometimes just

71

a memory or an image can trigger these responses. For example, try this simple exercise: Imagine that you are holding a big, bright yellow lemon slice. You hold it close to your nose and smell its strong citrus aroma. Now you bite into the lemon. It's juicy! The juice fills your mouth and dribbles down your chin. Now you begin to suck on the lemon and its tart juice. What happens? The body responds. Your mouth puckers and starts to water. You may even smell the scent of the lemon. All of these reactions are triggered by the mind and the memory of your experience with a real lemon.

This example shows the power which the mind has over the body. It also gives us a good reason to develop the mental abilities which will help us to manage our symptoms. With training and practice, we can use the mind to relax the body, to reduce stress and anxiety, and to reduce the discomfort or unpleasantness caused by our physical and emotional symptoms. Your mind can also greatly help relieve the pain and shortness of breath associated with various diseases and may even help you depend less on medications.

In this chapter we describe several ways in which you can begin to use your mind to manage symptoms. These are sometimes referred to as *thinking* or *cognitive* techniques because they involve the use of our thinking abilities to make changes in your body. As you read, keep some key principles in your mind:

- Symptoms have many causes: This means that there are many ways to manage most symptoms. If you understand the nature of your symptoms and what causes them, you will be able to manage things better.

- Not all management techniques work for everyone: It is up to you to experiment and find out what works best for you. Be flexible. This includes trying different techniques and checking the results. Doing this will help you to determine which management tool is most helpful, for which symptoms, and under what circumstances.

- Learning new skills to gain control of your situation takes time: Give yourself several weeks to practise before you decide if a new tool is working for you.

- Don't give up too easily: As with exercise and other new skills, using your mind to manage your health condition will require practise and time before you notice any benefits. So even if you feel you are not accomplishing anything, don't give up. Be patient and keep on trying.

- These techniques should not have negative effects: If you become frightened, angry, or depressed when using one of the tools we suggest, do not continue to use it. Try another tool instead.

Relaxation Techniques

Many of us have heard a lot about relaxation, yet we are still confused as to what it actually is, what its benefits are and how to do it. It's simple, relaxation involves using thinking techniques to reduce or eliminate tension from the body and the mind. This usually gives you improved sleep quality, less stress less pain and less shortness of breath. Whilst relaxation is *not a cure-all*, it can be an effective part of a treatment plan.

There are a variety of different relaxation techniques. Each has specific guidelines and uses. Some techniques are used mostly to achieve muscle relaxation, whereas others are aimed at reducing anxiety and emotional stress or diverting attention. All of these outcomes help in symptom management.

The term *relaxation* means different things to different people. However, we can all identify things we do that help us to relax. For example, we may walk, watch TV, listen to music, knit, or garden. These approaches however, are different from the techniques discussed in this chapter. In particular, they include some form of physical activity, or a stimulant like music, which provides something outside of your mind. The relaxation tools we are discussing here involve us in using our *mind* to help the body relax. The goal of relaxation is to turn off the outside world so that the mind and body are at rest. This allows you to reduce those tensions that can increase the intensity and severity of your symptoms.

Here are some guidelines to help you practise relaxation:

▪ *Pick a quiet place and time* when you will not be disturbed for at least 15 to 20 minutes. If this seems too long, then start with five minutes. The fact that in some homes the only quiet place is the bathroom is just fine, so practise there!

▪ *Try to practise the technique* twice daily and for not less than four times a week.

▪ *Don't expect miracles.* Some of these techniques take practice. Sometimes it takes three or four weeks of consistent application before you start to notice benefits.

▪ *Relaxation should be helpful.* At worst, you may find it boring, but if it is an unpleasant experience or it makes you more nervous or anxious, you might switch to one of the other symptom management tools described in this chapter.

Relaxation Quick and Easy

Some types of relaxation are so easy, so natural and effective that people do not think of them as *relaxation techniques* at all. For example, why not:

▪ Take a nap or a hot, soothing bath.

▪ Curl up and read or listen to a good book.

▪ Watch a funny film.

▪ Get a massage.

▪ Enjoy an occasional glass of wine.

▪ Start a small garden or grow a beautiful plant indoors.

▪ Do some crafts such as knitting, pottery, or woodworking.

▪ Watch a favourite TV show.

▪ Read a poem or reflect on an inspirational saying.

▪ Go for a walk.

▪ Start a collection of stamps, coins, folk art, shells, or something in miniature.

▪ Listen to your favourite music.

▪ Sing around the house.

▪ Crumble paper into a ball and imagine the wastebasket is a basketball hoop.

▪ Look at water, for example ocean waves, a lake, or a fountain.

- Watch the clouds in the sky.

- Put your head down on your desk and close your eyes for five minutes.

- Rub your hands together until they're warm, and then cup them over your closed eyes.

- Vigorously shake your hands and arms for ten seconds.

- Ring a friend or a family member to chat.

- Smile and introduce yourself to someone new.

- Do something nice and unexpected for someone else.

- Play with the cat.

- Visit a holiday place in your mind.

Relaxation Tools that Take 5 to 20 Minutes

Whilst these techniques take a bit longer they can be very effective:

Body scanning (a muscle relaxation technique

To relax your muscles, you need to know how to scan your body and recognise where you are tense. Then you will be able to release the tension. The first step is to become familiar with the difference between the feeling of tension and the feeling of relaxation. This exercise will allow you to compare these feelings and, with practice, you will be able to spot and release tension anywhere in your body. It is best done lying down on your back, but any comfortable position can be used. A body relaxation scan script can be found on page 76.

The Relaxation Response

In the early 1970s a physician named Herbert Benson studied what he calls the *relaxation response*. According to Benson, our bodies have several natural states. One example is the *fight or flight* response experienced by people when they are facing some great danger. The body becomes quite tense, and this tenseness is then followed by the body's natural tendency to relax. This is what Benson calls the *relaxation response*. As our lives become more and more hectic, our bodies tend to stay tense for long periods of time. We can lose our natural ability to relax.

The *relaxation response* helps to change this. So try this: Find a quiet place where there are few distractions. Find a comfortable position. You should be comfortable enough to remain in the same position for 20 minutes. Choose a word, an object, or a pleasant feeling. For example, repeat a word or sound, like the word *one*, gaze at a symbol, or a flower, perhaps, or concentrate on a *feeling* like *peace*. Adopt a passive attitude. This is of the utmost importance. Empty your mind of all your thoughts and distractions. You may become aware of thoughts, images and feelings, but don't concentrate on them. Just allow them to pass you by.

Here's what you should do to elicit the *relaxation response*:

- Sit quietly in a comfortable position.

- Close your eyes.

- Relax all your muscles, beginning at your feet and progressing up to your face. Keep them relaxed.

- Breathe in through your nose. Become aware of your breathing. As you breathe out through your mouth, say the word you chose silently to yourself. Try to empty all thoughts from your mind; concentrate on your word, sound, or symbol.

- Continue this for ten to 20 minutes. You may open your eyes to check the time, but do not use an alarm. When you finish, sit quietly for several minutes, at first with your eyes closed. Then, stay sitting for a few more minutes.

- Maintain a passive attitude, and let relaxation occur at its own pace. When distracting thoughts occur, ignore them by not dwelling on them, and return to repeating the word you chose. Do not worry about whether you are being successful in achieving a deep level of relaxation.

- Practise this once or twice every day.

Distraction

Our minds have trouble focusing on more than one thing at a time. It follows, that we can lessen the intensity of our symptoms by training our minds to focus attention on something *other than our body and its sensations*. This technique, called *distraction* or *attention re-focusing*, is particularly helpful for people who feel that their symptoms are painful, or overwhelming, or who worry that every bodily sensation might indicate a new or worsening health problem. It is important to emphasise that with distraction you are not *ignoring* the symptoms but simply choosing not to dwell on them.

Sometimes it may be difficult to put anxious thoughts out of your mind. When you try to suppress any thought, you may end up thinking more about it. For example, if we ask you to try not thinking about a tiger charging toward you and that whatever you do, don't let the thought of the tiger enter your mind. You'll probably find it nearly impossible not to think about the tiger.

Whilst you can't easily stop thinking about something, you can *distract* yourself and re-direct your attention elsewhere. For example, think about the charging tiger again. Now stand up suddenly, slam your hand on the table, and shout *"Stop!"* What happened to the tiger? It's gone ... at least for the moment.

Distraction works best for short activities or at the times when symptoms may be anticipated. For example, if you know climbing stairs will be painful or cause discomfort, or that falling asleep at night is likely to be difficult, you might try one of the following distraction techniques:

- *Make plans for exactly what you will do after the unpleasant activity passes:* For example, if climbing stairs is uncomfortable or painful, think about what you need to do once you get to the top. If you have trouble falling asleep, try making plans for some future event, being as detailed as possible.

- *Think of a person's name, a bird, a flower, or whatever, for each letter of the alphabet:* If you get stuck on one letter, go on to the next. This is a good distraction for pain and for sleep problems.

- *Challenge yourself to count backwards:* Say, from 100 reducing by threes in sequence, 100, 97, 94 and so on.

Body-Scan Script

As you get into a comfortable position, let yourself begin to sink comfortably into the surface below you, you may perhaps allow your eyes gradually to close . . . from there, turn your attention to your breath . . . breathing in, allow the breath gradually to go all the way down to your belly and then breathing out . . . and again, breathing in . . . and out . . . noticing the natural rhythm of your breathing . . .

Now let your attention focus on your feet. Starting with your toes, notice whatever sensations are there . . . warmth, coolness, whatever's there . . . simply feel it. Using your mind's eye, imagine that as you breathe in, the breath goes all the way down into your toes, bringing with it new refreshing air . . . and now notice the sensations elsewhere in your feet. Not judging or thinking about what you're feeling but simply becoming aware of the experience of your feet as you allow yourself to be fully supported by the surface below you . . .

Next, focus on your lower legs and knees. These muscles and joints do a lot of work for us, but often we don't give them the attention they deserve. So now, breathe down into the knees, calves, and ankles, noticing whatever sensations appear . . . see if you can simply stay with the sensations . . . breathing in new fresh air, and as you exhale, releasing tension and stress and allowing the muscles to relax and soften . . .

Now move your attention to the muscles, bones, and joints of the thighs, buttocks, hips . . . breathing down into the upper legs, noticing whatever sensations you experience. It may be warmth, coolness, a heaviness or lightness. You may become aware of the contact with the surface beneath you, or perhaps the pulsing of your blood . . . whatever's there . . . what matters is that you are taking time to learn to relax . . . deeper and deeper, as you breathe . . . in . . . and out.

Move your attention now to your back and chest . . . feeling the breath fill the abdomen and chest . . . noticing whatever sensations are there . . . not judging or thinking, but simply observing what is right here, right now. Allowing the fresh air to nourish the muscles, bones, and joints as you breathe in, and then . . . exhaling any tension and stress.

Now focus on the neck, shoulders, arms, and hands . . . Inhaling, down through the neck and shoulders, all the way down to the fingertips. Not trying too hard to relax, but simply becoming aware of your experience of these parts of your body in the present moment . . . turning now to your face and head, notice the sensations beginning at the back of your head, up along your scalp, and down into your forehead . . . then become aware of the sensations in and around your eyes and down into your cheeks and jaw . . . continue to allow your muscles to release and soften as you breathe in nourishing fresh air, and allow tension and stress to leave as you breathe out . . . As you drink in fresh air, allow it to spread throughout your body, from the soles of your feet all the way up through the top of your head . . . And then exhale any remaining stress and tension . . . and now take a few moments to enjoy the stillness as you breathe in . . . and out . . . Awake, relaxed, and still . . . now as the body scan comes to a close, coming back into the room, bringing with you whatever sensations of relaxation . . . comfort . . . peace . . . whatever's there . . . knowing that you can repeat this exercise at any appropriate time and place of your choosing . . . And when you're ready, open your eyes.

■ *Use your imagination:* To get through unpleasant daily chores such as sweeping, mopping, or using the vacuum cleaner, imagine your floor as a map of the UK. Try naming all the counties, moving east to west and north to south. If geography does not appeal to you, imagine your favourite department store and where each retail section is located.

■ *Use your memory:* Try to remember the words to favourite songs, or the events in an old story.

■ *Try the Stop! technique:* If you find yourself worrying or entrapped in endlessly repeating negative thoughts, stand up suddenly, slap your hand on the table or your thigh, and shout *Stop!* Practise this technique whenever your mind endlessly repeats negative thoughts. With practice, you won't have to shout out too loud. Just whispering *Stop!* or tightening your vocal cords and moving your tongue as if saying *Stop!* will often work. Some people imagine a large halt sign. Others put a rubber band on their wrist and snap it hard to break the chain of negative thinking. You could just pinch yourself. Do *anything* that redirects your attention.

■ *You might redirect your attention to a pleasurable experience:* Look outside at something in nature, perhaps flowers or birds. Try to identify all the sounds around you. Massage your hand. Smell a sweet or pungent odour.

There are, of course, many variations on these examples, all of which help you re-focus attention away from your problem.

So far, we have discussed short-term re-focusing strategies that involve using only the mind for distraction. Distraction also works well for longer lasting problems or symptoms, such as depression and some forms of chronic pain. In these cases, the mind must be focused not internally, but externally on some type of activity. If you are somewhat depressed or have continuous unpleasant symptoms, then find an activity that interests you which will distract you from the problem. The activity can be almost anything, from gardening to cooking to reading or going to a film, or doing volunteer work. One of the marks of a successful self-manager is that he or she has a variety of interests and always seems to be *doing* something.

Positive Thinking and Self-Talk

It is a fact that we all talk to ourselves all the time. For example, when you wake up in the morning, you may think, *"I really don't want to get out of bed. I'm tired and don't want to go to work today."* Or, at the end of an enjoyable evening, we think, *"That really was fun. I should get out more often."* What we think, or say to ourselves, is called our *self-talk.* The way we talk to ourselves tends to come from how and what we think of ourselves. Our thoughts can be positive or negative, and so is our *self-talk.* Therefore, self-talk can be an important self-management tool when it's positive or a weapon that hurts or defeats us when it's habitually negative.

All of our self-talk is learned from others and becomes a part of us as we grow older. It comes in many forms but tends to be mostly negative. Negative self-statements are usually in the form of phrases that begin with something such as *"I just can't do . . . ,"* or *"If only I could . . . ,"* or *"If only I didn't . . . ,"* or *"I just don't have the energy . . . ,"* or *"How could I be so stupid?"* This negative thinking represents the doubts and fears we have about ourselves in general and about our ability to deal with our condition and its symptoms. It damages our self-esteem, and worsens our attitude, and mood. Negative self-talk makes us feel bad and makes our symptoms worse.

What we say to ourselves plays a major role in determining our success or failure in becoming good self-managers. Negative thinking tends to *limit* our abilities and actions. If we tell ourselves *"I'm not very clever"* or *"I can't"* all the time, we probably won't try to learn new skills because this just doesn't fit in with what we think about ourselves. Soon we become prisoners of our own negative beliefs.

Fortunately, self-talk is not something fixed in our biological make-up, and therefore it is not completely out of our control. We can learn new, healthier ways to think about ourselves so that our self-talk can work for us instead of against us. By changing negative, self-defeating statements into positive ones, we can manage symptoms more effectively. This change, like any habit, requires practice and includes the following steps:

1. *Listen carefully to what you say to or about yourself, both out loud and silently:* If you find yourself feeling anxious, depressed, or angry, try to identify some of the thoughts you were having just before these feelings started. Then, write down all the negative self-talk you can remember. Pay special attention to the things you say during times that are particularly difficult for you. For example, what do you say to yourself when you get up in the morning feeling pain?; or while doing those exercises you don't really like?; or when you are feeling blue? Challenge these negative thoughts by asking yourself questions to identify what is really true or untrue. For example, are you exaggerating the situation, generalising, worrying too much, or assuming the worst? Are you thinking in *black and white* terms? Could there be grey, instead? Maybe you are making an unrealistic or unfair comparison, assuming too much responsibility, taking something too personally, or expecting perfection. Are you making assumptions about what other people think about you? What do you know for a fact? Look at the evidence so that you are better able to change these negative thoughts and statements.

2. *Next, work on changing each negative statement to a more positive one:* Try finding a positive statement, or two which might replace the negative one. Write these down. For example, take negative statements such as *"I don't want to get up," "I'm too tired and I am in pain," "I can't do the things I like anymore, so why bother?"* or *"I'm good for nothing."* These can become positive messages such as *"I'm feeling really good today, and I'm going to do something I enjoy," "I may not be able to do everything I used to do, but there are still a lot of things I can do," "People really like me, and I feel good about myself,"* or *"Other people need and depend on me; I'm worthwhile."*

3. *Read and rehearse these positive statements, mentally or with another person:* It is this conscious repetition or memorisation of positive self-talk that will help you replace those old, negative, habitual statements.

4. *Practise these new statements in real situations:* This practise, along with time and patience, will help your new patterns of thinking become automatic.

5. *Rehearse success:* When you aren't happy with the way you handled a particular situation, try this exercise:

   ◆ Write down three ways that it could have gone better.

   ◆ Write down three ways it could have been worse.

   ◆ If you can't think of alternatives to the way *you* handled it, imagine what someone you greatly respect might have done.

◆ Or think what advice you would give to someone else facing a similar situation.

Remember that mistakes aren't failures. They're great opportunities to learn. Mistakes give you the chance to rehearse other ways of handling things. This is important practice for future crises. At the very start, you may find it hard to change negative statements into more positive ones. A shortcut is to use either a *thought stopper* or a *positive affirmation*. A thought stopper can be anything that is meaningful to you, for example, a puppy, a polar bear, or an oak tree. When you have a negative thought, replace it with your thought stopper. We know it sounds silly, but try it. A positive affirmation is a positive phrase that you can use over and over again. For example, *"I am getting better every day"* or *"I can do this."* Again, you use this mantra to replace your negative thoughts.

Imagery

You may think that *imagination* is all in your mind. But the thoughts, words, and images that flow from your imagination can have real effects on your body. Your brain often cannot distinguish whether you are imagining something or it is really happening. Perhaps you've experienced a racing heartbeat, rapid breathing, or tension in your neck muscles while you are watching a movie thriller. These sensations were all produced by images and sounds *on a film*. During a dream, maybe your body responded with fear, joy, anger, or sadness. All of these have been triggered by your imagination. If you close your eyes and vividly imagine yourself by a still, quiet

pool, or relaxing on a warm beach, your body responds to some degree as though you were actually there.

Guided imagery and *visualisation* allows you to use your imagination to relieve symptoms. These techniques will help you to focus your thoughts on healing images and suggestions.

Guided Imagery

This tool is like a guided daydream. It allows you to divert your attention, refocusing your mind away from your symptoms and transporting you to another time and place. It has the added benefit of helping you to achieve deep relaxation by picturing yourself in a peaceful environment.

With *guided imagery*, you focus your mind on a particular image. Imagery usually involves your sense of sight and focusing on visual images. Adding other senses, such as smells, tastes, and sounds, makes the guided imagery even more vivid and powerful.

Some people are highly visual and easily see images with their *mind's eye*. But, if your images aren't as vivid as scenes from a great film, don't worry; it's normal for the intensity of imagery to vary. The important thing is to focus on as much detail as possible and to strengthen the images by using all your senses. Adding some real background music can also increase the impact of guided imagery.

With guided imagery, you are always completely in control. You're the film director. You can project whatever thought or feeling you want onto your mental screen. If you don't like a particular image, thought, or feeling, you can redirect your mind to something more comfortable; you can use other images to get rid of unpleasant thoughts. For example, you might put them on a raft and watch them float away, or you could sweep them away with a large brush, or erase them with a giant rubber; or you can open your eyes and stop the exercise.

The guided imagery scripts presented on pages 78 and 79 can help take you on a mental stroll. Here are some ways to use imagery:

- *Read the script over several times until it is familiar:* Then sit or lie down in a quiet place and try to reconstruct the scene in your mind. The script should take 15 to 20 minutes to complete.

- *Have a family member or friend read you the script slowly:* Ask them to pause for about ten seconds wherever there is a series of full stops . . .

- *Make a recording of the script:* Then play it over whenever it's convenient.

- *Use a pre-recorded tape, CD, or digital audio file:* Choose one that has a similar guided imagery script. There are examples in the *Other Resources* section at the end of this chapter.

Visualisation

Visualisation is similar to guided imagery. However, it allows you to *create your own images*, which is different from guided imagery, where the images are suggested to you. It is another way of using your imagination to create a picture of yourself in any way you want; doing the things you want to do. All of us use a form of visualisation every day, as we we dream, worry, read a book, or listen to a story. In all these activities the mind creates images for us to see. We also use visualisation intentionally when making plans for the day, considering the possible outcomes of the decisions we have to make, or rehearsing for an event or activity. Visualisation can be done in different ways and can be used for long periods of time or when you are also engaged in other activities.

One way to use visualisation to manage your symptoms is to remember pleasant scenes from your past or create new ones. To practise visualisation, try to remember every detail of a special holiday or a party that made you happy. Who was there? What happened? What did you do or talk about? You can also try this by remembering some other memorable and pleasant event.

Visualisation can be used to plan the details of some future event or fill in the details of a fantasy. For example, how would you spend a million pounds? What would be your ideal romantic encounter? What would your ideal home or garden look like? Where would you go and what would you do on your dream holiday?

Another form of visualisation involves using your mind to think of symbols that you can use to represent the discomfort or pain felt in different parts of your body. For example, a painful joint might be coloured red or a tight chest might have a constricting band around it. After forming these images, you then try to change them. The red colour might fade until there is no more colour, and the constricting band can stretch and stretch until it snaps; these new images can then change the way you think of the pain or discomfort..

Visualisation helps to build confidence and skill and therefore is a useful technique to help you set and accomplish personal goals as you saw in Chapter 2. After you write your *weekly action plan,* take a few minutes to imagine yourself taking a walk, doing your exercises, or taking your medications. You are, in effect, mentally rehearsing the steps you need to take in order to achieve your goal.

Imagery for Different Conditions

You have the ability to create special imagery to help, though not cure, specific symptoms or illnesses. Use any image that is strong and vivid for you. This often involves using all your senses to create the image and it should be one

that is meaningful to you. However, the image does not have to be accurate for it to work. Just use your imagination and trust yourself. Here are examples of images that some people have found useful:

Images for tension and stress:

A tight, twisted rope slowly untwists.

Wax softens and melts.

Tension swirls out of your body and down the drain.

Images for healing of cuts and injuries:

Plaster is being used to cover over a crack in a wall.

Cells and fibres stick together with very strong glue.

A shoe is laced up tightly.

Jigsaw puzzle pieces come together.

Images for arteries and heart disease:

A miniature *Dyno-Rod* truck speeds through your arteries and cleans out the clogged pipes.

Water flows freely along a wide, open river.

The crew in a small boat row together, easily and efficiently pulling the slender boat across a smooth water surface.

Images for asthma and lung disease:

The tiny elastic rubber bands that constrict your airways pop open.

A vacuum cleaner gently sucks the mucus from your airways.

Waves calmly rise and fall on the ocean surface.

Images for diabetes:

Small insulin keys unlock doors to hungry cells and allow nourishing blood glucose in.

An alarm goes off, and a sleeping pancreas gland awakens to the smell of freshly brewed coffee.

Images for cancer:

A shark gobbles up the cancer cells.

Tumours shrivel up like raisins in the hot sun, and then evaporate completely into the air.

The tap that controls the blood supply to the tumour is turned off, and the cancer cells starve.

Radiation or chemotherapy enters your body like healing rays of light and destroy cancer cells.

Images for infections:

White blood cells with flashing red sirens arrest and imprison harmful germs.

An army equipped with powerful antibiotic missiles attacks enemy germs.

A hot flame chases germs out of your entire body.

Images for a weakened immune system:

Sluggish, sleepy white blood cells wake up, put on protective armour, and enter the fight against the virus.

White blood cells rapidly multiply like millions of seeds bursting from a single ripe seed pod.

Images for an overactive immune system which has led to allergies, arthritis and psoriasis:

Over-alert immune cells in the fire station are reassured that the allergens have triggered a false alarm, and they go back to playing their game of poker.

A civil war ends with the warring sides agreeing not to attack their fellow citizens.

Images for pain:

All of the pain is placed in a large, strong metal box, it is closed, sealed tightly and locked with a huge padlock.

You grasp the TV remote control and slowly turn down the pain volume until you can barely hear it; then it disappears entirely.

The pain is washed away by a cool, calm river flowing through your entire body.

Images for depression:

Your troubles and feelings of sadness are attached to big colourful helium balloons which are floating off into a clear blue sky.

A strong, warm sun breaks through dark clouds.

You feel a sense of detachment and lightness, enabling you to float easily through your day.

Use any of these images, or make up your own. Remember, the best ones are vivid and have meaning for you. Use your imagination for health and healing.

A Guided-Imagery Script: *A Walk in the Country*

You're giving yourself some time to quieten down your mind and body. Allow yourself to settle comfortably, wherever you are right now. If you wish, you can close your eyes. Breathe in deeply, through your nose, expanding your abdomen and filling your lungs; now, pursing your lips, exhale through your mouth slowly and completely, allowing your body to sink heavily into the surface beneath you . . .

And once again, breathe in through your nose and all the way down to your abdomen, and then breathe out slowly through pursed lips . . . letting go of tension, letting go of anything that's on your mind right now, just allowing yourself to be present in this moment . . .

Imagine yourself walking along a peaceful old country road. The sun is gently warming your back . . . the birds are singing . . . the air is calm and fragrant . . .

With no need to hurry, you notice your walking is relaxed and easy. As you walk along in this way, taking in your surroundings, you come across an old gate. It looks inviting and you decide to take the path through the gate. The gate creaks as you open it and go through.

You find yourself in an old, overgrown garden, the flowers are growing where they've seeded themselves, vines climbing over a fallen tree, soft green wild grasses, and shady trees.

You notice yourself breathing deeply . . . smelling the flowers . . . listening to the birds and insects . . . feeling a gentle breeze cool against your skin. All of your senses are alive and responding with pleasure to this peaceful time and place . . .

When you're ready to move on, you follow the path out behind the garden, eventually coming to a more wooded area. As you enter this area, your eyes find the trees and plant life restful. The sunlight is filtered through the leaves. The air feels mild and a little cooler . . . you savour the fragrance of trees and earth . . . and gradually become aware of the sound of a nearby stream. Pausing, you allow yourself to take in the sights and sounds, breathing in the cool and fragrant air . . . and with each breath, you notice how refreshed you are feeling . . .

Continuing along the path for a time, you come to the stream. It's clear and clean as it flows and tumbles over the rocks and some fallen logs. You follow the path easily along the creek, and after some time, you come out into a sunlit clearing, where you discover a small waterfall emptying into a quiet pool of water.

You find a comfortable place to sit for a while, a perfect niche where you can feel completely relaxed . . .

You feel good as you allow yourself to enjoy the warmth and solitude of this peaceful place . . .

After a little time, you become aware that you need to return. You rise and walk back down the path in a relaxed and comfortable way . . . through the cool and fragrant trees, out into the sun-drenched, overgrown garden . . . one last smell of the flowers, and out through the creaking gate.

You leave this country retreat for now and retrace your steps down the road. You notice you feel calm and rested. You feel grateful and remind yourself that you can visit this special place whenever you wish to take some time to refresh yourself and renew your energy.

And now, preparing to bring this period of relaxation to a close, you may want to take a moment to picture yourself carrying this experience of calm and refreshment with you into the ordinary activities of your life . . . and when you're ready, take a nice deep breath and open your eyes.

A Guided-Imagery Script: *A Walk on the Beach*

Begin by getting into a comfortable position, whether you are seated or lying down. Loosen any tight clothing to allow yourself to be as comfortable as possible. Uncross your legs and allow your hands to fall by your sides or rest in your lap, and if you are at all uncomfortable shift to a more comfortable position.

When you are ready, you may allow your eyes to close gradually and then turn your attention to your breathing. Allow your belly to expand as you breathe in, bringing in fresh new air to nourish your body and then breathing out. Notice the rhythm of your breathing . . . in . . . and out . . . without trying to control it in any way. Simply attend to the natural rhythm of your breath . . .

And now in your mind's eye, imagine yourself standing on a beautiful beach. The sky is a brilliant blue, and as some fluffy white clouds float slowly by, you drink in the beautiful colours . . . the temperature is not too hot and not too cold. The sun is shining, and you close your eyes, allowing the warmth of the sun to wash over you . . . You notice a gentle breeze caressing your face, the perfect complement to the sunshine.

Then you find yourself turn turning and looking out over the vastness of the ocean . . . you become aware of the sound of the waves gently washing up on shore . . . You notice the firmness of the wet sand beneath your feet, or if you decide to take off your shoes, you may enjoy the feeling of standing, in the cool, wet sand . . . perhaps you allow the surf to roll up and gently wash across your feet, or perhaps you stay just out of its reach . . .

In the distance you hear some seagulls calling to one another. You look out to see the birds gracefully gliding through the air. And as you stand there, notice how easy it is to be here, perhaps feeling some sensations of relaxation, comfort, or peace . . . whatever's there . . .

Now take a walk along the shore. Turn and begin to stroll casually along the beach, enjoying the sounds of the surf, the warmth of the sun, and the gentle massage of the breeze. As you move along, taking your time, your stride becomes lighter and easier . . . you notice the scent of the ocean . . . you pause to take in the freshness of the air . . . and then you continue on your way, enjoying the peacefulness of this place.

After a time, you decide to rest, and find a comfortable place to sit or lie down . . . and simply allow yourself to take some time to enjoy this, your special place . . .

And now, when you feel ready to return, you stand and begin walking back down the beach in a comfortable, leisurely way, taking with you any sensations of relaxation, comfort, peace and joy . . . whatever's there . . . noticing how easy it is to be here. You continue until you reach the place where you began your walk . . .

And now pausing to take one last long look around, enjoy the vibrant colours of the sky and the sea . . . the gentle sound of the waves washing up on the shore . . . the warmth of the sun . . . the cool of the breeze . . .

And as you prepare to leave this special place, taking with you any sensations of joy, relaxation, comfort, peace . . . whatever's there . . . knowing that you can return at any appropriate time and place of your choosing.

And now, bringing your awareness back into the room, focusing on your breathing . . . in and out . . . take a few more breaths . . . and when you're ready, open your eyes.

Prayer and Spirituality

Many people find spirituality through religion. Some find it through music, art, or a connection with nature. Others find it in their values and principles. Many people are religious and share their religion with others. Many may not have a specific religion but do have spiritual beliefs. Our religion and beliefs can bring a sense of meaning and purpose to our life, helping us to put things into perspective, and set priorities. Our beliefs may help us find comfort during difficult times. They can help us with acceptance and motivate us to make difficult changes. Being part of a spiritual or religious community can offer a source of support when needed, and provides the opportunity to help others.

Some scientifically conducted trials in the laboratory have demonstrated that people experience the *relaxation response* when they pray or meditate. Their blood pressure, heart rate and levels of stress hormones drop. There are also other physiological changes which can reduce anxiety. All these reactions have a positive effect on your health management. If you are someone who prays and has strong religious beliefs there are opportunities in NHS hospitals to share this information with your health care professionals. They will respect your beliefs and try to assist you in whatever way is appropriate.

If you are not religious you might consider taking up some form of meditation which might help you with relaxation and allow you to enjoy some of the health benefits of this.

Other Techniques That Use Your Mind

There are other valuable techniques you can consider which can clear your mind and positively shift your emotional state. These will also reduce your tension and stress.

Using Mindfulness

Mindfulness involves simply keeping your attention in the present moment, without judging it as happy or sad, good or bad. It encourages living each moment, even the painful ones, as fully and as mindfully as possible. Mindfulness is more than a relaxation technique; it is an attitude toward living. It is a way of calmly and consciously observing and accepting whatever is happening, moment by moment. This may sound simple enough, but our restless, judging minds make it surprisingly difficult. Just as a restless monkey jumps from branch to branch, our mind seems to jump from thought to thought.

In mindfulness, you focus your mind on the present moment. The *goal* of mindfulness is simply to observe, with no intention of changing or improving anything. Nevertheless, people *are* often positively changed by this practice. Observing and accepting life just as it is, with all its pleasures, pains, frustrations, disappointments and insecurities, will often enable you to become calmer, more confident and better able to cope with whatever comes along.

To develop your capacity for mindfulness, sit comfortably on the floor or on a chair with your back, neck and head straight, but not stiff. Then try this:

- *Concentrate on a single object, such as your breathing:* Focus your attention on the feeling of the air as it passes in and out of your nostrils with each breath. Don't try to control your breathing by speeding it up or slowing it down. Just observe it as it is.

- *If you lose concentration consider where your mind has gone:* Even when you resolve to keep your attention on your breathing, your mind will quickly wander off. When this occurs, observe where your mind went: perhaps to a memory, a worry about the future, a bodily ache, or a feeling of impatience. Then gently return your attention to your breathing.

- *Use your breath as an anchor:* Each time a thought or feeling arises, momentarily acknowledge it. Don't analyse it or judge it. Just observe it, and return to your breathing.

- *Let go of all thoughts of getting somewhere, or having anything special happen:* Just keep stringing moments of mindfulness together, breath by breath.

- *Practise and prolong:* At first, practise this for just five minutes, or even one minute at a time. You may wish to gradually extend the time to ten, 20 or 30 minutes.

Because the practice of mindfulness is simply the practice of *moment-to-moment awareness*, you can apply it to anything: eating, showering, working, talking, running errands, or playing with your children. Mindfulness takes no extra time. Considerable research has demonstrated the benefits of practising mindfulness in relieving stress, easing pain, improving concentration, and relieving a variety of other symptoms.

Using the Quieting Reflex

This technique was developed by a physician named Charles Stroebel. It will help you deal with short-term stresses such as the urge to eat or smoke, road rage, and other annoyances. It relieves muscle tightening, jaw clenching, and holding your breath by activating the sympathetic nervous system.

It should be practised frequently throughout the day, whenever you start to feel stressed. It can be done with your eyes opened or closed. Have a try now:

1. *Become aware of what is annoying you:* a ringing phone, an angry comment, the urge to smoke, a worrisome thought, whatever it is.

2. *Repeat the phrase "Alert mind, calm body"* to yourself.

3. *Smile inwardly with your eyes and your mouth.* This stops facial muscles from forming a fearful or angry expression. The inward smile is a *feeling*. It cannot be seen by others.

4. *Inhale slowly to the count of three while imagining that the breath comes in through the bottom of your feet.* Then exhale slowly. Feel your breath move back down your legs and out through your feet. Let your jaw, tongue, and shoulder muscles go limp.

With several months of practice the quieting reflex will become an automatic skill.

Trying Nature Therapy

Many of us suffer from what has been called *nature deficit disorder*. This can be readily cured by regular doses of the *great outdoors*. For thousands of years exposure to natural environments has been recommended for healing. Taking a break from artificial lighting, excessive computer and TV screen time, and indoor environments can all be restorative. A brief walk in a park or a longer planned visit to a beautiful outdoor environment can restore the mind and body. Or, you can bring nature indoors with plants, pets, and nature photography. Even a few minutes of playing with or stroking a pet can lower blood pressure and calm a restless mind.

Working with Worry Time

Worrying negative thoughts will feed anxiety. Problems we try to ignore also have a way of thrusting themselves back into our consciousness. You'll find it easier to set aside worries if you make time to deal with them. Set aside 20 or 30 minutes a day as your *worry time*. Whenever a worry pops into your mind, write it down and tell yourself that you'll deal with it during your worry time. Jot down the little things, such as *"Did Linda take her lunch to school?"* along with the big worries such as *"Will our children be able to find jobs?"* During your scheduled worry time, don't do anything except worry, think freely, and write down possible solutions. For each of your worries, ask yourself the following questions:

- What is the problem?

- How likely is it that the problem will occur?

- What's the worst that could happen?

- What's the best that could happen?

- How will I cope with the problem?

- What are the possible solutions?

- What is my plan of action?

Be specific. Instead of worrying about what might happen if you lose your job, ask yourself real questions. Questions such as: *"How likely it is that I will lose my job?"* and *"If I lose my job what will I do?"* Consider who else you would involve and how and when. Write down a plan for a job search.

If you're anxious about getting seasick on a ferry and not making it to the toilet in time, imagine how you would deal with the situation. Ask yourself if any of this is really unbearable. Tell yourself that although you might feel uncomfortable or embarrassed, you will survive.

Remember, if a new worry pops up during the rest of the day, jot it down. Then distract yourself by re-focusing intently on whatever you are doing. Scheduling a definite worry time seems to cut the amount of time spent worrying by at least a third. If you look at your list of worries later on, you'll find that the vast majority of them never materialised. Almost all of them were not nearly as bad as you anticipated.

Developing a Healthy Perspective

Sometimes you can relieve stress and break a cycle of negative thoughts by shifting your perspective. If you are upset, ask yourself *"How important will this be in an hour, a day, a month, or in a year?"* This reframing often helps to bring to the surface things that are really important and need action rather than minor, less significant annoyances.

Practising Thankfulness

One of the most effective ways to improve your mood and overall happiness is by focusing your attention on what's going well in your life. What are you most thankful for? Psychologists have done research to demonstrate that people can increase their happiness by *gratitude exercises*. We encourage you to try these three:

1. *Write a letter of thanks:* Write and then deliver a letter of thanks to someone who has been especially kind to you but has never been properly thanked. Perhaps it's a teacher, a mentor, a friend, or a family member. Express your appreciation for this person's kindness. The letter will have more impact if you include some specific examples of what the recipient has done for you. Describe how their actions made you feel.

2. *Acknowledge at least three good things every day:* Each night before bed, write down at least three things that went well today. No event or feeling is too small to note. By putting your thanks into words, you increase appreciation and enhance the memory of your blessings. Knowing that you will need to write down these good things each night will change your mental filters during the whole day. You will tend to seek out, look for, and specially note the good things that happen. If doing this daily is too much or it begins to seem like a routine chore, do it once a week.

3. *Make a list of the things you take for granted:* For example, if your condition has affected your lungs, you can still be grateful that your kidneys are working. Perhaps you can celebrate a day in which you don't have a headache or backache? Counting your

blessings can add up to a better mood and greater happiness.

Compiling a List of Strengths

Make a personal inventory of your talents, skills, achievements, and qualities, big or small. Celebrate your accomplishments. When something goes wrong, consult your list of positives, and put the problem in perspective. The *problem* then becomes just one specific experience, not something that defines your whole life.

Putting Kindness into Practice

This world is plagued by acts of violence. When something bad happens, it is front-page news. As an antidote to this misery, despair, and cynicism, you can practise acts of kindness. Look for opportunities to give without expecting anything in return. Here are some examples:

- Hold the door open for the person behind you.
- Give an unexpected gift of theatre or concert tickets.
- Send an anonymous gift to a friend who needs cheering up.
- Help someone with a heavy load.
- Tell positive stories you know about helping and kindness.
- Cultivate an attitude of thankfulness for the kindnesses that you have received.
- Plant a tree.
- Pick up litter.

Be creative. Such kindness is contagious and it has a ripple effect. In one study, people who were given an unexpected treat of biscuits were later more likely to help others.

Writing Stress Away

It's hard work to keep our deep, negative feelings hidden. Over time, this cumulative stress undermines our body's defences and seems to weaken our immunity. Confiding our feelings to others, or writing them down puts them into words and helps us sort them out. Words help us to understand and absorb a traumatic event and eventually put it behind us. It gives us a sense of release and control.

The psychologist Jamie Pennebaker described in his book *Opening Up*, a series of studies which looked at the healing effects of *confiding* or *writing*. One group was asked to express their deepest thoughts and feelings about something bad that had happened to them. Another group wrote about ordinary matters such as their plans for the day. Both groups wrote for 15 to 20 minutes a day for three to five consecutive days. No one involved read what members of either group had written.

The results were surprisingly powerful. When compared with the people who wrote about ordinary events, those who wrote about their bad experiences reported fewer symptoms, fewer visits to the doctor, fewer days off work, improved mood, and a more positive outlook. Their immune function was enhanced for at least six weeks after writing. This was especially true for those who expressed previously undisclosed painful feelings.

Try this *writing approach* when something is bothering you: for example, when you find yourself thinking or dreaming too much about a bad experience; or when you avoid thinking about something because it is too upsetting; or when there's something you would like to tell others but can't because you fear either embarrassment or punishment.

Here are some guidelines for writing as a way to deal with traumatic experiences:

■ *Set a specific schedule for writing*: For example, you might write 15 minutes a day for four consecutive days, or one day a week for four weeks.

■ *Choose your place*: Write in a place where you won't be interrupted or distracted.

■ *Don't plan to share your writing*: Doing so could stop your honest expression. Save what you write or destroy it, as you decide.

■ *Explore your very deepest thoughts and feelings*: Do some analysis about why you feel the way you do. Write about your negative feelings such as sadness, hurt, anger, hate, fear, guilt, or resentment.

■ *Write continuously*: Don't worry about grammar, spelling, or making sense. If clarity and coherence do come as you continue to write, so much the better. If you run out of things to say, just reflect on what you have already written.

■ *Keep going*: Even if you find the writing awkward at first, it gets easier. If you just cannot write these things down, try talking into a tape recorder for 15 minutes about your deepest thoughts and feelings.

■ *Don't expect to feel better immediately*: You may feel sad or depressed when your deepest feelings begin to surface. This usually fades in an hour or two, or maybe a day or two. The overwhelming majority of people report feelings of relief, happiness, and contentment soon after writing for a few consecutive days.

■ *Writing may help you clarify what actions you need to take:* However, don't use writing as a substitute for taking action or as a way of avoiding things.

Once established, relaxation, imagery, and positive thinking can be some of the most powerful tools you can add to your self-management tool box. They will help you manage symptoms and master the other skills discussed in this book.

As with exercise and other acquired skills, using your mind to manage your health condition requires both practice and time before you begin to notice the benefits. So if you feel you are not accomplishing anything, don't give up. Be patient and keep on trying.

Suggested Further Reading

Burgess, M. and Chalder, T. *Overcoming Chronic Fatigue Syndrome.* London: Robinson, 2009.

Cole, F., Howden-Leach, H. et al. *Overcoming Chronic Pain: A Self-Help Guide Using Cognitive Behaviour Therapy Techniques.* London: Constable and Robinson, 2005.

Cleave, G. *Introducing Positive Psychology: A Practical Guide.* London: Totem Books/Icon Books, 2012.

Lyubomirsky, S. *The How of Happiness: A New Approach to Getting the Life You Want.* New York: Penguin, 2008.

Moorey, S, and Greer, S. *Cognitive Behaviour Therapy for People with Cancer.* Oxford: Oxford University Press, 2002.

Selak, J, and Overman, S. *You don't look sick: Living Well with Invisible Chronic Illness.* New York and London: The Haworth Medical Press, 2005.

Wiseman, R. *59 Seconds: Think a Little, Change a Lot.* New York: Borzoi Books, 2009.

Audio Visual and Other Resources

☐ *The British Association of Behavioural Psychotherapies* (BABCP). This organisation maintains a register of CBT practitioners. Tel: 0161 705 4304. Their website also provides information on CBT. www.babcp.com.

☐ Naparstek, B. *Health Journeys Guided Imagery* [audio CDs]. www.healthjourneys.com.

☐ *Oxford Cognitive Behaviour Centre* (OCTC). This website gives details of how to order a number of self-help booklets with a CBT approach for conditions such as OCD, anxiety, panic, depression and phobias. www.octc.co.uk.

☐ Regan, C. and Seidel, R. *Relaxation for Mind and Body: Pathways to Healing* [audio CD]. Boulder, Colo.: Bull Publishing, 2012.

☐ Weil, A. and Rossman, M. *Self-Healing with Guided Imagery* [audio CD]. Louisville, Colo.: Sounds True, 2006.

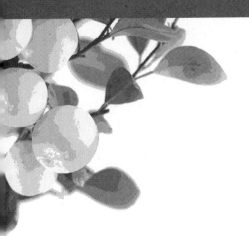

CHAPTER **6**

Exercise and Physical Activity for Every Body

ACTIVE PEOPLE ARE HEALTHIER AND HAPPIER than people who are not. This is true for all ages and conditions. Not moving enough can sometimes cause or worsen the condition or symptoms.

You have probably heard that regular physical activity is important, but if you have a chronic health problem, you may not know what to do and worry that you will do the wrong thing. Just 30 years ago, if you had arthritis, diabetes, or lung disease, it was hard to learn how to exercise. Now there is a lot of information about this. We will help you to get started and be successful. Many countries have public health programmes to help people understand the importance of physical activity and offer programmes to get you going. There are guidelines for children, young and older adults, people with long-term conditions, and people with disabilities. These guidelines clarify what kinds of exercise or physical activity is best and how much you need. In this and the following three chapters, you will learn about these guidelines and about wise exercise choices. Of course, *learning about* this is not enough. It is up to you to make your life more enjoyable, more comfortable, and healthier through physical activity. *However, you should note that this advice is not intended to take the place of medical advice.* If you have a prescribed exercise plan that differs from the suggestions here, take this book to your doctor or physiotherapist and ask what they think about this programme. We provide additional information and helpful exercise ideas for people with specific conditions in separate chapters later in this book.

Why Exercise?

Regular exercise can prevent or manage heart disease and diabetes. It improves blood pressure, blood sugar levels, and blood fat levels like cholesterol. You will find more information about the different types of cholesterol in Chapter 11 on *Healthy Eating*. Exercise can help you maintain a good weight, which takes stress off weight-bearing joints. Exercise is also part of keeping bones strong and treating osteoporosis. There is evidence that regular exercise can also help prevent blood clots. Indeed, this is one of the reasons exercise can be of particular benefit to people with heart and vascular diseases. Regular exercise improves levels of strength, energy, and self-confidence and lessens feelings of stress, anxiety, and depression. Regular exercise can help you sleep better and feel more relaxed and happy.

In addition, strong muscles help people with arthritis protect their joints by improving stability and absorbing shock. Regular exercise also helps nourish joints and keeps cartilage and bone healthy. Regular exercise has been shown to help people with chronic lung disease to improve their endurance and reduce the trips they make to A&E. Many people with leg pain resulting from poor circulation can walk further and more comfortably with a regular exercise programme. Studies of people with heart disease show that exercise improves the health f their heart and their quality of life.

The good news is that it doesn't take hours of painful, sweat-soaked exercise to achieve health benefits. Even short periods of moderate physical activity can improve health and fitness, reduce disease risk, and boost your mood. Being active also helps you to feel more in control of your life and less at the mercy of your health condition. You don't have to kill yourself to save your life!

Developing an Exercise Programme

For most people who are not already active, starting a regular exercise programme means creating a new routine in your life. This usually involves setting aside a period of time on most days of the week so that exercise becomes a part of your day. Exercise programmes that are recommended in guidelines today distinguish four types of fitness:

1. **Flexibility**: Being flexible means you can move comfortably to do everything you need or want to do. Limited flexibility can cause pain, lead to injury, and make muscles work harder and tire more quickly. You lose flexibility when you are inactive and also as a result of some conditions and disabilities. However, you can increase flexibility by doing gentle stretching exercises such as those described in Chapter 7.

2. **Strength**: Muscles need to be exercised in order to maintain their strength. When inactive, muscles weaken and shrink. When your muscles are weak, you feel weak and get tired quickly. Much of the disability and lack of mobility people with chronic conditions experience is due to muscle weakness. Exercise programmes that ask muscles to do more work, like lifting a weight, strengthen them.

3. **Endurance**: Feeling energetic depends on the fitness of your heart, lungs, and muscles. The heart and lungs must work efficiently to send oxygen-rich blood to the muscles. The muscles must be fit enough to use the oxygen. *Aerobic exercise* uses the large muscles of your body in continuous activity such as walking, swimming, dancing, mowing the lawn, and riding a bike. The word *aerobic* simply means *with oxygen*. Aerobic exercise improves cardiovascular fitness, reduces heart attack risk, and helps to control your weight. Aerobic exercise also promotes a sense of well-being, eases depression and anxiety, promotes restful sleep, and improves your mood and energy levels.

4. **Balance**: Good balance helps to keep you from falling. Strong and co-ordinated muscles in your trunk and legs are an important part of good balance. Flexibility, strength, and endurance also contribute to balance. Of course, you can fall for many reasons such as poor vision, poor lighting, tripping over rugs, or getting dizzy, but being strong and co-ordinated is an important factor. Certain exercises are especially good for improving balance.

Establishing Your Exercise Programme

A complete programme combines exercises designed to improve all four aspects of fitness: *flexibility, strength, endurance,* and *balance.* Chapter 7 shows you a number of flexibility and strengthening exercises and includes specific exercises for your posture and balance. Chapter 8 explains and gives examples of aerobic exercise for improving endurance. If you haven't exercised regularly for some time or have pain, stiffness, shortness of breath, or weakness that interferes with your daily activities, be careful. Discuss exercise with your health care professionals. Begin your exercise programme by choosing some flexibility and strengthening exercises that you are willing to do *every other* day. Once you are able to exercise comfortably for at least ten minutes at a time, you are ready to start adding some endurance or aerobic activities.

You may wonder how to choose the right exercises. The truth is that the best exercises for you are the ones that will help you do what you want to do. Often the most important decision to start a successful exercise programme is to choose a goal that exercise will help you to reach. Your *goal* is simply something you want to do. For example, walk for ten minutes so that you can go to your nearest local shop. Once you have a goal in mind, it is much easier to choose exercises that make sense. There is no doubt that we are all more successful exercisers when we know where we want the exercise to take us. If you can't see how exercise can be helpful, then it's hard to get excited about adding yet another task to your daily routine.

Choose your goal and make a plan

- *Choose something that you want to do but don't because of your physical condition:* For example, you might want to enjoy a shopping excursion or a fishing trip with your friends, or mow the lawn, or take a family holiday.

- *Think about why you don't do it or don't enjoy doing it now:* It might be that you get tired before everybody else, or that it's too hard to get up from a low chair or bench, or that climbing steps is too painful, or that your shoulders are too weak or stiff to cast a fishing line or carry a small overnight bag.

- *Decide what it is that makes it hard to do what you want:* For example, if getting up from a low seat is difficult, it may be that your hips or knees are stiff and your leg muscles are weak. In this case, look for flexibility and find some strengthening exercises for hips and knees. If you decide that a major problem is that your shoulders are stiff and your arms are too weak to carry a small overnight bag onto the train, then choose flexibility and strengthening exercises for your shoulders and arms.

- *Design your exercise plan:* Read Chapter 7 and choose no more than ten to 12 exercises. Begin by doing each exercise five times. As you get comfortable, you will be able to do more. If you want to improve your endurance, read Chapter 8 about aerobic exercise. Start off with short times and build up gradually. Health and fitness take time, but every day you exercise you are healthier and becoming more successful. That's why it is so important to make sure you keep it up.

Overcoming Your Exercise Barriers

Health and fitness make sense. Yet, when faced with being more physically active, people often come up with lots of excuses, concerns, and worries. These barriers can prevent you from taking the first step. Here are some common barriers and possible solutions:

- *"I don't have enough time."* We all have the same amount of time; we just use it differently. It's a matter of priorities. Some people find time for television but not for exercise. Exercise doesn't take a lot of time. Just 15 minutes a day is a good start, and it's much better than nothing. You may be able to work exercise into your day: for example, why not watch television whilst pedalling a stationary bicycle or arrange a *walking meeting* to discuss business or family matters. If you take three 10-minute walks each day, you have 30 minutes of daily exercise.

■ *"I'm too tired."* When you're unfit or depressed, you can feel tired. You have to break out of the *too tired* cycle. Try an experiment: next time you are too tired, take a short walk, just for five minutes, or even two minutes will do! You may be surprised that this *gives* you energy. As you get fitter, you will recognise the difference between *feeling listless* and *feeling physically tired*. The more you do the easier it is to see things change.

■ *"I'm too old."* You're never too old for physical activity. No matter what your level of fitness or your age, you can always find ways to increase your activity, raise your energy level, and heighten your sense of wellbeing. Fitness is increasingly important as we get older.

■ *"I'm too ill."* It may be true that you are too ill for a vigorous or strenuous exercise programme, but you can usually find ways to be more active. Remember, you can start with exercise for only one minute at a time, several times a day. Better fitness will help you to cope with your illness and prevent further problems.

■ *"I get enough exercise."* This may be true, but for most people, their jobs and daily activities do not provide enough sustained exercise at a moderate level to keep them fit and energetic.

■ *"Exercise is boring."* You can always make it more interesting and fun. Exercise with other people. Entertain yourself with a headset and musical tapes, or an MP3 player, or listen to the radio. Vary your activities and your walking routes. You might find that exercise time is also good thinking time.

■ *"Exercise is painful."* The old saying *"No pain, no gain"* is simply wrong. Health benefits come from moderate-intensity physical activity. If you feel more pain when you finish than before you started, take a close look at what you are doing. You may be exercising incorrectly, or over-doing it. Talk with your instructor, physiotherapist, or doctor. You may simply need to be less vigorous or perhaps change the type of exercise that you're doing. For some conditions, such as arthritis, exercise actually reduces pain.

■ *"I'm too embarrassed."* Some people have put on weight over the years and wear baggy track suit bottoms to avoid showing all their lumps and bumps. They are not very fit and don't want to look like fools in front of other people. This is not a problem, because the options for physical activity range from exercise in the privacy of your own home to group social activities. You will be able to find something that suits you.

■ *"I'm afraid I might fall."* Check that you will exercise somewhere where you are unlikely to fall. This means good lighting, well-maintained parking and pavements, handrails, and uncluttered floors. Choose exercises that feel safe, like chair exercise, water exercise, or recumbent bicycling. The last of these involves a bicycle ridden in a reclining position. All of these activities will provide a lot of support as you get started. Remember, strong and flexible legs and ankles will help you to stay active and co-ordinated. This will reduce the risk of falls. Your doctor or therapist may also recommend a cane, walking stick, or walker to enhance your balance. However, it is important to have a physiotherapist fit it for you and teach you how to use it safely. Using a cane, walking stick or walker that doesn't fit or is used incorrectly can even cause a fall.

- *"I'm afraid I'll have a heart attack."* In most cases, the risk of a heart attack is greater for people who are not physically active than for those who exercise regularly. But if you are worried about this, check with your doctor. It's probably safer to exercise than not to exercise, especially if your condition is under control. Check with your hospital cardiology team if you can join a special exercise class for patients with cardiac problems.

- *"It's too cold, hot, dark . . ."* If you are flexible and vary your exercise, you can generally work around changes in the weather that make certain types of exercise more difficult. Consider indoor activities when the weather is a barrier. Try exercises such as stationary cycling, swimming, or walking in an enclosed shopping area.

- *"I'm afraid I won't be able to do it right or won't be good at it."* Many people don't even start because they are afraid they will fail. If you feel this way, remember two things. *First,* whatever activities you are able to do, no matter how short or easy, will benefit you more than doing nothing. Be proud of what you can do rather than guilty about what you haven't done. *Second,* whilst new projects can sometimes seem overwhelming, it's certainly better to get on with it and learn to enjoy each day's adventures and successes.

Perhaps you have some other barriers. Be honest with yourself about your worries. Talk to yourself and others to develop positive thoughts about exercise. If you get stuck, ask others for suggestions. You could use some of the positive thinking discussed in Chapter 5.

Achieving Better Balance

Sometimes people decide that the best way to avoid a fall is to spend more time sitting. At first you might think that as you are not walking around, you won't be at risk of falling. However, inactivity causes weakness, stiffness, slower reflexes, inadequate muscles, and even social isolation and depression. All of these can harm your balance and cause an increase in your risk of falling. Even simple things such as getting up or sitting down in a chair, going to the bathroom, or going down a step can cause problems.

Other physical conditions such as weakness, dizziness, stiffness, poor eyesight, loss of feeling in your feet, or inner ear problems can cause a fall. So too, can the side-effects of medications. Falls can also be caused by the nature of the space around you: poor lighting, uneven ground, rugs, and cluttered floors. To avoid falls, reduce all of these risks and keep yourself strong, flexible, and co-ordinated. Research shows that people who have strong legs and ankles, are flexible, and do things that require them to balance, have less fear of falling and actually fall less.

If you have fallen or are afraid that you may fall, then talk with your health care professional or your GP and get your balance checked. Make sure there are no vision or inner ear problems or medication problems that need attention. Make sure that your home is safe. Exercising to keep yourself strong, flexible and active will also help protect you from falling. Look at Chapter 7 for the balance exercises marked "BB" and, particularly exercises 27–32.

Preparing to Exercise

Committing to regular exercise is a big deal for everyone. If you have a long-term condition, you may also have many daily challenges and special exercise needs. People with arthritis, for example, must learn how to adapt exercise to changes in their arthritis and their joint problems. People with heart or lung disease should not continue to *exercise through* serious symptoms such as chest pain, palpitations, shortness of breath, or excessive fatigue. They should seek the doctor's advice if these things happen or new symptoms appear. If your illness is not under good control, or if you have been inactive for more than six months, or if you have questions about starting an exercise

programme, it is best to check with your doctor or physiotherapist. Take this book with you and discuss your exercise ideas. Make a list of your questions before you go.

We hope this chapter helps you to learn how to meet your needs and enjoy the benefits of physical activity. Start by knowing your own needs and limits and respect your body. Talk to other people like yourself, who take exercise. Talk with your doctor and other health professionals who understand your chronic condition. Always pay attention to your own experience. That helps you to know your body and make wise choices.

Physical Activity Guidelines

Many countries now have guidelines about the kind and amount of physical activity, people should do to be healthy. These guidelines are pretty much the same all over the world

and include advise for adults with and without chronic conditions and disabilities. *When you read these guidelines, it is important to remember that they are goals to work towards; they are not the starting point.* On average, only about 25% of people in any country exercise enough to satisfy the guidelines. So don't worry that everyone else can do these but you can't.

Your goal is to gradually and safely increase your physical activity to a level that is right for you. You may be able to get to exercise up to that level, but maybe you won't. The important point is to use the information in order to get started on the pathway to being more active and healthier, but to do so in a way that is right for you. Start doing what you *can*. Even a few minutes of activity several times a day is a good beginning. The important thing is to do something that works for *you*. Make your exercise a habit, and gradually increase the time or number of days a week you spend on it. Chapters 7 and 8 will give you more information to help you get started on your exercise plan.

In July 2011 the four *Chief Medical Officers* in the UK published the new physical activity guidelines in a Report. This Report was entitled *Start Active, Stay Active* and covers all the age groups from children to those over 65. Here are summaries taken from *Factsheets 4* and *5* of this guidance:

Guidelines for 19–64 Year Olds Taken from Factsheet 4

1. Over a week, activity should add up to at least 150 minutes of moderate intensity activity in brief bouts of ten minutes or more. There are various combinations for achieving this. For example by doing 30 minutes a day for five days.

2. Alternatively, and if it is appropriate for you, comparable benefits can be achieved by doing 75 minutes of vigorous intensity activity spread across the week.

3. Physical activity should also be undertaken to improve muscle strength on at least two days a week.

4. The amount of time spent sitting down should be minimised.

Examples of activities which meet the guidelines:

Moderate Activity
- Brisk walking
- Cycling

Vigorous Activity
- Running
- Sports such as swimming or football

Muscle strengthening activity
- Exercising with weights
- Carrying heavy loads such as shopping

Minimising sedentary behaviour
- Reducing time watching television
- Taking regular breaks at work
- Breaking up bus or car journeys by walking part of the way

Guidelines for 65+ Years Taken from Factsheet 5

1. Older adults should aim to be active daily. Over a week activity should add up to at least 150 minutes of *moderate intensity* activity in bouts of ten minutes or more. There are various combinations for achieving this as for example doing 30 minutes a day for five days.

2. For those who are already regularly active at the *moderate intensity* level, comparable benefits can be achieved by doing 75 minutes of *vigorous intensity* activity spread across the week or a combination of moderate and vigorous activity.

3. Physical activity should also be undertaken to improve muscle strength on at least two days a week.

4. Older adults at risk of falling should incorporate physical activity to improve balance and co-ordination on at least two days a week.

5. The amount of time spent sitting should be minimised.

Examples of activities which meet the guidelines:

Moderate Activity

■ Brisk walking

■ Ballroom dancing

Vigorous Activity

■ Climbing stairs

■ Running

Muscle strengthening activity

■ Carrying heavy loads such as shopping

■ Dancing

■ Chair aerobics

Activities to improve balance

■ Tai Chi

■ Yoga

Minimising sedentary behaviour

■ Reducing time watching television

■ Taking regular breaks by walking around the garden or the street

■ Breaking up bus or car journeys by walking part of the way

Seeking Opportunities in Your Community

Many people who exercise regularly do so with at least one other person. Two or more people can keep each other motivated, and a whole *exercise class* can become a circle of friends. On the other hand, exercising alone gives you more freedom. You may feel that there are no classes that would work for you and that you have no close friend with whom to exercise. If so, start your own programme; as you progress, you may find that these feelings change.

Most local community organisations offer a variety of exercise classes, including: special programmes for people over 50, adaptive exercises, healthy walks, tai chi, and yoga. Check with the local community and day centres, parks and recreation programmes, adult education classes, community colleges, and organisations for specific conditions such as arthritis, diabetes, cancer and heart disease. There is a great deal of variation in these programmes, as well as in the expertise of the exercise instructors. By and large, these classes are inexpensive, and the staff who are in charge of planning are willing to respond to individual needs. Your local authority or NHS often makes free or subsidised classes available. For example, you could try the *Healthy Walks Scheme,* and your GP, local library and newspaper may have information on a variety of other possibilities.

Hospitals sometimes have medically supervised classes for people with heart or lung disease, called cardiac or pulmonary rehabilitation classes. There is similar provision for other long term medical conditions. Private health and fitness clubs usually offer aerobic classes, weight training, cardiovascular equipment, and sometimes a heated pool. However they do charge membership fees. The following list describes some things to think about when you search for community programmes:

- *Are classes designed for moderate and low-intensity exercise for beginners?* Ask if you can observe some classes and participate in at least one class before signing up and paying.

- *Are there safe and effective endurance, strength, balance, and flexibility components?* Ask if these can be tailored to meet your needs.

- *Are the instructors qualified and have they experience of working with people such as you?* Knowledgeable instructors are more likely to understand special needs and be willing and able to work with you.

- *Are there flexible membership policies* that allow you to pay by the class or for a short series of classes or let you freeze your membership at times when you can't participate? Some fitness facilities offer different rates depending on how many services you use.

- *Are the facilities easy to get to and enter and is there nearby parking?* Car parking, dressing rooms, and exercise locations should be accessible and safe, with professional staff available on site.

- *Is there a pool that allows "free swim" times when the water isn't crowded?* Also, find out about the policy concerning children in the pool; small children playing and making lots of noise may not be good for your needs.

- *Is it a friendly location?* Are the staff and other members friendly and easy to talk to?

- *Is there an emergency management protocol?* Also are the instructors certified in CPR and first aid?

Note that there are many excellent exercise DVDs for use at home. These programmes vary in intensity, from very gentle chair exercises to more strenuous aerobic exercise. Ask your doctor, physiotherapist, or voluntary organisation for suggestions. *Age UK* in particular offers exercise classes in England under the name *Fit as a Fiddle* at www.fitasafiddle.org.uk and *Age Cymru* in Wales offers a different exercise programme at www.agecymru.org.uk. In Northern Ireland and Scotland contact *Age Northern Ireland* or *Age Scotland* to find out what exercise classes they can offer.

Putting Your Programme Together

The best way to enjoy and stick with your exercise programme is to *suit yourself*. Choose what you want to do, a place where you feel comfortable, and an exercise time that fits your schedule. If you want to have your meal on the table at 6:00 p.m., don't choose an exercise programme that requires you to attend a 5:00 p.m. class. If you are retired and enjoy lunch with friends and an afternoon nap, it is wise to choose an early or mid-morning exercise time.

Pick two or three activities that you think you would enjoy and that would be comfortable. Choose activities that can be easily worked into your daily routine. If an activity is new, try it out before going to the expense of buying equipment, or joining a health club. By having more than one exercise option, you can keep active and work round holidays, seasons, and changes in your condition. Variety also helps to prevent over-use injuries and keeps you from getting bored.

Having fun and enjoying yourself are benefits of exercise that often go unmentioned. Too often we think of exercise as a serious business. However, most people who stick with an exercise programme do so because they come to enjoy it and also how they feel because of it. They think of their exercise as recreation or as a positive part of their life rather than a chore. Start off with success in mind. Allow yourself time to get used to doing something new and meeting new people. If you do this you'll probably find that you look forward to exercise.

Follow the self-management steps in Chapter 2 to make starting your programme easier.

Experience, practice, and success all help build a habit, so keep these issues in mind:

■ *Keep your exercise goal in mind:* Review *"Choose Your Goal and Make a Plan"* discussed earlier in this chapter.

■ *Choose exercises you want to do:* Combine activities that move you toward your goal and those recommended by your health professionals. Select exercises and activities from the next two chapters to get you started.

■ *Choose the time and place to exercise:* Tell your family and friends about your plan.

■ *Make an action plan with yourself:* Decide how long you'll stick with these particular exercises; six to eight weeks is a reasonable time for any new programme.

■ *Start your programme:* Remember to begin doing what you can and proceed slowly, especially if you haven't exercised for a while.

■ *Keep an exercise diary or calendar:* A diary lets you write more. Some people enjoy having a record of what they did and how they felt. Others like a simple calendar on which they can note each exercise session.

■ *Use self-tests to keep track of your progress:* You will find these tests at the end of the next two chapters. Record the date and results of the ones you choose.

■ *Repeat self-tests at regular intervals:* Record the results, and check the changes.

■ *Revise your programme:* At the end of your six or eight weeks, decide what you liked, what worked, and what made exercising difficult. Make changes and draw up an action plan for another few weeks. You may decide to change some of the exercises, or alter the place and time you exercise, or you may change your exercise partner or group.

■ *Reward yourself for a job well done:* Rewards from improved health and endurance come in many forms: enjoyable family outings, refreshing walks, trips to concerts and museums, or a day out fishing. These are all great rewards, and so to are pats on the back, and a new exercise shirt can be fun too!

Keeping It Up

If you haven't exercised recently, you'll probably experience some new feelings and perhaps some discomfort. When exercising, it's normal to feel *some* muscle soreness, tenderness in your joints and to be more tired in the evenings. However, muscle or joint pain that lasts more than two hours after the exercise or feeling tired into the next day means that you probably did too much, or worked too fast. Don't stop; just don't work so hard the next day or work for a shorter time.

When you do aerobic exercise, it's natural to feel your heart beating faster, your breathing speeding up, and your body getting warmer. But, chest pain, feeling sick, feeling dizzy, or being severely short of breath is an indication that you should contact your doctor. If this happens, stop exercising until you check with your doctor. Take a look at Table 6.1.

People who have a long-term condition or disability often have additional sensations to sort out. It can be difficult to separate out whether it is the condition, the exercise, or anxiety that is causing concern. You can find out a lot if you talk to someone like yourself who has already started an exercise programme. Once you've sorted out these new feelings, you'll be able to exercise with more confidence.

Expect setbacks. During the first year, people often have two to three interruptions in their exercise schedule, often because of family needs, minor injuries, or illnesses not related to exercise. You may get off track for a while. Don't be discouraged. You may need a rest, or a revised schedule, or different activities. When you are feeling better and start again, begin at a lower, gentler level. It can take you the same length of time to get back into shape as the period you had off. For instance, if you missed three weeks, it may take at least that long to get back to your previous level. Go slowly. Be kind to yourself. You are learning to exercise for the long-term and there is no pressure to make immediate, dramatic improvements.

With exercise experience you develop a sense of control over yourself and your condition. You learn how to choose your activity to fit in with your needs. You know when to do less

Table 6.1 **If Exercise Problems Occur**

Problem	Advice
Irregular or rapid heartbeat. Pain, tightness or pressure in the chest, jaw, arms, or neck. Shortness of breath lasting past the exercise period.	Stop exercising. Talk with your doctor right away. Don't exercise until you have been cleared by your doctor.
Light-headedness, dizziness, fainting, cold sweat, or confusion.	Lie down with feet up or sit down with head between knees. Seek medical advice immediately.
Shortness of breath or calf pain from circulation or breathing problems.	Warm up by going slowly at first. Take short rests to recover and keep going. Discuss these Issues with your doctor
Excessive tiredness after exercise, especially if you are still tired the next day.	Exercise less hard next time. If tiredness persists, check with your doctor.

and when to do more. You know that a change in symptoms or a period of inactivity is usually only temporary and doesn't have to feel like a disaster. You know you have the tools to get back on track. Give yourself a chance to succeed. What follows in Chapters 7 and 8 will give you more information to help you get started on your exercise plan.

Suggested Further Reading

Dahm, D. and Smith, J., eds. *Mayo Clinic Fitness for Everybody*. Rochester, Minn.: Mayo Clinic Health Information, 2005.

Daley, D. *Exercises to Improve your Health.* London: CICO Books, 2011.

Dagleish, J. *Health and Fitness Handbook.* London: Longman, 2001.

Other Resources

Physical activity guidelines: Nearly every individual patient organisation has guidelines for exercising. So go to their websites for information or publications on specific exercise for your condition. Here are just a few examples:

☐ *Arthritis Care* has specific information on exercise. www.arthritiscare.org.uk.

☐ *Epilepsy Society* contains information on exercise for those diagnosed with epilepsy. www.epilepsy.society.org.uk.

☐   *MS Society* has information for those diagnosed with Multiple sclerosis and a free exercise DVD. www.mssociety.org.uk.

☐   *Parkinson's Society* has information for those diagnosed with Parkinson's and a free exercise DVD called *The Keep Moving Parkinson's Exercise Programme.* www.parkinsons.org.uk.

NHS: There is a NHS *life change* initiative operating across the UK, to help us live a healthier lifestyle focusing on exercise and nutrition:

☐   This is the website for *England.* www.nhs.uk/change4life.

☐   This is the website for *Wales.* www.change4lifewales.org.uk.

☐   This is the website for *Scotland.* www.takelifeon.co.uk.

☐   This is the website for *Northern Ireland.* www.getalifegetactive.com.

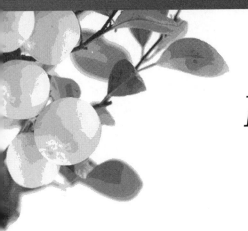

CHAPTER 7

Exercising for Flexibility, Strength, and Balance: Making Life Easier

You CAN USE THE EXERCISES IN THIS CHAPTER in several ways: to get ready for aerobic exercise; to improve your flexibility, strength, and balance; to stretch and strengthen your back and chest for better posture and breathing; and to warm up for or cool down from your aerobic exercise routines.

The exercises are arranged in a logical order starting from the head and neck and running down to the toes. Most of the upper-body exercises may be done either sitting or standing. Exercises done lying down can be performed on the floor or on a firm mattress. We have labelled the exercises that are particularly important for breathing and good posture with the letters VIP, standing for Very Important for Posture. Exercises to improve balance by strengthening and loosening legs and ankles are marked BB, standing for Better Balance. There is also a section of balance exercises that are designed to give you practice in balancing skills.

105

If you see this symbol next to an exercise, it means that you can add weights, such as hand or ankle weights to this exercise. This will make it a harder strengthening exercise. If you can do an exercise easily at least ten times, you can add more weight. Start with one to two pounds (0.5 to 1.0 kg), and add weight gradually as you get stronger and the exercise gets easier for you. You can use home-made weights such as tins, bags of dried beans or packets of rice for lighter weights and plastic milk bottles filled with water or sand for heavier ones. Alternatively, you can buy weights in different sizes.

You can make up a routine of exercises that flow together. Arrange them so you don't have to get up and down too often. Exercise to music if you wish.

The following tips apply to all the exercises in this chapter:

- *Move at a comfortable speed:* Do not bounce or jerk.

- *Stretch just until you feel tension:* This will loosen tight muscles and joints. Hold it for 10 to 30 seconds, and then relax. Remember to breathe in and out.

- *Stop if your body starts to hurt:* Stretching should feel good, not painful.

- *Start with no more than five repetitions of any exercise:* Increase gradually as you make progress.

- *Keep to the same number of exercises on each side:* Always do the same number for your left and right sides.

- *Breathe naturally:* Do not hold your breath. Count out loud to make sure that you are breathing.

- *If you have more symptoms, like pain, that lasts more than two hours after exercising:* do less next time. If an exercise gives you problems, stop and try another exercise. Don't stop exercising.

The following exercises are for both sides of the body and a full range of motion. If you are limited by muscle weakness or joint tightness, go ahead and do the exercise as completely as you can. Remember, the benefit of doing an exercise comes from moving toward a certain position, not from being able to complete the movement perfectly. In some cases, you may find that after a while you can complete the movement and increase your available range of motion. At other times, keep doing it your own way.

Neck Exercises

1. Heads Up (VIP)

This exercise relieves jaw, neck, and upper back tension or pain. It is the start of good posture. You can do it while you are sitting at a desk, sewing, reading, or exercising. Just sit or stand straight and gently slide your chin back. Keep looking forward as your chin moves backward. You'll feel the back of your neck lengthen and straighten. To help, put your finger on your nose and then draw straight back from your finger. Don't worry about a little double chin.

You really do look much better with your neck straight!

Clues for Finding the Correct Position

- Your ear should be over your shoulder, not out in front.
- Your head should be balanced over your neck and trunk, not in the lead.
- Back of neck more vertical, not leaning forward
- Bit of double chin

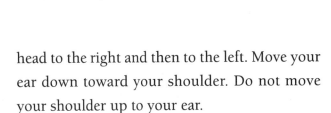

2. Neck Stretch

In the heads-up position, as in Exercise 1 and with your shoulders relaxed, turn slowly to look over your right shoulder. Then turn slowly to look over your left shoulder. Next, tilt your head to the right and then to the left. Move your ear down toward your shoulder. Do not move your shoulder up to your ear.

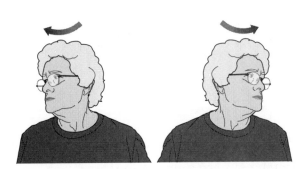

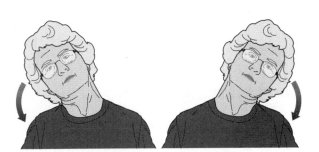

Hand and Wrist Exercises

A good place to do hand exercises is at a table that supports your forearms. Do these exercises after washing up the dishes, after bathing or showering, or when taking a break from handwork. At these times your hands are warmer and more supple.

3. Thumb Walk

Holding your wrist straight, form the letter O by lightly touching your thumb to each fingertip. After each O, straighten and spread your fingers. Use the other hand to help if needed.

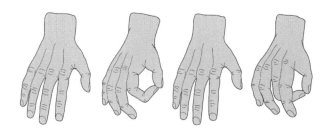

Shoulder Exercises

4. Shoulder Shape Up

In the heads-up position, as in Exercise 1, slowly raise your shoulders to your ears; hold the position, and then drop them. Next, raise the shoulders again to the ears and then begin to slowly rotate them backward by pinching the shoulder blades together; bring your shoulders down and forward to complete a circle. Return to the heads-up position. Finally, reverse the direction of the shoulder circles.

This is a good exercise if the neck stretch, Exercise 2, is difficult for you.

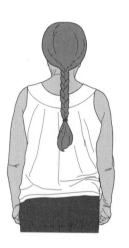 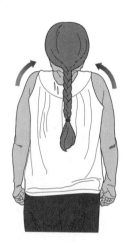 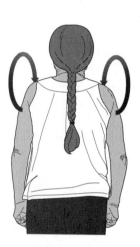

5. Good Morning (VIP)

Start with your hands in gentle fists, palms down, and wrists crossed. Breathe in and stretch out your fingers while you uncross your arms and reach up for the sky. Breathe out as you stretch your arms, and then relax.

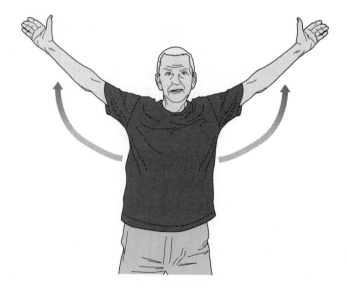

6. Wand Exercise

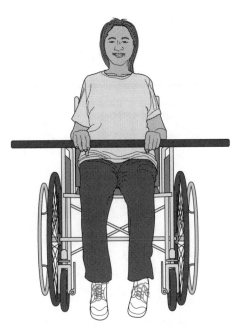

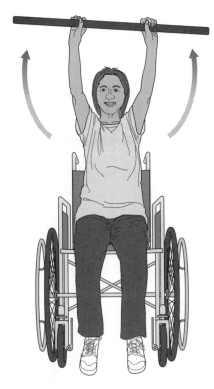

If one or both of your shoulders are tight or weak, you may want to give yourself a helping hand. This shoulder exercise allows the arms to help each other. Exercise 7 will also help this.

Use a long-handled brush, or a mop handle, or cane as your wand. Place one hand toward each end, and raise the wand as high overhead as possible. You might try this in front of a mirror. This exercise can be done standing, sitting, or lying down.

7. Pat and Reach

This double-duty exercise helps to increase the flexibility and strength for both your shoulders. Raise one arm up over your head, and bend your elbow to pat yourself on the back. Move the other arm to your back, bend the elbow, and reach up toward the other hand. Can your fingertips touch? Relax, and switch arm positions. Can you touch on that side?

For most people, one position will work better than the other. Don't worry if you cannot touch. Many people can't do this, but you will get closer as you practise. If you wish, you can use a towel as if you were drying your back; this will provide you with feedback and assist in the motion.

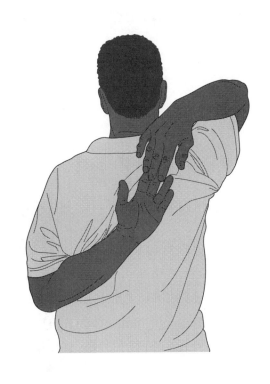

8. Shoulder Blade Pinch (VIP)

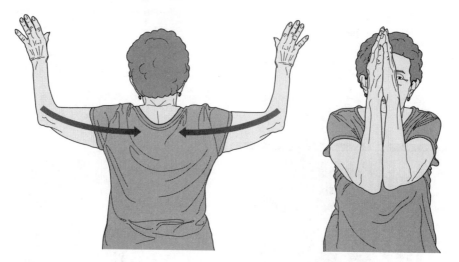

This is a good exercise to strengthen the middle and upper back and to stretch your chest. It can be especially good for individuals with breathing problems. Sit or stand with your head in the heads-up position, as in Exercise 1, with your shoulders relaxed. Raise your arms out to the sides with your elbows bent. Pinch your shoulder blades together by moving your elbows as far back as you can. Hold it briefly, and then slowly move your arms forward together in order to allow your elbows to touch. If this position is uncomfortable, lower your arms or rest your hands on your shoulders.

Back and Abdominal Exercises

9. Knee to Chest Stretch

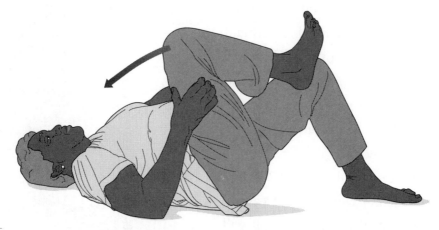

For a low back stretch, lie on the floor with your knees bent and feet flat. Bring one knee toward your chest, using your hands to help. Hold your knee near to your chest for ten seconds, and lower the leg slowly. Repeat this with the other knee. You can also tuck both legs at the same time, if you wish. Relax and enjoy the stretch.

10. Pelvic Tilt (VIP)

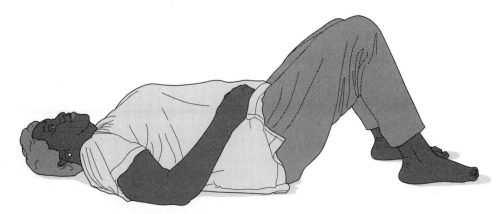

This is an excellent exercise for the low back and can help relieve low back pain. Lie on your back with knees bent and feet flat. Place your hands on your abdomen. Flatten the small of your back against the floor by tightening your stomach muscles and your buttocks. When you do this exercise, you will be tilting your tailbone forward and pulling your stomach back. Think about trying to pull your stomach in enough to zip up a tight pair of trousers. Hold the tilt for five to ten seconds. Then relax. Arch your back slightly. Relax again, and then repeat the pelvic tilt. Keep breathing. Count the seconds out loud. Once you've mastered the pelvic tilt lying down, practise it sitting, standing, and walking.

11. Back Lift (VIP)

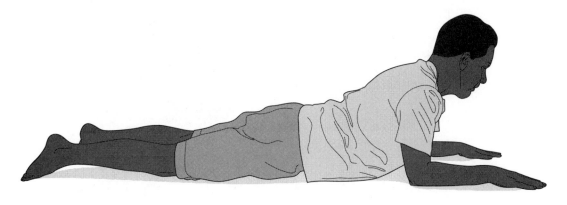

This exercise improves flexibility along your spine and helps you to lift your chest for easier breathing. Lie on your stomach, and rise up on to your forearms. Keep your back relaxed, and keep your stomach and hips down. If this is comfortable, straighten your elbows. Breathe naturally and relax for at least ten seconds. If you have moderate to severe low back pain, do not do this exercise unless it has been specifically prescribed for you.

To strengthen back muscles, lie on your stomach with your arms at your side or overhead. Lift your head, shoulders, and arms. Do not look up. Keep looking down with your chin tucked into that double-chin position. Count out loud as you hold for a count of ten. Then relax. You can also lift your legs off the floor, instead of your head and shoulders.

Note that lifting both ends of your body at once is a fairly strenuous exercise. It may not be helpful for a person with back pain.

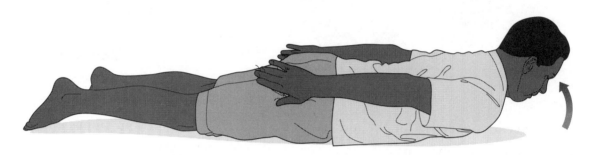

12. Low Back Rock and Roll

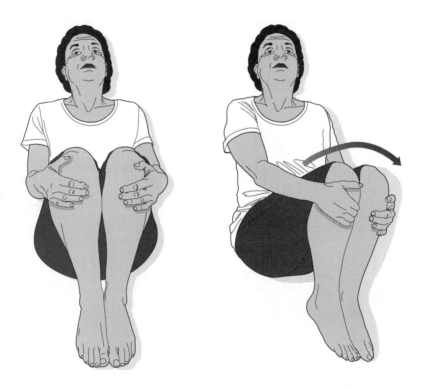

Lie on your back, and pull your knees up to your chest. You can keep holding on to your legs with your hands behind your thighs or you can stretch your arms out to your sides to lie on the floor at shoulder level. Rest in this position for ten seconds, and then gently roll your hips and knees to one side and then the other. Rest and relax as you roll to each side. Keep your upper back and shoulders flat on the ground.

13. Curl-Up (BB)

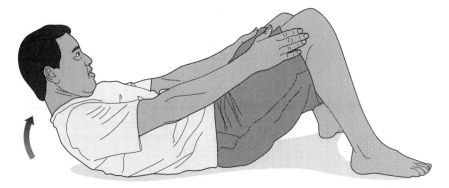

A curl-up, as shown here, is a good way to strengthen stomach muscles. Lie on your back, knees bent, feet flat. Do the pelvic tilt, look back at Exercise 10. Slowly curl up in segments. Tuck your chin as you roll your head up and begin to lift your shoulders off the floor. Slowly uncurl back down, or hold for ten seconds and slowly lower. Breathe out as you curl up, and breathe in as you go back down. Don't hold your breath. If you have neck problems or if your neck hurts when you do this exercise, try the next one instead. Never tuck your feet under a chair or have someone hold your feet!

14. Roll-Out

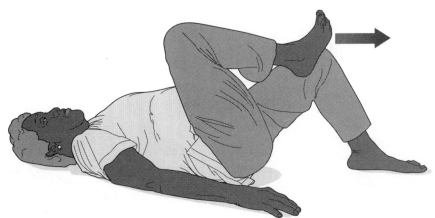

This is another good stomach strengthening exercise, and it's easy on the neck. Use it instead of Exercise 13, the curl-up, or if neck pain is not a problem, do them both.

Lie on your back with your knees bent and feet flat. Now, do Exercise 10, the pelvic tilt, and hold your lower back firmly against the floor.

Slowly and carefully, move one leg away from your chest as you straighten your knee. Move your leg out until you feel your lower back start to arch. When this happens, tuck your knee back to your chest. Reset your pelvic tilt and roll your leg out again. Breathe out as your leg rolls out. Do not hold your breath. Now repeat with the other leg.

You are actually strengthening your abdominal muscles by holding your pelvic tilt against the weight of your leg. As you get stronger, you'll be able to straighten your legs out farther and move both legs together

Hip and Leg Exercises

15. Straight Leg Raises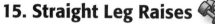

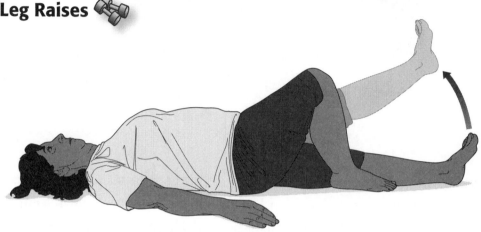

This exercise strengthens the muscles that bend the hip and straighten the knee. Lie on your back, knees bent, feet flat. Straighten one leg. Tighten the muscle on the upper surface of that thigh, and straighten the knee as much as possible. Keeping the knee straight, raise your leg a foot or two (up to 50 cm) off the ground. Do not arch your back. Hold your leg up, and count out loud for 10 seconds. Relax. Repeat with the other leg.

16. Hip Hooray (standing only)

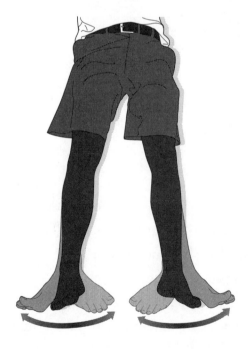

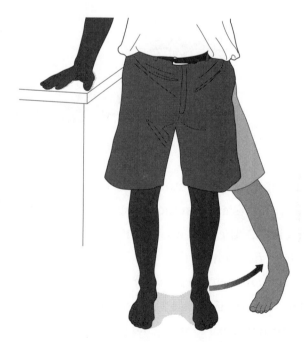

This exercise can be done standing or lying on your back. If you lie down, spread your legs as far apart as possible. Roll your legs and feet outwards like a duck, then inwards so that you become pigeon-toed. Then move your legs back together. If you are standing, move one leg out to your side as far as you can. Lead out with the heel and in with the toes. Hold on to a counter for support. You can make the muscles work harder while you are standing by adding a weight to your ankle.

17. Back Kick (VIP) (BB)

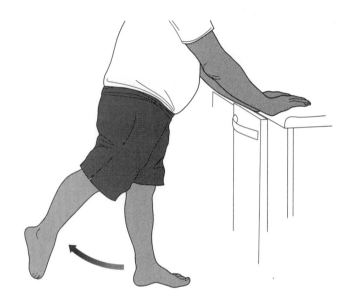

This exercise increases the backward mobility and strength of your hip. Hold on to a surface for support. Move your leg up and back, knee straight. Stand tall, and do not lean forward.

18. Knee Strengthener (BB)

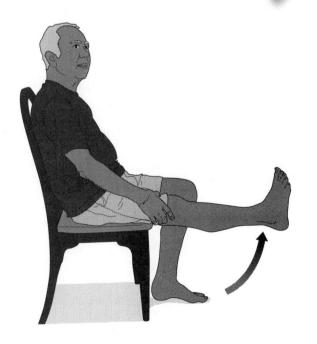

Strong knees are important both for walking and standing comfortably. This exercise strengthens the knee. Sitting in a chair, straighten your knee by tightening up the muscle on the upper surface of your thigh. Place your hand on your thigh and feel the muscle work. If you wish, make circles with your toes. As your knee strengthens, see if you can build up to holding your leg out for 30 seconds. Count out loud. Do not hold your breath.

19. Power Knees

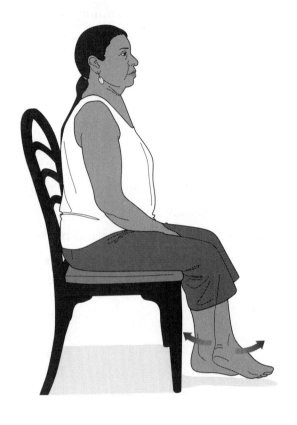

This exercise strengthens the muscles that bend and straighten your knee. Sit in a chair and cross your legs at the ankles. Your legs can be almost straight, or you can bend your knees as much as you like. Try several positions. Push forward with your back leg, and press backward with your front leg. Exert pressure evenly, so that your legs do not move. Hold and count out loud for ten seconds. Relax. Now, switch leg positions. Be sure to keep breathing. Repeat.

20. Ready-Go (BB)

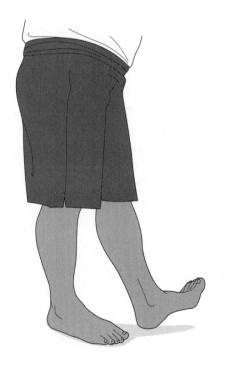

Stand with one leg slightly in front of the other with your heel on the floor, as if ready to take a step forward with the front foot. Now tighten the muscles on the front of your thigh, making your knee firm and straight. Hold to a count of ten. Relax. Now, repeat with the other leg.

21. Hamstring Stretch

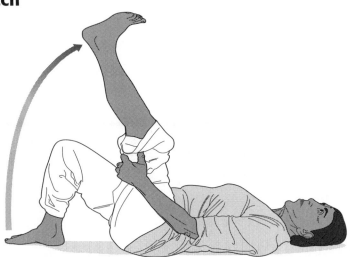

Do the self-test for hamstring tightness. Look on page 124 to see if you need to do this exercise. If you have unstable knees or a back knee do not do this exercise. A back knee is one that curves backward when you stand up.

If you do have tight hamstrings, lie on your back, with your knees bent and feet flat. Grasp one leg at a time behind the thigh. Holding your leg out at arm's length, slowly straighten the knee. Hold the leg as straight as you can as you count to ten. You should feel a slight stretch at the back of your knee and thigh.

Be careful with this exercise. It's easy to overstretch and end up sore.

22. Achilles Stretch (BB)

This exercise helps to maintain flexibility in the Achilles tendon which is the large tendon at the back of your ankle. Good flexibility helps to reduce the risk of injury, calf discomfort, and heel pain. The Achilles stretch is especially helpful for cooling down after walking or cycling and for people who get cramps in the calf muscles. If you have trouble with standing balance or muscle jerk spasticity, you can do a sit-down version of this exercise. Sit in a chair with your feet flat on the floor. Keep your heel on the floor and slowly slide your foot, one foot at a time, backwards to bend your ankle and feel some tension on the back of your lower leg.

Stand at a counter surface or against a wall. Place one foot in front of the other, toes pointing

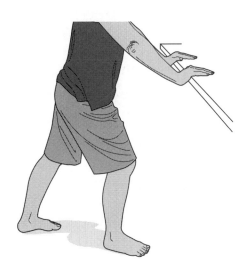

forward and heels on the ground. Lean forward, bend the knee of your forward leg, and keep the back knee straight, heel down. You will feel a good stretch in the calf. Hold the stretch for ten seconds. Do not bounce, just move gently. You can adjust this exercise to reach the other large calf muscle by slightly bending your back knee while you stretch the calf. Can you feel the difference?

It's easy to get sore doing this exercise. If you've worn shoes with high heels for a long time, be particularly careful.

23. Tiptoes (BB)

This exercise will help strengthen your lower leg muscles and make walking, climbing stairs, and standing less tiring. It may also improve your balance. Hold on to a cupboard or counter surface for support and rise up on your tiptoes. Hold for ten seconds. Now, lower slowly. How high you go is not as important as keeping your balance and controlling your ankles. It is easier to do both legs at the same time. If your feet are too sore to do this standing up, start doing it while sitting down. If this exercise makes your ankle jerk, stop doing it and talk to your therapist about other ways you might strengthen these calf muscles.

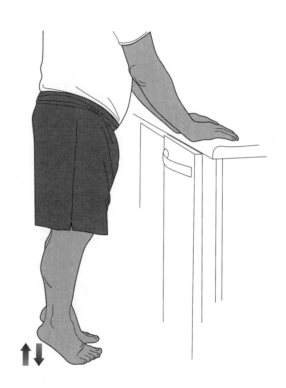

Ankle and Foot Exercises

Do these exercises sitting in a straight-backed chair with bare feet. Have a bath towel and ten marbles next to you. These exercises are aimed at flexibility, strength, and comfort. This is a good time to examine your feet and toes for any signs of circulation or skin problems and to check your nails to see if they need trimming.

24. Towel Grabber

Spread a towel out in front of your chair. Place your feet on the towel, with your heels near the edge closest to you. Keep your heels down and your foot slightly raised. Push the towel back, underneath your feet, by pulling it with your toes. When you have done as much of this as you can, you can reverse the toe motion, and push the towel out again.

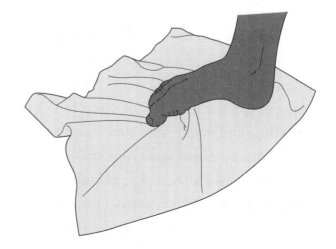

25. Marble Pickup

Do this exercise one foot at a time. Place several marbles on the floor between your feet. Keep your heel down, and pivot your toes toward the marbles. Pick up one marble with your toes, and pivot your foot to drop it as far away as possible from where you picked it up. Repeat this until all the marbles have been moved. Reverse the process and return all the marbles to the starting position. If you find marbles difficult, try other objects, such as jacks, dice, or balls of paper.

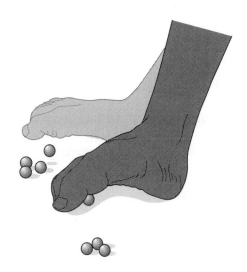

26. Foot Roll

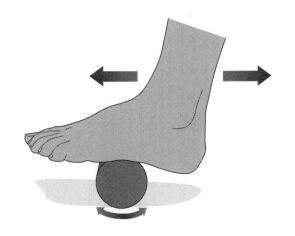

Place a rolling pin, or a similarly shaped stick, under the arch of your foot and roll it back and forth. It feels great and stretches the ligaments in the arch of the foot.

Balance Exercises

The exercises here are designed to let you practise balance activities in a safe and progressive way. The exercises are provided in order of difficulty, so start with the first exercises and work up to the more difficult ones as your strength and balance improve. If you feel that your balance is particularly poor, exercise with someone else close by who can give you a supporting hand if needed. Always practise by a counter surface or stable chair that you can hold on to if necessary. Signs of improving balance are indicated by being able to hold a position for longer, or without extra support. Better balance is also shown when you can do the exercise or hold the position with your eyes closed. There may also be some balance exercise classes in your community to help continue your progress. Tai chi is a wonderful programme to help you work on balance and strength. It is low-impact and gentle on your joints. Age UK offers an exercise guide and DVD that includes other balance exercises, but you can use what we offer here to get started.

27. Beginning Balance

Stand quietly with your feet comfortably apart. Place your hands on your hips, and turn your head and trunk as far to the left as possible.

Then do the same to the right. Repeat this five to ten times. To increase the difficulty, do the same thing with your eyes closed.

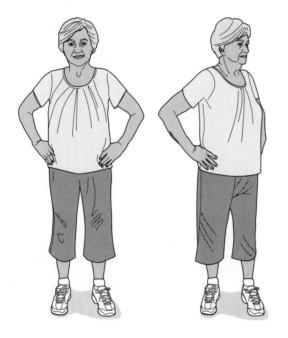
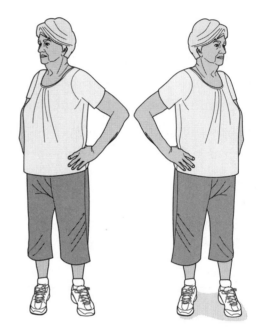

28. Swing and Sway

Using a cupboard or the back of a stable chair for support, do each of the following five to ten times:

1. Rock back on your heels and then go up on your toes.

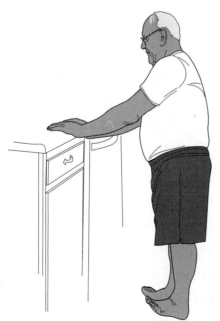
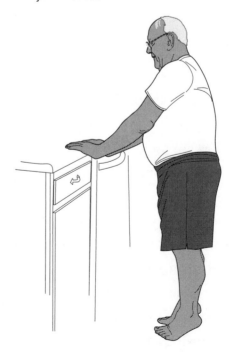

2. Do the box step (like dancing the waltz).

3. March in place, first with eyes open and then with eyes closed.

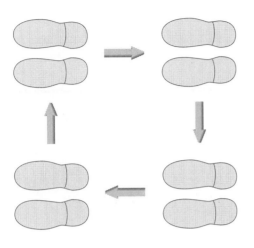

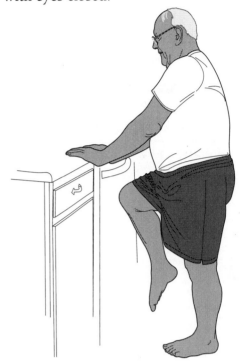

29. Base of Support

Do these exercises with standby assistance or standing close to a cupboard for support. The purpose is to help you improve your balance by going from a larger to a smaller base of support. Aim on being able to hold each position for ten seconds. When you can do that with your eyes open, then practise it with your eyes closed. Look at the numbered illustration below.

1. Stand with feet together.

2. Stand with one foot out in front and the other back.

3. Stand heel to toe.

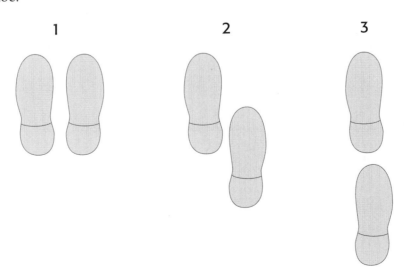

30. Toe Walk

The purpose of this exercise is to increase ankle strength and to give you practice balancing on a small base of support while moving. Stay close to a counter or support. Rise up on your toes and walk up and back along the counter. Once you are comfortable walking on your toes without support and with your eyes open, try it with your eyes closed.

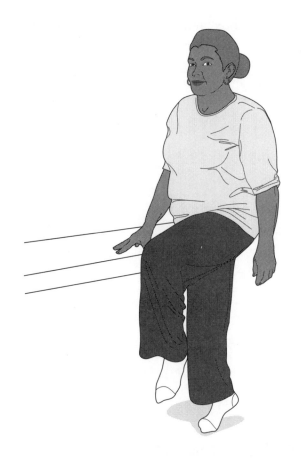

31. Heel Walk

This exercise is designed to increase your lower leg strength and give you practice moving on a small base of support. Stay close to a counter surface or cupboard for support. Raise your toes and forefoot and walk up and back along the counter on your heels. Once you are comfortable walking on your heels without support and with your eyes open, try it with your eyes shut.

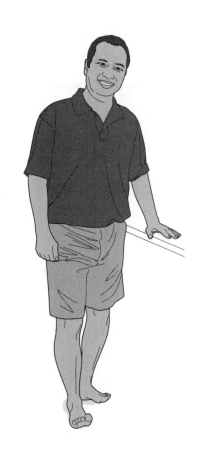

32. One-Legged Stand

Holding on to a counter surface or chair, lift one foot completely off the ground. Once you are balanced, lift your hand. The goal is to hold this position for ten seconds. Once you can do this without holding on, practise it with your eyes closed. Now, repeat for the other leg.

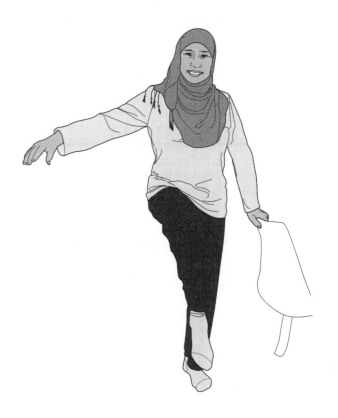

The Whole Body

33. The Stretcher

This exercise is a whole-body stretch and is to be done lying on your back. Start the motion at your ankles as explained in what follows, or reverse the process if you want to start with your arms first.

1. Point your toes, and then pull your toes toward your nose. Then relax.

2. Bend your knees first and then flatten your knees and let them relax.

3. Arch your back. Do Exercise 10, the pelvic tilt. Then relax.

4. Breathe in and stretch your arms above your head. Now breathe out, lower your arms and relax.

5. Stretch your right arm above your head, and then stretch your left leg by pushing away with your heel. Hold for a count of ten. Now, switch to the other side and repeat.

Using Self-Tests to Check Progress

Whatever your goals, we all need to see that our efforts make a difference. Because an exercise programme produces gradual change, it is often hard to tell if the programme is working and to recognise improvement. So, you can choose several of these flexibility and strength tests to measure your own progress. Not everyone will be able to do all the tests. Just choose those that work best for you. Perform each test before you start your exercise programme, and record the results. After every four weeks, do the tests again and check for any improvement.

Self Test 1: Arm Flexibility

Do Exercise 7, Pat and Reach, for both sides of the body. Ask someone to measure the distance between your fingertips. *The Goal:* A smaller distance between your fingertips.

Self Test 2: Shoulder Flexibility

Stand facing a wall with your toes touching it. For one arm at a time, reach up the wall in front of you. Hold a pencil, or have someone mark how far you reached. Also do this sideways, standing about three inches, or eight centimetres away from the wall. *The Goal:* To reach higher.

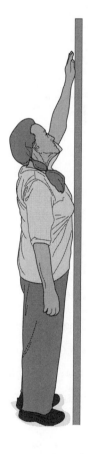 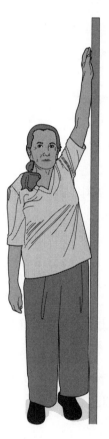

Self Test 3: Hamstring Flexibility

Do the Hamstring Stretch, Exercise 21, one leg at a time. Keep your thigh, or upper leg, perpendicular to your body. How much does your knee bend? How tight does the back of your leg feel? *The Goal:* A straighter knee and less tension in the back of the leg.

Self Test 4: Ankle Flexibility

Sit in a chair with your bare feet flat on the floor and your knees bent at a 90-degree angle. Keep your heels on the floor. Raise your toes and the front of your foot. Ask someone to measure the distance between the ball of your foot and the floor. *The Goal:* A distance of one to two inches, or three to five centimetres, between your foot and the floor.

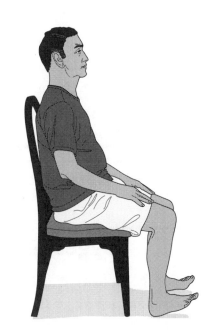

Self Test 5: Abdominal Strength

Do Exercise 13, the Curl-Up. Count how many repetitions you can do before you get too tired to do more, or count how many you can do in one minute. *The Goal:* To do more repetitions.

Self Test 6: Ankle Strength

This test has two parts. Stand at a table or counter surface for support.

First, do Exercise 23, Tiptoes, as quickly and as often as you can. How many can you do before you tire?

Second, stand with your feet flat. Put most of your weight on one foot, and quickly tap the floor with the front part of your other foot. How many taps can you do before you tire? *The Goal:* A total of ten to 15 repetitions of each movement.

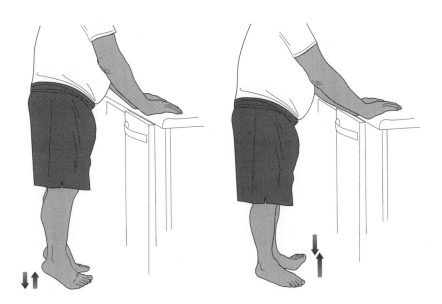

Self Test 7: Balance

Do Exercise 31, the Heel Walk, and record how long you can stand on each foot without needing to reach for support. Record your times with eyes open and eyes closed. When you are ready to test your balance again, see if you can stand without support for longer, or if you can balance with your eyes closed. *The Goal:* To be able to balance on one foot with your eyes open and closed for 30 or more seconds each way.

Suggested Further Reading

Durstine, J. M., Painter, G., Roberts, P. and Roberts, S. *Exercise Management for Persons with Chronic Disease,* 3rd Edition. American College of Sports Medicine. Champaign, Il.: Human Kinetics, 2009

Hooker, S. *Armchair Exercise for Fitness Phobics.* Bloomington, Ind.: Trafford Publishing, 2007. This is written in a very amusing way by a physiotherapist.

Jerome, J. *The Pleasures of Staying Supple.* London: Souvenir Press, 2000

Other Resources

☐ *Age UK*: Preventing Falls: Strength and Balancing Exercises for Healthy Ageing. www.ageuk.org.uk.

☐ American Lung Association: Asthma: Don't Let Exercise-Induced Asthma Keep You Side-lined. www.lungusa.org/about-us/our-impact/top-stories/active-exercise-asthma.html.

☐ Exercise: Arthritis Self-Management (two-CD Audio). Bull Publishing, 2006.

☐ Flexibility, strength, and balance DVDs: Sit and Be Fit. www.sitandbefit.org.

☐ Keep Fit Association. Tel: 01403 266000. www.keepfit.org.uk.

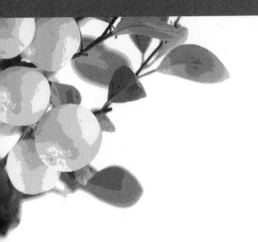

CHAPTER 8

Exercising for Endurance: Aerobic Activities

W HEN THINKING ABOUT AEROBIC (ENDURANCE) EXERCISE, many people are confused about what and how much to do. We described the guidelines for aerobic, flexibility, and strengthening exercises in Chapter 6. Going further and working out your very own programme may be a challenge. The guidelines recommend that adults exercise at a moderate intensity for at least 150 minutes spread over the week. There are many ways to work aerobic activities into your day. In this chapter you will learn about *exercise effort*, various aerobic activities, and how to put together a programme that works for you. The most important thing is that some activity is always better than none. If you start off doing what is comfortable and increase your efforts gradually, it is likely that you will build a healthy, lifelong habit. You will learn how to stay active and how to get back to activity, even when changes in your condition may slow you down for a time. Generally, it is better to begin your programme by under-doing rather than over-doing the level of activity.

You can adjust your *exercise effort* and work toward your goal by using the three basic building blocks: *frequency*, *time*, and *intensity*.

■ *Frequency is how often you exercise:* Most guidelines suggest doing at least some exercise most days of the week. Three to five times a week is a good choice for moderate-intensity aerobic exercise. Taking every other day off gives your body a chance to rest and recover.

■ *Time is the length of each exercise period:* According to the guidelines, it is best if you can exercise at least ten minutes at a time. You can add up ten-minute exercise periods all week to work toward your 150 minutes. For example, three ten-minute walks a day for five days gets you to 150 minutes for the week. If ten minutes is too much at first, start with what you *can* do and work toward it as a target.

■ *Intensity is your exercise effort:* This is how hard you are working. Aerobic exercise is safe and effective at a moderate intensity. When you exercise at this intensity, you'll feel warm, you'll breathe more deeply and faster than usual. Your heart will beat faster than normal, as well. Maybe you will feel that you can continue for a little longer. This is because exercise intensity is relative to your fitness. For an athlete, running a mile in ten minutes is probably low-intensity exercise. For a person who hasn't exercised in a long time, a brisk ten-minute walk may be moderate to high intensity. And indeed, for someone with severe physical limitations, a slow walk may be high intensity. The trick, of course, is to work out what is moderate intensity for you. There are several easy ways to do this.

Use the Talk Test

When exercising, talk to another person, or to yourself, or recite poems out loud. Moderate-intensity exercise allows you to speak comfortably. If you can't carry on a conversation because you are breathing too hard or are short of breath, you're working at a high intensity. If so, slow down to a more moderate level. The *talk test* is an easy and quick way to recognise your effort and regulate intensity. If you have lung disease, the talk test might not be appropriate for you. If that is the case, try using the *perceived-exertion scale*.

Use the Perceived Exertion Scale

Another way to monitor intensity is to rate how hard you're working on a *scale of perceived exertion*. There are two scales: 0 to 10 and 6 to 20. On the 0-to-10 scale, 0 is at the low end of the scale, lying down, or doing no work at all, and 10, by contrast, is equivalent to working as hard as possible, so hard, in fact, that you can't do it for more than a few seconds. A good level for moderate aerobic exercise on the 0-to-10 scale is between 4 and 5.

On the 6-to-20 scale, 6 is considered to be the same as sitting quietly and 20 involves working as hard as possible. On the 6-to-20 scale, moderate intensity is between 11 and 14. Use whichever scale you like better.

Your Heart Rate

Checking your heart rate is another way to measure exercise intensity. If you're taking heart-regulating medicine (such as the beta blocker *propranderol*), this has the effect of slowing down your heart rate. So, in this case the *British Heart Foundation* suggests that it might be better for you to use the *Talk Test* rather than calculating your heart rate. The faster your heart beats, the harder you're working. However, you should note that your heart also beats fast when you are frightened or nervous.

In the context of exercise, what we are talking about here is how your heart responds to physical activity. Endurance exercise at moderate intensity raises your heart rate to a range between 50% and 70% of your *safe maximum heart rate*. The safe maximum heart rate declines with age, so your safe exercise heart rate is lower when you get older. You can follow the general guidelines in Figure 8.1 or you can calculate your own exercise heart rate using the formula provided. Either way, you need to know how to take your pulse.

Take your pulse by placing the tips of your index and middle fingers at your wrist below the base of your thumb. Move your fingers around, but don't push them down, until you feel the pulsations of blood pumping with each heartbeat. Count how many beats you feel in

15 seconds, and then multiply this number by four. Start by taking your pulse whenever you think of it, and you'll soon learn the difference between your resting and exercise heart rates. Most people have a resting heart rate between 60 and 100 beats per minute.

Figure 8.1: **Calculating your personal exercise heart rate**

Here's how to calculate your personal exercise heart rate range

1. Subtract your age from 220:

Example (Age 60 years old): 220 − 60 = 160

You: 220 − _____ = _____

2. Multiply the figure for Step 1 by 0.50: This gives you the ***low end*** of your exercise heart rate range.

Example: 160 × 0.50 = 80

You: _____ × 0.50 = _____

3. Multiply your answer in step 1 by 0.7: This gives you the ***upper end*** of your moderate intensity range.

Example: 160 × 0.7 = 112

You: _____ × 0.7 = _____

The exercise heart rate range for moderate intensity in our example is from 80 to 112 beats per minute. What is yours?

You only need to count your pulse for 15 seconds, not a whole minute. To find your 15-second pulse rate for exercise, simply divide both the lower-end and upper-end numbers by four. The person in our example should be able to count between 20, which is *80 divided by 4* and 28, which is *112 divided by 4*, beats in 15 seconds when exercising.

The most important reason for knowing your exercise heart rate range is so that you can learn not to exercise too vigorously. After you've done your warm-up and five minutes of endurance exercise, take your pulse. If it's higher than the upper rate, don't panic. Just slow down a bit. You don't need to work so hard.

Note that these calculations for predicted heart rate are based on averages. This means that your personal maximum may be higher or lower than 220 minus your age.

As mentioned previously if you are taking medicine that regulates your heart rate, or have trouble feeling your pulse, or think that keeping track of your heart rate is a bother, then try the other methods. You can easily use the *talk test* or the *perceived-exertion scale* to monitor your exercise intensity. The *Department of Health Guidelines* suggest that the physical guidelines for older adults which have been written for healthy adults should be used cautiously. They suggest including a statement to recognise that physical activity guidelines written for healthy adults should be *tailored* for individuals based on their needs and abilities; this is particularly so for those with disabilities or any special health issues. This is something you should discuss with your doctor or hospital consultant.

Be FIT

You can design your own programme by using the *FIT* approach. FIT covers the three elements of your exercise programme:

F = *Frequency*; how often you exercise.

I = *Intensity*; how hard you work.

T = *Time*; and how long you exercise each day.

The guidelines recommend that you exercise at moderate intensity for a minimum of 150 minutes a week.

You can build your own exercise programme by varying the frequency, time, and activities as you decide. We are recommending *moderate-intensity exercise*, so that you are able to start slowly and increase frequency and time as you work toward, or even beyond, 150 minutes each week. You can use different combinations of exercises. The following are three programmes of moderate intensity that will let you reach 150 minutes each week:

1. A ten-minute walk at moderate intensity three times a day, five days a week.

2. A 20-minute bike ride at moderate intensity, which means mostly on level ground,

three days a week and a 30-minute walk, three days a week.

3. A 30-minute aerobic dance class at moderate intensity twice a week and three ten-minute walks, three days a week.

If you are just starting out, you could begin more cautiously like this:

■ Take a five-minute walk around the house three times a day, six days a week.
Total = 90 minutes.

■ Take a water aerobics class for 40 minutes twice a week and two ten-minute walks on two other days a week.
Total = 120 minutes.

■ Take a low-impact 50 minute aerobic class once a week, mow the lawn for 30 minutes, and take two 20-minute walks.
Total = 120 minutes.

An easy way to remember the guideline goal for minimum physical activity is that you should accumulate 30 minutes of moderate physical activity on most days of the week. This could

Be FIT

Here's a quick way to remember the three building blocks of your exercise programme:

F = Frequency (how often)

I = Intensity (how hard)

T = Time (how long)

be a combination of walking, stationary cycling, dancing, swimming, or household chores that require moderate-intensity activity.

It is important to remember that 150 minutes is your goal, but is not necessarily your starting point.

So, if you begin exercising just two minutes at a time, you are likely to be able to reach the recommended ten minutes three times a day. Almost everyone can reach these guideline goals and achieve important health benefits. If you have a set-back and stop exercising for a period, just start again, exercising for less time and less vigorously than when you stopped. It takes some time to work back up again; be patient with yourself.

Warming Up and Cooling Down

If you are going to exercise at moderate intensity, it is important to warm up first and cool down afterwards.

Warming Up

Don't exercise cold. Before building to moderate intensity, you must prepare your body to do more strenuous work. This means doing at least five minutes of low-intensity activity to allow your muscles, heart, lungs, and circulation to

gradually increase their work. For example, if you are going for a brisk walk, warm up with five minutes of slow walking. Or, if you are riding a stationary bike, warm up on the bike with five minutes of easy pedalling. In an aerobic exercise class, you will warm up with a gentle routine before getting into more vigorous activity. Warming up reduces the risk of injuries, soreness, and an irregular heartbeat.

Cooling Down

A cool-down period after moderate-intensity exercise helps your body return to its normal resting state. So, repeating the five-minute warm-up activity or taking a slow walk, will help your muscles to gradually relax and your heart and breathing to slow down again. Gentle flexibility exercises during the cool-down can be relaxing, and gentle stretching following exercise will help to reduce muscle soreness and stiffness.

Aerobic (Endurance) Exercises

We will examine a few common *low-impact* aerobic exercises. All of these exercises can condition your heart and lungs, strengthen your muscles, relieve tension, and help you to manage your weight. Most of these exercises can also strengthen your bones. However, swimming and aqua-aerobics are the main exceptions to this.

Walking

Walking is easy, inexpensive, and safe, and it can be done almost anywhere. You can also walk by yourself or with others. Walking is safer than jogging or running and puts less stress on the body. It's an especially good choice if you have been sedentary for some time or have joint or balance problems.

If you already walk to do shopping, household chores or visit friends, then you can walk for exercise, too. Using a cane, walking stick or walker need not stop you from getting into a walking routine. However, if you are a wheelchair user or use crutches, or you experience more than mild discomfort when you walk a short distance, then you should consider some other type of aerobic exercise. Ask your doctor or physiotherapist for help.

Be cautious during the first two weeks of walking. If you haven't been doing much for some time, five or ten minutes may be enough. You can alternate brisk walks and slow walks to build up your time. Each week, increase the brisk walking interval by no more than five minutes until you are up to 20 or 30 minutes. Remember that your goal is to walk most days of the week, at moderate intensity, and to get up to at least ten minutes each time. Before starting, read our suggested *walking tips*, which follow.

Four walking tips

1. *Choose your ground:* Walk on a flat, level surface. Walking on hills, or uneven ground, soft earth, sand, or gravel is hard work and can often lead to hip, knee, or foot pain. Fitness trails, shopping centres, parks, streets with pavements, and quiet neighbourhoods are good places.

2. *Always warm up and cool down with a stroll:* Walk slowly for five minutes to prepare your circulation and muscles for a brisker walk. Again, you should finish up with the same slow walk to let your body calm down gradually. Experienced walkers know they

can avoid shin and foot discomfort if they begin and end with a stroll.

3. *Set your own pace:* It takes practice to find the right walking speed. To find your personal speed, start walking slowly for a few minutes and then increase your speed to a pace that is slightly faster than normal for you. After five minutes, check your exercise intensity by using a *perceived-exertion* or *talk test.* If you are working too hard or feel out of breath, slow down. If you are below your desired intensity, then try walking a little faster. Walk another five minutes and check your intensity again. If you are still below your target intensity, keep on walking at a comfortable speed and simply check your intensity in the middle, and at the end, of each walk.

4. *Increase your arm work:* You can use your arms to raise your heart rate into the target exercise range. However you should note that many people with lung disease may want to avoid arm exercises, as they can cause more shortness of breath than other exercises. Bend your elbows a bit, and swing your arms more vigorously. You might carry a 1 or 2 pound weight in each hand. You can purchase hand weights for walking, but you can easily hold a tin of food in each hand, or put sand, dried beans, or pennies in two small plastic bottles or socks. The extra work you do with your arms increases your intensity of exercise without forcing you to walk faster than you will find comfortable.

Suitable Shoes

Wear shoes of the correct length and width with shock-absorbing soles and insoles. Make sure particularly that they're roomy enough in the toe area. It's best if there is a thumb-width space between the end of your longest toe and the end of the shoe. You shouldn't feel pressure on the sides or tops of your toes. The heel counter, which is a piece of leather forming the back of a shoe, should also hold your heel firmly when you walk.

Wear shoes with a continuous composite sole. Be sure your shoes are in good repair. Shoes with laces or Velcro allow you to adjust width as needed and will give you more support than slip-ons. If you have problems tying laces, consider Velcro closers or elastic shoelaces. Shoes with leather soles and a separate heel don't absorb shock as well as sports and casual shoes. Good shoes do not need to be expensive; any shoes that meet the criteria we have just described will serve your purpose.

Many people prefer shoes with removable insoles that can be exchanged for more shock-absorbing ones. You can find insoles in some sport shops and in shoe shops. When you shop for insoles, take your walking shoes with you. Try on the shoe with the insole inserted to make sure there's still enough room for your foot to be comfortable. Insoles come in different sizes and can be trimmed with scissors for a custom fit. If your toes take up extra room, try the *three-quarter insoles* that stop just short of your toes. If you have prescribed inserts in your shoes already, ask your doctor about insoles.

Avoid purchasing shoes that are too heavy or that have very thick, rubbery, or sticky soles. These may create a tripping hazard for you.

Dealing with Possible problems

If you have pain around your shins when you walk, it may be because you are not spending enough time warming up. Try *Exercises 24–26* in Chapter 7, before you start your programme. Start your walk at a slow pace for at least five minutes. Keep your feet and toes relaxed.

Sore knees are another common problem. Certainly, fast walking puts more stress on knee joints. To slow your speed and keep your heart rate up, try to do more work with your arms, as described earlier. Do *Exercises 18 and 20* in Chapter 7, during your warm-up. These are the *knee strengthener* and *ready-go exercises*.

Cramps in your calf and pain in the heel can be reduced by starting with the *Achilles stretch*, *Exercise 22* in Chapter 7. A slow walk to warm up is also helpful. If you have circulation problems in your legs and get cramps or some pain in your calves while walking, then try to alternate between comfortably brisk and slow walking. Slow down and give your circulation a chance to catch up before the pain is so intense that you *have* to stop. As you will see, such exercises may help you gradually to walk further with less cramping or pain. If this doesn't help, then you should discuss the problem with your doctor.

Maintain a good posture. Remember the *heads-up position* we described in Chapter 7? Keep your shoulders relaxed to help reduce neck and upper back discomfort.

Swimming

Swimming is another good aerobic exercise. The buoyancy of the water lets you move your joints through their full range of motion, so that you can strengthen your muscles and cardiovascular system with less stress than on dry land. Because swimming involves the arms, it can lead to excessive shortness of breath. This is especially true for people with lung disease. However, for people with asthma, swimming may be a preferred exercise, as the moisture helps to reduce shortness of breath. People with heart disease who have severely irregular heartbeats and have had an *implantable defibrillator (ICD)*, should avoid swimming. For most people with a chronic condition, however, swimming is excellent exercise. It uses the whole body. If you haven't been swimming for a period, consider a refresher course.

To make swimming an aerobic exercise, you will eventually need to swim continuously for ten minutes. Try different strokes, changing your stroke after each lap or two. This lets you exercise all your joints and muscles without over-tiring any one area.

Note that although swimming is an excellent aerobic exercise, it does not improve balance, nor does it provide essential weight-bearing exercise for healthy bones. Incorporating swimming as one part of your overall fitness regime is recommended.

Swimming tips

- The breast stroke and crawl normally require a lot of neck motion and may be uncomfortable. One way of solving this problem is to use a mask and snorkel so that you can breathe without twisting your neck. However not all swimming pools will allow you to use them.

- Chlorine can be irritating to the eyes. Consider a good pair of goggles. You can even have swim goggles made in your glasses prescription.

- A hot shower, or soak in a hot bath, after your workout helps reduce stiffness and muscle soreness. Remember not to work too hard or get too tired. If you're sore for more than two hours, go easier next time.

- Always swim where there are qualified lifeguards or with a friend. Never swim alone.

Aquacising

If you don't like to swim or feel uncomfortable learning strokes, you can walk laps in the pool or join the millions who are *aquacising,* or exercising in the water.

Aquacise is comfortable, fun, and effective as a flexibility, strengthening, and aerobic activity. The buoyancy of the water takes weight off your hips, knees, feet, and back. Because of this, exercise in water is generally better tolerated than walking by people who have pain in these areas. Exercising in a pool also allows you a degree of privacy in doing your own routine. No one can see you much below shoulder level.

Getting started

Joining a water exercise class with a good instructor is an excellent way to get started. Many local authority swimming baths have classes for those with a disability and for the over 60's. Your local library will also be able to help you find a suitable class in your area.

If you have access to a pool and want to exercise on your own, there are many water exercise books available that can guide you. Water temperature is always a concern when people talk about water exercise. Most public swimming baths retain the pool temperature of 84°F or 29–30°C. But for disabled swimming classes they may sometimes adopt a higher temperature of 32°C, with the surrounding air temperature in the same range. Except in warm climates, this will mean a heated pool. If you are just starting to aquacise, find a pool with the water around this higher temperature. If you can exercise more vigorously and aren't too sensitive to the cold, you can probably aquacise in cooler water. Many pools where people swim laps are about 80–83°F or 27–28°C. It feels quite cool when you first get in, but starting off with water walking, jogging, or another whole-body exercise will help you to warm up quickly.

The deeper the water you stand in, the less stress there is on joints; however, water above the chest can make it hard to keep your balance. You can let the water cover more of your body just by spreading your legs or bending your knees a bit.

Aquacising tips

- If you need to wear something on your feet to protect them from rough pool floors and provide traction in the pool and at poolside, check with your pool that these are permitted. Some footgear is especially designed to wear in the water, and some of these also have Velcro straps to make them easier to put on. Beach shoes with rubber soles and mesh tops also work well.

- If you are sensitive to the cold or have *Raynaud's syndrome*, wear a pair of disposable latex surgical gloves. Boxes of gloves are available at most pharmacies. The water trapped and warmed inside the glove seems to insulate your hand. In addition, if your body gets cold in the water, wear a T-shirt or full-leg pair of Lycra exercise tights for warmth. Again, if using public swimming pools check that these are allowed.

- Wearing a flotation belt, or a life vest adds extra buoyancy and comfort by taking weight off your hips, knees, and feet.

- As on land, moving slower makes your exercise easier. However, another way to regulate the exercise intensity is to change how much water you push when you move. For example, when you move your arms back and forth in front of you under water, it becomes hard work if you hold your palms facing each other and clap. It is easier if you turn your palms down and slice your arms back and forth with only the narrow edge of your hands pushing against the water.

- Be aware that additional buoyancy allows for greater joint motion than you are probably used to, especially if you are exercising in a warm pool. Start slowly and do not over-extend your time in the pool because it feels good, wait until you discover how your body will react the next day.

- If you have asthma, exercising in water can help you to avoid making the symptoms worse. This is probably due to the beneficial effect of water vapour on the lungs. Remember though, that for many people with lung disease, exercises involving the arms can cause more shortness of breath than leg exercises. You may therefore want to focus most of your exercises on your legs.

- If you have had a stroke or have another condition that may affect your strength and balance, make sure that you have someone to help you in and out of the pool. Find a position close to the wall or stay close to a friend who can lend a hand if needed. This will add to your safety and security. Ask the instructor to help you design the best exercise programme, and to select the equipment, and facilities which are best suited to your specific needs.

Stationary Bicycling

Stationary bicycles offer the fitness benefits of bicycling without any outdoor hazards. They're better for people who don't have the flexibility, strength, or balance to be comfortable pedalling and steering on the road. Even people with paralysis of one leg or arm can sometimes exercise on stationary bicycles. Indeed, there are special attachments which can allow for their paralysed limbs. The indoor use of stationary bicycles may also be preferable to outdoor cycling for people who live in a cold or hilly area.

The stationary bicycle is a particularly good alternative to other forms of exercise. It doesn't put excess strain on your hips, knees, and feet; you can easily adjust how hard you work; and the weather doesn't matter. So, why not use the cycle on those days when you don't want to walk or do more vigorous exercise, or when you can't exercise outside?

Making it interesting

The most common complaint about riding a stationary bicycle is that it's boring. But, if you pedal as you watch television, or read, or listen to music, you can become fit without becoming bored. One woman keeps herself interested by mapping out tours of places she would like to visit. She charts her progress on a map as she rolls off the miles. Other people set their cycle time for the half hour of soap opera or news that they watch every day. There are also DVDs of exotic bike tours that put you in the rider's position. Book racks that you can clip onto the handlebars can also make reading easier and riding more interesting.

Riding tips

■ Stationary bicycling uses different muscles from those used in walking. Consequently, until your leg muscles get used to pedalling, you may be able to ride for only a few minutes. Start off with no resistance. Then, increase the resistance slightly as your riding gets easier. Increasing the resistance has the same effect as cycling up hills. If you use too much resistance, your knees will begin to hurt, and you'll have to stop. Later on, you will earn the benefit of greater endurance!

■ Pedal at a comfortable speed. For most people, 50 to 70 revolutions per minute is a good place to start. Some cycles tell you the rpm rate, or you can simply count the number of times your right foot reaches its lowest point in a minute. As you get used to cycling, you can increase your speed. However, faster is not necessarily better. Listening to music at the right tempo makes it easier to pedal at a consistent speed. Experience will tell you the best combination of speed and resistance.

■ Set your goal at 20 to 30 minutes of pedalling at a comfortable speed. Build up your time by alternating intervals of brisk pedalling with periods of less exertion. Use your heart rate or the perceived exertion or the talk test to make sure you aren't working too hard. If you're alone, then reciting poems or telling a story to yourself as you pedal, can make the time pass more quickly. If you get out of breath, slow down.

Stationary Bicycle Checklist

■ Check that the bicycle is steady when you get on and off.

■ Check that the resistance is easy to set and can be set to zero.

■ Check that the seat is comfortable and can be adjusted for full knee extension when the pedal is at its lowest point.

■ Check that the large pedals and loose pedal straps will allow your feet to move slightly while you pedal.

■ Check that there is ample clearance from the frame for your knees and ankles.

■ Check that the handlebars allow good posture and a comfortable arm position.

- Keep a record of your bike trips and the times and distances you cover. You'll be amazed at how much you can do.

- On bad days, maintain your exercise habit by pedalling with no resistance, at a lower rpm, or cycle for a shorter period of time.

Other Exercise Equipment

If you have trouble getting on or off a stationary bicycle, or don't have room for one where you live, then you might try a restorator or arm crank. Ask your physiotherapist or doctor, or phone a medical supply shop for more information on these useful exercise machines.

A restorator is a small piece of equipment with foot pedals that can be attached to the foot of your bed or placed on the floor in front of a chair. It allows you to exercise by pedalling. Resistance can be varied, and placement of the restorator lets you adjust for your leg length and knee bend. A restorator can be a good alternative to a stationary bicycle for people who have problems with balance, weakness, or paralysis. People with other chronic conditions, such as lung disease, may also find the restorator to be an enjoyable way to start an exercise programme.

Arm cranks, sometimes called arm ergometers, are bicycles for the arms. They are mounted on a table. People who are unable to use their legs for active exercise can improve their cardiovascular fitness and upper body strength by using the arm crank. It's important to work closely with a physiotherapist to set up your programme, because using only your arms for endurance exercise, rather than your bigger leg muscles, will require a different approach to monitoring your exercise intensity. As mentioned previously, many people with lung disease may find arm exercises to be less enjoyable than leg exercises because they may experience shortness of breath.

There are many other types of exercise equipment available. These include treadmills, self-powered and motor-driven *rowing machines*, *cross-country skiing machines*, *mini-trampolines*, and *stair-climbing and elliptical machines*. The latter machines are designed to ensure a workout for both your upper and lower body. Most of these devices are available in both commercial and home models. If you're thinking about exercise equipment, be sure you know what you want to achieve. For cardiovascular fitness and endurance, you want equipment that will help you exercise as much of your body at one time as possible. The motion should be rhythmic, repetitive, and smooth. The equipment should be comfortable, safe, and not stressful on your joints. If you're interested in a new piece of equipment, try it out for a week or two before buying it.

Exercise equipment that requires you to use weights usually will not improve cardiovascular fitness, unless some individualised circuit training can be designed. Most people will find that the flexibility and strengthening exercises in this book will help them safely achieve significant increases in strength as well as flexibility. Be sure that you consult your doctor, physiotherapist, or trained fitness instructor if you want to add strengthening exercises involving weights or weight machines to your programme.

Low-Impact Aerobics

Most people find low-impact aerobic dance good fun and a safe form of exercise. *Low-impact* means that one foot is always on the floor and there is no jumping. However, low-impact exercise does not necessarily mean low intensity, nor do the low-impact routines protect all your joints. If you participate in a low-impact aerobics class, you'll probably need to make some changes to suit your needs. You can also get low-impact aerobic exercise in classes that include dancing. Regular dancing such as *salsa, ballroom,* and *line dancing* will provide good aerobic exercise.

Getting Started

Let the instructor know who you are and explain that you may need to modify some movements to meet your needs, and that you may require some advice. It is probably easier to start off with a newly formed class than it is to join an on-going one. If you don't know people, try to get acquainted. Be open about why you may sometimes do things a little differently. You'll be more comfortable and you may find others who also have special needs.

Most instructors use music or count to a specific beat and do a set number of repetitions. You may find that the movement is too fast or that you don't want to do as many repetitions. Modify the routine: by moving to every *other* beat; or by keeping up with the beat until you start to tire and then slowing down or stopping. If the class is doing an exercise that involves arms and legs and you get tired, you can try resting your arms and doing only the leg movements, or just walking on the spot until you are ready to go again. Most instructors will be able to instruct you in *chair aerobics* should you need some time off your feet.

Some low-impact routines use a lot of arm movements at or above shoulder level in order to raise the heart rate. Remember, that for people with lung disease, hypertension, or shoulder problems, too much arm exercise *above shoulder level* can worsen your shortness of breath, increase your blood pressure, or cause pain. Modify the exercise by lowering your arms or taking a rest break.

Of course, being different from the group, in a room walled with mirrors will take courage, conviction, and a sense of humour. The most important thing you can do for yourself is to choose an instructor who encourages everyone to exercise at their own pace, and operates so that the people in the class are friendly and having fun. Observe the classes you are considering, speak with the instructors, and participate in at least one class session before making any financial commitment.

Aerobics tips

■ *Wear shoes:* Many studios have cushioned floors and soft carpet that might tempt you to go bare-foot. Don't do it. Shoes help protect the small joints and muscles in your feet and ankles by providing a firm, flat surface on which to stand.

- *Protect your knees:* Stand with your knees straight but relaxed. Many low-impact routines are done with bent, tensed knees and a lot of bobbing up and down. This can be painful and is unnecessarily stressful. Avoid this by remembering to keep your knees relaxed. Your aerobics instructor may call this *soft knees.* Watch in the mirror to see that you keep the top of your head steady as you exercise. Don't bob up and down.

- *Don't overstretch:* The beginning warm-up and the end cool-down for the session will feature stretching and strengthening exercises. Remember to stretch only as far as you comfortably can. Hold the position and don't bounce. If the stretch hurts, then don't do it. Instead, ask your instructor for a less stressful substitute, or choose one of your own.

- *Change movements:* Do this often enough so that you don't get sore muscles or joints. It's normal to feel some new sensations in your muscles and around your joints when you start a new exercise programme. However, if you feel discomfort doing the same movement after some time, change movements or stop for a rest.

- *Alternate different kinds of exercise:* Many exercise facilities have a variety of exercise opportunities: equipment rooms with cardiovascular machines, pools, and aerobics studios. If you have trouble with an hour-long aerobics class, see if you can join the class for the warm-up and cool-down and use a stationary bicycle or a treadmill for your main aerobics activity. Many people have found that this routine gives them the benefits of both an individualised programme, and group exercise.

Self-Tests for Aerobic Fitness and Endurance

For some people, just the feeling of increased endurance and well-being are enough to indicate progress. Others may need proof that their exercise programme is making a measurable difference. You can use one or both of these aerobic fitness tests. Not everyone will be able to do both tests, so pick the one that works best for you. Record your results. After four weeks of exercise, repeat the test and check your improvement. Measure yourself again after another four weeks.

Self-Testing by Distance

- *Use a pedometer:* One of the least expensive pieces of equipment you can use for distance measuring is a *pedometer.* Because distance can be difficult to set, the best pedometers measure your steps. If you get into the habit of wearing a pedometer, it is easy to motivate yourself to add a few extra steps each day. You will be surprised at how these add up.

■ *Measure the distance:* Find a place to walk, cycle, swim, or water-walk in places where you can measure the distance easily. A running track works well. On a street you can measure distance using your car. Also a stationary bicycle with an odometer, an instrument that measures distance for equipment with wheels, works well. If you plan on swimming or water-walking, you can count lengths of the pool.

■ After your warm-up, note your starting point and then cycle, swim, or walk as briskly as you comfortably can for five minutes. Try to move at a steady pace for the full time.

■ At the end of five minutes: mark your spot or note the distance or the number of laps; take your pulse; or rate your perceived exertion from zero to ten. Continue at a slow pace for three to five more minutes to cool down. Then record the distance, your heart rate, and your perceived exertion.

■ For people who have difficulty working out their heart rate while exercising, it is possible to buy heart monitors to do this. These can vary in price starting from around £15 and up to several hundreds. The simple one will do the job perfectly well.

■ *Repeat the test after several weeks of exercise:* There may be a change even within a four week period. However, it often takes eight to 12 weeks to see improvement.

Your Goal: To cover more distance, or to lower your heart rate, or to lower your perceived exertion.

Self-Testing by Time

■ *Set a time:* Measure a given distance to walk, cycle, swim, or water-walk. Estimate how far you think you can go in one to five minutes. You can pick a number of streets, the actual distance, or number of lengths in a pool. Spend three to five minutes warming up. Start timing and begin moving steadily or briskly, and comfortably. At the finish, record: how long it took you to cover your course; your heart rate; and your perceived exertion.

■ *Repeat the test:* After several weeks of exercise, test yourself again just as you would for distance.

Your Goal: To complete the distance in less time, with a lower heart rate, or with a lower perceived exertion.

Conclusion

Exercising to improve endurance has a central role in keeping muscles and other systems conditioned. When faced by the challenges of a chronic condition, your *conditioned* body will be better able to resist and overcome them.

Suggested Further Reading

Beevers, D. G., *Understanding Blood Pressure.* Poole: Family Doctor Publications Ltd. Revised ed. 2011

Gibson, T. and Spitzer, A. *Water aerobics for Fitness and Wellness*, 3rd Edition. Belmont, California: Wadsworth, 2002

Fortmann, S. P. and Breitrose, P. E, *The Blood Pressure Book: How to Get It Down and Keep It Down*, 3rd ed. Boulder, Colorado: Bull Publishing, 2006.

White, M. *Water Exercise: 78 Safe and Effective Exercises for Fitness and Therapy.* Champaign, Illinois: Human Kinetics, 1995.

Sit and Be Fit (Chair Exercise). www.sitandbefit.org.

CHAPTER 9

Communicating with Family, Friends, and Health Care Professionals

"You just don't understand!"

HOW OFTEN HAS THIS STATEMENT concluded a frustrating discussion? Whenever we talk to someone, we expect the other person to understand what we are saying. When they don't understand we become frustrated. This failure to communicate effectively can then lead to anger, helplessness, isolation, and depression. Such feelings can be even worse when we have a long-term health problem. When communication breaks down, our symptoms may increase. Pain can be worse, blood glucose and blood pressure levels may rise, and there is an increased strain on the heart. Worry caused by conflict and misunderstanding can make us irritable, interfere with our concentration, and sometimes lead to accidents. Clearly, *poor communication* is bad for our physical, mental, and emotional health.

Healthy communication is the lifeblood of relationships, and relationships are a lifeline for healthy functioning. Poor communication is the biggest single reason for poor relationships between spouses, partners, family members, friends, co-workers, and members of your health care team.

Good communication is a necessity when you have a long-term condition. In particular, it is vital that your doctors, nurses and other health care professionals understand you and that equally you understand them. When you don't understand advice or recommendations from your doctor or health team, the resulting lack of clarity can be life-threatening. So, for a self-manager, effective communication skills are essential.

In this chapter we discuss a number of tools which can improve communication. Specifically, these are tools to help you express your feelings in a positive way, so as to minimise conflict, to ask for help, and sometimes to say *no*. We will also discuss how to listen, how to

recognise body language and different styles of communication, and how to get more information from other people.

Keep in mind that communication is a *two-way process*. Whilst you may feel uncomfortable about expressing your feelings or asking for help, the chances are that others are also feeling the same way. It may be up to *you* to make sure the lines of communication are open. Here are two key elements of better communication:

1. *Do not make assumptions regarding others because 'they should know':* People are not mind readers. If you want to be sure they know something, tell them.

2. *You cannot change the way other people communicate:* What you can do is to change *your* way of communicating to make sure that you are understood.

Expressing Your Feelings

When communication is difficult, take the following steps:

- First, review the situation.

- Next, decide exactly what is bothering you.

- Then, ask yourself what you are feeling.

Here is an example. John and Steve had agreed to go to a football match. When John came to pick him up, Steve was not ready. In fact, he was not sure he wanted to go because he was having trouble with the pain in his knees caused by his arthritis. The following conversation took place.

Steve: *I don't think you really understand. If you had pain like I do, you wouldn't be so quick to criticise. You don't think of anyone but yourself.*

John: *Well, I think it's probably better if I just go by myself.*

In this conversation, neither John nor Steve had stopped to think about what the trouble really was, or how he felt about it. Each blamed the other for an unfortunate situation.

The following is the same conversation but with both people using more thoughtful communication.

John: *When we have already made plans and then at the last minute you are not sure you can go, I feel frustrated and angry. I don't know what to do, do I go on without you, stay here and change our plans, or just not make any plans to do things with you in the future?*

Steve: *When my arthritis acts up at the last minute, I am also confused. I keep hoping I can go and so I don't phone you because I don't want to disappoint you and I do really want to go. I keep hoping that my knees will get better as the day wears on.*

John: *That makes sense.*

Steve: *Let's go to the game. You can drop me off at the gate before parking so I won't have to walk as far. Then, I can take the steps slowly and be at our seats when you arrive. I really do want to go to the game with you. In future, I will let you know sooner if I think my arthritis is acting up.*

John: *Sounds good to me. I really enjoy your company and knowing how I can help. It is just that being caught by surprise sometimes makes me angry.*

In this dialogue, John and Steve talked about the situation and how they felt about it. Neither blamed the other.

Unfortunately, we are often in situations where the other person uses blaming communications. Maybe we are not listening and get caught out. Then we blame the other person. Even in this situation, thoughtful communication can be helpful. Look at the following example.

Jan: *Why do you always spoil my plans? At least you could have called. I am really fed up of trying to do anything with you.*

Sandra: *I understand. When my anxiety acts up at the last minute, I get confused. I keep hoping I can go and so I don't call you because I don't want to disappoint you. I really want to go. I keep hoping that I will feel less anxious as the day wears on.*

Jan: *Well, I hope that in the future you will call. I don't like being caught by surprise.*

Sandra: *I understand. If it is OK with you, let's go shopping now. If I start feeling too anxious, I'll take a break in the coffee shop with my book while you carry on shopping. I do want us to keep making plans. In future, if I am too anxious, I will let you know sooner.*

In this example, only Sandra is using thoughtful communication, while Jan continues to blame. The outcome, however, is still positive. Both people got what they wanted.

What follows provides some suggestions for using good communications and creating supportive relationships:

■ *Show respect:* Always show respect and regard for the other person. Try not to preach or be excessively demanding. Avoid demeaning or blaming comments such as *"Why do you always spoil my plans?"* The use of the word *you* provides a clue that your communication might be blaming. A bit of tact and courtesy can go a long way in defusing problem situations. Look at the section on *Anger* on page 58–60 in Chapter 4.

■ *Be clear:* Describe a specific situation and your observations should stick to the facts. Avoid words such as *always* and *never.* For example, Sandra does not use these words, *"When my anxiety acts up at the last minute, I get confused. I keep hoping I can go and so I don't call you because I don't want to disappoint you and I really want to go. I keep hoping that I will feel less anxious as the day wears on."*

■ *Don't make assumptions:* Ask for more details. Jan did not do this. She assumed that Sandra was rude because she did not call. It would have been better if she had asked Sandra why she hadn't called earlier. Assumptions are the enemy of good communication. Many arguments arise from one person expecting the other person to be a mind reader. One sign that you are making assumptions is thinking, *"This person should know . . ."* Don't rely on mind reading; express your own needs and feelings directly and clearly; ask questions if you don't understand something.

■ *Open up:* Try to express your feelings openly and honestly. Don't make others guess what you are feeling. The chances are that they may be miles out. Sandra did the right thing. She talked about wanting to go, and not wanting to disappoint Jan, and

hoping that her anxiety would get better. Bottling up our feelings, particularly anger, can sometimes lead to chronic stress. As we know, this can have an effect on our physical health. Take a look at the discussions on *anger* and *stress* in Chapter 4.

■ *Accept the feelings of others:* Try to understand them. This is not always easy. Sometimes you need to think about what has been said, rather than answering at once. You can always stall a bit by saying *"I understand"* or *"I'm not sure I understand; could you explain some more?"*

■ *Use humour, but sparingly:* On the other hand don't use sarcasm or demeaning humour, and know when to be serious.

■ *Avoid the role of victim:* You become a victim when you do not express your needs and feelings or expect that someone else ought to act in a certain way. Unless you have done something to hurt another person, you should not apologise. Apologising on a regular basis is a sign that you view yourself as a victim. You deserve respect, and you have a right to express your wants and needs.

■ *Listen first:* Good listeners seldom interrupt. Wait a few seconds when someone has finished talking before you respond. This person may have more to say.

"I" Messages

Many of us are uncomfortable expressing our feelings, especially when it may seem that we are being critical of someone else.

If emotions are running high, attempts to express frustration can be full of 'you' messages. These suggest blame, causing the other person to feel under attack. At once, the other person is on the defensive, and the barriers go up. The situation escalates from there, leading to anger, frustration, and bad feelings.

"I" statements are direct, assertive expressions of your views and feelings; whereas 'you' can be accusative and confrontational. For example, *"I try very hard to do the best work I can"* rather than *"You always criticise me."* Or, you might say *"I appreciate it when you turn down the television while I talk"* rather than *"You never pay attention"* Notice, that saying *"I feel that you are not treating me fairly"* is actually a disguised 'you' statement. A true "I" statement would be, *"I feel angry and hurt"* Here are some more examples:

■ *You* message: *"Why are you always late? We never get anywhere on time."*

■ "I" message: *"I get really upset when I'm late. It's important to me to be on time."*

■ *You* message: *"There's no way you can understand how lousy I feel."*

■ "I" message: *"I'm not feeling well. I could do with a little help today."*

Watch out for the hidden "you" messages with "I feel . . ." stuck in front of them. Here's an example to think about:

■ *You* message: *"You always walk too fast."*

■ Hidden *you* message: *"I feel angry when you walk so fast."*

■ "I" message: *"I have a hard time walking fast."*

The trick to "I" messages is to avoid the use of the word *you* and instead report your personal feelings using "*I.*" Naturally, like any new skill, using "I" messages takes practice. Start by really listening, to yourself and to others. Supermarkets are a good place to hear lots of *you* messages as parents talk to their children. In your head, take some of the *you* messages you hear and turn them into "I" messages. You'll be surprised at how fast "I" messages become a habit. If using "I" statements seems difficult, try adopting this format:

"I notice . . ." – stating just the facts

"I think . . ." – stating your opinion

"I feel . . ." – stating what your feelings are

"I want . . ." – stating exactly what you'd like the other person to do

For example, you make a special cake to take as a gift for a friend. Somebody comes into your kitchen, sees the cake on the table, and cuts out a large slice. You're upset because, with a piece missing, the gift is spoilt. You might say to the cake eater: *"You cut into my special cake (observation). You should have asked me about it first (opinion). I'm really upset and disappointed because I can't give it as a gift now (feeling). I'd like an apology, and I'd like you to ask me first next time (want)."*

Here are some cautions about using "I" messages:

1. They are not a cure-all. Sometimes the listener has to have time to hear them. This is especially true if the person often hears blaming *you* messages. If using "I" messages do not work at first, just persevere and continue to use them. Things will change as you gain skill and you begin to break down old patterns of communication.

2. Some people can use *"I"* messages as a means of manipulation. They may often express that they are sad, angry, or frustrated in order to gain sympathy from others. If used in this way, problems can escalate. Effective *I* messages must report *honest* feelings.

3. Note finally, that *I* messages are an excellent way to express positive feelings and deliver compliments. For example, *"I really appreciate the extra time you gave me today, doctor."*

Good communication skills can help make life easier for everyone, especially those with long-term health problems. Try this exercise:

Exercise: Creating *"I"* Messages

Change the following statements into *"I"* messages. Be careful, and watch out for hidden *you* messages.

1. *"You expect me to wait on you, hand and foot!"*

2. *"Doctor, you never have enough time for me. You're always in a hurry."*

3. *"You hardly ever touch me anymore. You haven't paid any attention to me since my heart attack."*

4. *"Doctor, you didn't tell me the side effects of all these drugs or why I have to take them."*

Minimising Conflict

Besides *"I"* messages, there are other ways to reduce conflict. For example, consider:

- *Shifting the focus:* If a discussion gets off the topic and emotions are running high, shift the focus of the conversation. That is, try bringing the discussion back to the agreed topic. For example, you might say something like *"We're both getting upset now and drifting away from what we agreed to discuss."* Or perhaps, *"I feel like we are bringing up things other than the ones we agreed to talk about and this is upsetting me. Can we discuss these extra things later and just talk about what we originally agreed on?"*

- *Buying time:* For example, you might say, *"I think I understand your concerns, but I need more time to think about it before I can respond."* Or what about, *"I can hear what you are saying, but I am too frustrated to respond now. I need to find out more about this before I can respond properly."*

- *Making sure you understand each other's viewpoints:* You do this by summarising what you have heard and asking for clarification. You can also switch roles. Try arguing from the other person's position as thoroughly and thoughtfully as you can. This will help you understand all sides of the issue, as well as conveying that you respect and value the other person's point of view. It will also help you to develop greater tolerance and empathy for others.

- *Looking for compromise:* You may not always find the perfect solution to a problem or reach total agreement. Nevertheless, it may be possible to compromise. Find something on which you can both agree. For example, you can do it your way this time and the other person's way the next time. Or, you can agree to part of what you want and part of what the other person wants. Or you can decide what you'll do and then suggest what the other person might do in return. These are all forms of compromise that can help you through some difficult times.

■ *Saying you're sorry:* We have all said or done things that have hurt others, either intentionally or unintentionally. Many relationships are hurt, sometimes for years, because people have not learned the powerful social skill of apologising. Often all it takes is a simple, sincere apology to restore a relationship. Rather than a sign of weakness, saying you are sorry shows great strength. To be effective, an apology must do all of the following:

- ◆ Admit to the specific mistake and accept responsibility for it.

- ◆ Name the offence. Do so with no *glossing over* by just saying *"I'm sorry for what I did."* Be specific. You might say, "I'm very sorry that I talked behind your back."

- ◆ Explain the particular circumstances that led you to do what you did. But don't offer excuses or side-step responsibility.

- ◆ Express your feelings about the situation. A genuine, heartfelt apology can be painful. Your sadness shows that the relationship matters to you.

- ◆ Acknowledge the impact of wrong-doing. You might say, *"I know that I hurt you and that my behaviour cost you a lot. For that I am very sorry."*

- ◆ Offer to make amends. Ask what you can do to make the situation better, or volunteer some specific suggestions.

Making an apology is not fun, but it is an act of courage, generosity, and healing. It brings the possibility of a renewed and stronger relationship, and it can also bring peace for you.

Asking for Help

Getting and giving help is a part of life, but it is something that can cause many problems. Even though most of us will need help on some occasions, few of us like to ask for it. We may not want to admit that we are unable to do things for ourselves. We may not want to be a burden on others. We may hedge or make a very vague request: *"I'm sorry to have to ask this . . ."* or *"I know this is asking a lot . . ."* or *"I hate to ask this, but . . . ."* Hedging like this tends to put the other person on the defensive, and they might think: *"Gosh, what's he going to ask that's such a big deal?"* To avoid this response, be specific. A general request can lead to misunderstanding. The person being asked to help may react negatively, if the request is not clear. This leads to a further breakdown in communication and may mean that there will be no help. A specific request is more likely to have a positive result:

General request: *"I know this is the last thing you want to do, but I need help moving. Will you help me?"*

Reaction: *"Uh . . . well . . . I don't know. Um . . . can I get back to you after I check my diary?"*

Specific request: *"I'm moving next week, and I'd like to move my books and kitchen stuff ahead of time. Would you mind helping me load and unload the boxes in my car on Saturday morning? I think it can be done in one trip."*

Reaction: *"I'm busy Saturday morning, but I could give you a hand on Friday night."*

People with health problems sometimes have to deal with offers of help that are neither needed nor desired. In most cases, these offers come from important people in your life. These people care for you and genuinely want to help. A well-worded *I* message allows you to decline the help without embarrassing the other person. *"Oh that's really kind of you, but today I think I can manage it myself. I hope I can take you up on your offer another time."*

Saying 'No'

Let's look at the other side, when you are the one being asked for help. It is probably best not to answer right away. You may need more information. If a request leaves you feeling negative, trust your feelings.

The example we considered about helping a person to move is a good one. *"Help me to move"* can mean anything from moving a chair upstairs to moving a complete household. Using your skills that help you to get at the specifics will avoid problems. It is important to understand any request fully before you respond. Asking for more information or restating the request will often bring clarification: Starting with *"Before I answer, . . ."* will not only clarify the request but will also prevent the person making the request assuming that you are going to say *yes*.

If you decide to say *no*, it is still important to acknowledge the importance of the request. In this way, the person will see that you are rejecting the request rather than them as a person. Your turn-down should not be a put-down: *"That sounds like a worthwhile project you're doing, but it's beyond what I can do this week."* Again, specifics are the key. Try to be clear about the conditions of your turn-down: will you always turn down this request, or is it just that today or this week or right now that is a problem? If you are feeling overwhelmed and put on, saying *no* can be a useful tool. You may wish to make a counter offer such as *"I won't be able to drive today, but I will next week."* But remember, you always have a legitimate right to decline a request, even if it is a reasonable one.

Accepting Help

We often hear *"How can I help?"* Our answer is often *"I don't know"* or *"Thank you, but I don't need any help."* All the time we may be thinking, *"They should know . . ."* Be prepared to accept help by having a specific answer. For example, *"It would be great if we could go for a walk together once a week"* or *"Could you please take out the rubbish? I can't lift it."* Just remember that people cannot read your mind, so you'll need to tell them what help you want, and thank them for it. Think about how each person can help you. If possible, give people a task that they can easily accomplish. You are giving them a gift. People like being helpful and feel rejected when they cannot assist someone they care for. It is also beneficial to express thanks for the help you receive. Take a look at the section on *practising thankfullness*, on page 88, in Chapter 5.

Listening

Good listening is probably one of the most important communication skills. Most of us are much better at talking than we are at listening. When others talk to us, we are often preparing a response instead of just listening. There are several steps to becoming a better listener:

1. *Listen to the words, the tone of voice, and observe the body language:* There may be times when the words being used don't tell the whole story. Is the voice wavering? Is the speaker struggling to find the right words? Do you notice body tension? Does he or she seem distracted? Do you hear sarcasm? What is the facial expression? If you pick up on some of these signs, the speaker probably has something more on his or her mind. Take a look at page 144 for more on this.

2. *Let the person know you have heard what he or she said:* This may be a simple *"uh-huh."* Many times the only thing the other person wants is an acknowledgment or just someone to listen. Sometimes it is helpful for everyone just to talk to a sympathetic listener.

3. *Let the person know you heard both the content and the emotion behind what is said:* You can do this simply by re-stating the content. For example, *"Sounds like you are planning a nice trip."* Or, you can respond by acknowledging the emotions: *"That must be difficult"* or *"How sad you must feel."* When you respond on an emotional level, the results can be startling. These responses tend to open the gates for the expression of feelings and thoughts. Responding to either the content or the emotion can help communication. It discourages the other person from simply repeating what has been said. But don't try to talk people out of their feelings. They are real to them. Just listen and reflect.

4. *Respond by seeking more information:* This is especially important if you are not completely clear about is being said or what is wanted. Again, take a look at page 144.

Getting More Information

Getting more information is a bit of an art. It can involve both simple and more complicated techniques.

- *The simplest way to get more information is to ask directly:* "Tell me more" will probably get more information, as will "I don't understand; please explain," or "I would like to know more about . . . ," or "Could you put that another way?" or "How do you mean?" or "I'm not sure I understood that," or "Could you expand on that?"

- *Another way to get more information is to paraphrase what you have heard:* This means simply repeating what you heard in your own words. This is a good tool if you want to make sure you have understood what the other person means. This could be the *actual* meaning behind what has been said. Paraphrasing can help but sometimes it can hinder effective communication. This depends on the way the paraphrase is worded. It is important to remember to paraphrase in the form of a question, rather than a statement. For example, someone says:

> "I don't know. I'm really not feeling up to par. This party will be crowded, there'll probably be smokers, and I really don't know the hosts very well."

A *provocative paraphrase* would be:

> "Obviously, you're telling me you don't want to go to the party."

This paraphrase might provoke an angry response such as "No, I didn't say that! If you're going to be that way, I'll definitely stay at home." Or, it might simply lead to no response at all, in effect a total shut-down resulting from either anger or despair and a feeling that "He just doesn't understand." People really don't like being told what they meant.

Here's a better and softer paraphrase, expressed as a question:

> "Are you saying that you'd rather stay home than go to the party?"

The response to this paraphrase might be:

> "That's not what I mean. Now that I'm using oxygen, I'm feeling a little nervous about meeting new people. I'd appreciate it if you'd stay near me during the party. I'd feel better about it, and I might have a good time."

As you can see, the second paraphrase helps communication. You have discovered the real reason why they are expressing doubt about the party. In short, you get more information when you paraphrase with questions. Be specific. If you want specific information, you must ask specific questions. We often tend to speak in generalities. For example:

Doctor: *"How have you been feeling?"*

Patient: *"Not so good."*

The doctor has not got much information. "Not so good" isn't very useful. Here's how the doctor might get at more information:

Doctor: *Are you still having those sharp pains in your right shoulder?*

Patient: *Yes a lot.*

Doctor: *How often?*

Patient: *A couple of times a day.*

Doctor: *How long do they last?*

Patient: *A long time.*

Doctor: *About how many minutes would you say? . . .*

. . . and so it goes on.

■ *Avoid asking, 'Why?' which is far too general a question: 'Why?'* makes a person think in terms of cause and effect and can put people on the defensive. A person may respond at an entirely different level than you had in mind when you asked the question. Health care professionals are trained to get specific information from patients, although they sometimes do ask very general questions. Most of us are not trained, but we can learn to ask specific questions. Simply asking for specifics can usually work: *"Can you be more specific about . . ."* or, *"Are you thinking of something special?"*

Most of us have had the experience of being with a three-year-old who just keeps asking *"Why?"* over and over again. This goes on until the child gets the wanted information, or the parent runs from the room, screaming! The poor parent doesn't have the faintest idea what the child has in mind and answers *"Because . . ."* in an increasingly specific way until the child's question is answered. Sometimes, however, the parent's answers are just not what the child really wants to know and, as a result the child never gets the desired information. Rather than using *why,* begin your responses with *who, which, when,* or *where.* These words will produce more specific responses.

We should point out that sometimes we do not get the correct information because we do not know the best question to ask. For example, you may be seeking legal services from a Citizens Advice Bureau or community centre. You call and ask if there is a lawyer on the staff and hang up when the answer is *no.* If instead you had asked where you might get low-cost legal advice, you might have got some answers.

Body Language and Conversational Styles

Body Language

Body language is an important part of listening to what others are saying, but it also includes observing *how* they say it. Even when we say nothing, our bodies are talking; sometimes they are even shouting. Research shows that our body language provides more than half of what we communicate. If we want to communicate really well, we must be aware of body language, facial expressions, and tone of voice. These should match what we say in words. If we do not do this, we are sending mixed messages and creating misunderstandings. For example, if you want to make a firm statement, look at the other person, and keep your expression friendly. Stand tall and confident; relax your legs and arms, and breathe steadily. You may even lean forward to show your interest. Try not to sneer or bite your lips; this might indicate discomfort or doubt. Don't move away or slouch, as these communicate disinterest and uncertainty.

When you notice that the body language and words of others do not match, gently point this out. Ask for some clarification. For example, you might say, *"I hear you saying that you would like to go with me to the family picnic, but you look tired and you're yawning as you speak. Would you rather stay at home and rest while I go alone?"*

Expressing Ourselves

In addition to reading people's body language, it is also helpful if you recognise and appreciate that we all express ourselves differently. Our conversational styles vary according to where we were born, how we were brought up, our occupation, our cultural background, and especially our gender.

For example, women tend to ask questions that are more personal. These show interest and help form relationships. Men are more likely to offer opinions or suggestions and to state facts. They tend to discuss problems in order to find solutions, whereas women want to share their feelings and experiences. No one style is better or worse; they're just different. By acknowledging and accepting these differences, we can reduce some of the misunderstanding, frustration, and resentment we sometimes feel in our communication with others.

Communicating with Members of Your Health Care Team

Communication lies at the very heart of the management of your condition. Your health and circumstances may be complicated and certainly the lives and experiences of those you are working with, will be too. Think carefully about some aspects of these interactions:

1. *Consider good communication:* The key to making the health care system work for you is *good communication* with the professionals involved in your care, in particular with your doctor or hospital consultant. The *General Medical Council*, which defines

the standards for doctors, emphasises that patients receive the best care when they work in partnership with their doctors. In the case of patients with a long-term medical condition, this partnership may be a life-long one. Good communication is essential for these long-term partnerships to work.

2. *Think about achieving clarity:* One of the difficulties for many people is that medicine is a science which uses technical terms that we may not understand. Yet there is often a reluctance to ask for clarification. The General Medical Council published a short booklet in 2013 called, *What to expect from your doctor: a guide for patients.* It recognises that it can be difficult to take in all the information the doctor is sharing with you and recommends that you ask for clarification. It cites examples of questions surrounding your medication, how you should take it and how to prepare for any tests you may need to undergo.

3. *Ensure that members of your health team are feeling comfortable:* Your doctor probably knows more intimate details about you than anyone else, except perhaps your spouse, partner, or parents. You, in turn, should feel comfortable expressing your fears, even asking questions that you may think sound *stupid*, and negotiating a treatment plan that satisfies you both.

4. *Be clear and make good use of everyone's time:* Two things will help keep the lines of communication open.

     Firstly, you must be clear about what you want from your doctors and healthcare professionals. Many of us would like them to be like warm-hearted computers, gigantic brains, stuffed with knowledge about the human body and mind . . . and especially yours! We all want health providers who can analyse the situation, read our minds, make perfect diagnoses, come up with good treatment plans, and tell us what to expect. At the same time, we want them to be warm and caring and to make us feel as though we are their most important patient.

Most doctors and healthcare professionals wish they were just that sort of person. Unfortunately, no one person can be all things to all patients. Doctors, nurses and physiotherapists are all human. They have bad days, they get headaches, they get tired, and they get sore feet. They have families who demand their time and attention, and they may get frustrated by paperwork, electronic record keeping, and large bureaucracies.

Most doctors and other health care professionals have endured a gruelling training. They entered the health care system because they wanted to help people to get well. They are frustrated when they cannot cure someone with a long-term condition. Many times they must take their satisfaction from improvements rather than cures, or even from slowing the inevitable decline for some of the conditions they encounter. Undoubtedly, you have been frustrated, angry, or depressed from time to time about your condition. So, you should appreciate that your doctors have probably felt similar emotions about their inability to make you well. In this, you are truly partners.

Secondly, time is a threat to a good patient-provider relationship. We all know when we have an appointment to see our doctor that there is a limited time slot allocated to us. The effect of this is that sometimes we feel we don't have the opportunity to talk fully about the issues that concern us. The doctor probably feels the same way, because they are conscious they have a waiting room full of other patients with similar time slots.

One way to help you to get the most from a visit to your doctor is to use the take PART strategy. This acronym stands for Prepare; Ask; Repeat; Take action.

> **Take P.A.R.T.**
>
> **P**repare
>
> **A**sk
>
> **R**epeat
>
> **T**ake action

Prepare

Before your appointment you should prepare an agenda. What are the reasons for your visit? What do you expect from your doctor?

Take some time to make a written list of your concerns or questions. Have you ever thought to yourself, when leaving the doctor's surgery, *"Why didn't I ask about . . ."* or, *"I forgot to mention . . ."* Making a list beforehand helps to ensure that your main concerns are addressed. Be realistic. If you have 13 different problems, your doctor probably cannot deal with all of them in one visit. So, highlight your two or three most important items.

Give the list to your doctor at the beginning of the visit, and explain that you have highlighted your most important concerns. By giving your doctor the whole list, you let the doctor know which items are the most important to you; it also lets the doctor see everything, in case there is something medically important that you've not highlighted. By contrast, if you wait until the end of your appointment to bring up concerns, there may not be time to discuss them.

Here is an example: When your doctor asks *"What can I do for you today?"* You might say something like *"I have a lot of things I want to discuss in this visit."* Faced with this, your doctor may be looking at his or her watch and thinking of the appointment list and beginning to feel anxious. If you then continue, *". . . but I know that we have a limited amount of time, so I'll get to the point. The things that most concern me are my shoulder pain, my dizziness, and the side-effects from one of the medications I'm taking."* The doctor feels instantly relieved because the concerns are focused and potentially manageable in the appointment time available.

The final thing to prepare is your story, or response when the doctor asks *"What can I do for you today."* You should be able to present a clear summary of what you want. You should be prepared to describe your symptoms:

When they started

How long they last

Where they are located

What makes them better or worse?

Whether you have had similar problems before

Whether you have changed your diet, exercise, or medications in a way that might influence your symptoms

What worries you most about the symptoms?

What you think might be causing the symptoms

In addition, if you are on a new medication or treatment, be ready to report how it is going.

Also, in telling your story, talk about the *trends* you have noticed. Are you getting better or worse, or about the same? And talk about the *tempo* of your symptoms, are they more or less frequent or intense? For example, you might say *"In general, I am slowly getting better, although today I do not feel very well."*

Be as open as you can in sharing your thoughts, feelings, and fears. Remember, your doctor is not a mind reader. If you are worried, explain why: *"I am worried that I may not be able to work,"* or *"My father had similar symptoms before he died."* The more open you are, the more likely it is that your doctor can help you. If you have a problem, don't wait for the doctor to *discover* it. State your concern immediately. For example, *"I am worried about this mole on my chest."*

The more specific you can be, without overdoing it with irrelevant details, the clearer the picture the doctor will have of your problem, with less time being wasted for both of you.

Ask

Your most powerful tool in the doctor-patient partnership is the *question.* You can fill in vitally important missing pieces of information and close critical gaps in communication with your questions. And asking all your questions reflects your active participation in the care process, a critical ingredient in restoring your health. Getting answers and information that you understand is a cornerstone of self-management. Be prepared to ask questions about diagnosis, tests, treatments, and follow-up:

■ *Diagnosis:* Ask what's wrong, what caused it, if it is contagious, what the future

outlook is, and what can be done to prevent or manage it.

■ *Tests:* If the doctor wants to do tests, ask how the results are likely to affect treatment and what will happen if you are not tested. If you decide to have a test, find out how to prepare for it and what it will be like. Also ask how and when you will get the results.

■ *Treatments:* Ask if there are any choices in treatments and the advantages and disadvantages of each. Ask what will happen if you have no treatment. For a general discussion on treatments see Chapter 13 beginning on page 219.

■ *Follow-up:* Find out if, and when you should call or return for a follow-up visit. What symptoms should you watch for, and what should you do if they occur?

Repeat

One way to check that you have really understood everything is to briefly report back on the key points. For example, *"You want me to take this three times a day."* Repeating back like this, also gives your doctor a chance to quickly correct any misunderstandings and miscommunication.

If you don't fully understand or remember something which has been said, then admit that you need to go over it again. For example, *"I'm sure you told me some of this before, but I'm still confused about it."* Don't be afraid to ask even what you may consider a stupid question. Such questions are important and may prevent a misunderstanding.

Sometimes it is hard to remember everything. You may want to jot down some notes or bring another person with you to important visits. A second set of ears can be very useful in remembering what was said.

Take Action

At the end of a visit, you need to clearly understand what to do next. This includes treatments, tests, and when to come back. You should also know about any danger signs and what to do if they occur. If necessary, ask your health provider to write down instructions, or recommend reading material, or indicate other places where you can get help.

If for some reason you can't, or won't, follow the advice you have been given, then let the doctor know. For example, *"I didn't take the aspirin. It gives me stomach problems"* or *"I've tried to exercise, but I can't seem to keep it up."* If your doctor knows why you can't or won't follow the advice, it may be possible to offer alternative suggestions. If you don't share information about the barriers to taking actions, it's difficult for your doctor to help you.

Asking for a Second Opinion

Sometimes you may want to see another doctor or specialist for a second opinion. Asking for this can be hard. This is especially true if you have had a long and good relationship with your doctor. You may worry that asking for another opinion will anger your doctor, or that your doctor will interpret your request as questioning their competence. However, your GP does not have to do this for you. If it is thought to be unnecessary you do not have a legal right to a second opinion. Having said this, doctors are seldom hurt by requests for a second opinion. If your condition is complicated or difficult, your doctor may suggest it themselves. They may wish in any case to consult with another doctor, and indeed they may already have done so.

Asking for a second opinion is perfectly acceptable and providers are taught to expect such requests. Ask for a second opinion by using a non-threatening *"I"* message:

> *"I'm still feeling confused and uncomfortable about this treatment. I feel that another opinion might reassure me. Can you suggest someone I could see?"*

In this way, you have expressed your own feelings without suggesting that the provider is at fault. You have also confirmed that you have confidence in your provider by asking for his or her recommendation.

Giving Positive Feedback to Your Healthcare Professionals

Let your healthcare professional know how satisfied you are with your care. If you do not like the way you have been treated by any of the members of your health care team, let them know. In the same way, if you are pleased with your care, then also let them know. Everyone appreciates compliments and positive feedback. The members of your health care team are no different. They are human, and your praise can help nourish and console these busy, hardworking professionals. Letting them know that you appreciate their efforts is one of the best ways to improve your relationship with them, and it makes them feel good!

Making Decisions about Treatments

Making decisions about treatments can be difficult. For some suggestions on how to do this see page 18, and also Chapter 14 for help you on evaluating new treatments.

Working with the Health Care System

The National Health Service underwent many changes in 2013 and 2014 is when we are seeing the results of these changes. These can lead to problems for both patients and professionals. The stage of *transition* means that it will take some time before all the new services are well established. However, this transition stage should not interfere with vital services. Here are some of the problems you might encounter:

■ *A major change which affects us all is the abolition of Primary Care Trusts (PCTs) and the transfer of their commissioning role to Clinical Commissioning Groups (CCGs):* To find out about how local decisions are made you will need to contact your local Clinical Commissioning Group. An organisation has also been introduced called the *Local Health Watch Body*, which is to act as the local consumer champion for patients, service users and the public.

■ *The Practice Manager:* On a more personal level, if you have problems with your local GP surgery the best person to contact initially is the Practice Manager.

■ *Working with PALS:* If you have problems relating to your hospital, in whatever capacity, the *Patient Advice and Liaison Service* (PALS) is the best contact. Each hospital has a *PALS* office and has staff you can discuss your problems with.

■ *Health care has become more complex with the result that there are many more types of healthcare providers working with patients:* Health care may be better and more thorough, but getting that care can be more complicated. A good example of this is making a booking for an appointment with a hospital consultant. This now often involves your GP making the referral. You then receive a letter to contact the appointment office. This letter contains a *password* for you to use in making your booking, together with information about the choice of hospitals available to you. These hospitals can be in different locations, from five miles away to 40 miles away. The website *NHS Choices* may be helpful for you here. It is designed to give you as much information as possible, about different diseases and conditions and how and *where* you can get the best treatments. The web address is www.nhs.uk.

■ *The range of options for medication has also increased and this aspect can be bewildering:* Your local pharmacist is often in a good position to explain what your medications are and what they are used for, if you don't have the opportunity or are reluctant to ask your GP for the information, directly, then Chapter 13 provides more information for you on the role of your pharmacist.

Hints on Working with the Health Care Systems

The following are a few hints for working with the health care system to address some of the most common complaints made by patients.

Not all of these problems and suggestions will apply to every system, but most do:

- *"I hate the phone system"*: Often when we call for an appointment or information, we reach an automated system. This can be frustrating. Unfortunately, we cannot change this. However, phone systems do not change that often. If you can memorise the numbers, or the exact keys to press, you can move quickly from one part of the choice system to another. Sometimes pressing the hash key (#) or zero will get you to a real person. Once you do get through, ask the person answering if there is a way to do this faster next time.

- *"It takes too long to get an appointment"*: Delay in getting an appointment is one of the most frequent matters complained about at local NHS surgeries. Most GP surgeries have their own system for booking appointments and it pays to familiarise yourself with your doctor's system. The surgery should be able to offer you an appointment to see a GP or other health-care professional quickly if this is necessary. You should also be able to book appointments in advance and sometimes you can book on-line for routine appointments. The demand for appointments in some surgeries can be very high. So, it can be an incredibly frustrating experience trying to make an appointment whilst retaining your normal politeness! The staff are more likely to help you if you do not get aggressive or become rude. Remember the skills of good communication. Medical emergencies are very important so be sure not to waste time getting help. Dial 999 if you need an ambulance, for example when you suspect something such as a heart attack, or stroke, or serious bleeding. You can go straight to A&E at the hospital when this is appropriate.

- *"I don't understand the Electronic Medical Record (EMR)"*: There are changes in progress concerning your Electronic Medical Records. These have become known as your *NHS Summary Care Record (SCR)* and it is expected that approximately 50 million records will be uploaded onto the system by 2014. These records are held centrally and information on them can be transferred electronically for speed and efficiency. You should be aware that:

  - The new record will contain important information about the medicines you are taking, the allergies you suffer from, and any bad reactions you have had to medicines.

  - Your record will be available for use by all those directly involved in your care.

  - The users will need to have an *NHS Smartcard* to access the information.

  - Users will only see the information they require to do their job

  - All users will have their details recorded whenever they access your records.

One of the justifications for the SCR is that it will allow safe care in an emergency when your GP practice is closed or when you are in another part of the country.

Note that it is not compulsory to have a Summary Care Record. However, if this is not what you want then you must opt out of the system by completing a form and then returning it to your GP. You will automatically be included in the system if you do not complete an opt-out form.

Apart from ensuring you have safe care during an emergency the Summary Care Record also has other advantages. A very important advantage is the power it gives you personally to have a stronger and more effective voice in improving and personalising your care. This can be done by getting a print-out of your SCR from your GP surgery. This will give you the opportunity to inform your GP of any errors or inaccuracies in the records. More importantly you can also ask your doctor to add information which you consider crucial about your condition. You can also add information about your end of life wishes. Generally, the extra information you provide will then be used to personalise and improve the care you receive. As a consequence of this, patients have a more effective and stronger voice in their treatment. Many *Voluntary Patient Organisations* are raising awareness amongst their patients about the SCR and its potential use.

Medical Records

These are different from the Electronic Summary Care Records: they comprise a file of notes, letters, x-rays, test results and correspondence regarding any treatment you have received from the NHS.

Remember that you have a right, to see *anything* in your medical records and this can be arranged informally with your GP or hospital. You can also make a formal request to see them and it is not necessary to give a reason. Your request can sometimes be refused, if the relevant healthcare professional believes that giving you access might pose a serious risk to your mental or physical health. There will be a cost for accessing the records particularly if you require copies. You can consult *NHS Choices* for a detailed account of these conditions. See www.nhs.uk.

Parting Words of Advice

If something in the health care system is not working for you, why not ask how you can help make it work better? Very often, if you learn your way round the system, you can solve, or at least partially solve, some of your problems.

If you think that things should not be as they are and that it is not fair to place any extra burden on you as the patient, then many people will agree with you. Health systems should change to be more responsive and patient-friendly. But in the UK we have to acknowledge that the NHS is a vast and complicated organisation. It is working with a rapidly expanding population. Also, it must cope with an explosive increase in medical knowledge and of the technology necessary to apply it. There will inevitably be weaknesses which we all have to address in whatever way we can. In the meantime, we have offered you, in this chapter, some suggestions which will help you to deal with potential difficulties.

Suggested Further Reading

Beck, A. T. *Love Is Never Enough: How Couples Can Overcome Misunderstandings, Resolve Conflicts, and Solve Relationship Problems Through Cognitive Therapy.* New York: HarperCollins, 1989.

Gabor, D. *Talking with Confidence.* London: Sheldon Press, 1999.

Grimsley, A. *Vital Conversations: Making the Impossible Conversation Possible.* Princes Risborough, Buckinghamshire: Barnes Holland Publishing, 2010.

Jones, J., Alfred, G., Kreps, L. and. Phillips, G. M. *Communicating with Your Doctor: Getting the Most Out of Health Care.* Cresskill, N.J.: Hampton Press, 1995.

Tannen, D. *"You Just Don't Understand": Women and Men in Conversation.* New York: HarperCollins, 1990.

Other Resources

☐ Check health and care professional registration. Tel: 0845 300 4472. www.checktheregister.org.uk.

☐ *General Medical Council.* A Pamphlet *What to Expect from Your Doctor: A Guide for Patients.* April 2013. www.gmc-uk.org.

☐ *NHS Choices.* www.nhs.uk.

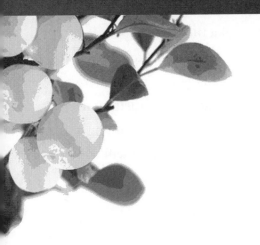

CHAPTER 10

Sex and Intimacy

LOVING RELATIONSHIPS WITH PHYSICAL INTIMACY and sexual pleasure are basic, human needs. However, many individuals and couples with physical or mental long-term conditions can face a challenge in maintaining this important part of their lives. Emotions, including fear of injury, of being unable to perform, or of causing a health emergency, can dampen desire in one or both partners. Likewise, fear of increasing the existing symptoms can frustrate couples, even if these symptoms occur only during sex itself. Sex, after all, is supposed to be joyful and pleasurable, not scary or uncomfortable.

For humans, sex is more than the act of sexual intercourse or achieving orgasm; it is also the sharing of our physical and emotional selves. There is a special intimacy when we make love. Believe it or not, having a health problem may actually offer the opportunity to *improve* your sex life by encouraging you to experiment with new types of physical and emotional stimulation. This process of exploring sensuality with your partner can open up communication and strengthen your relationship. Furthermore, when we have sex, natural *feel-good* hormones, including endorphins, are released into our bloodstream. These help us to achieve a deep sense of relaxation and feelings of well-being.

Facing Obstacles

For many people with long-term conditions, intercourse can be difficult because of the physical demands it places on our bodies. Intercourse increases the heart rate and breathing. It can therefore tax someone with limited energy or with breathing or circulatory problems. Some people can no longer find a sexual position which is comfortable. Others may find that pain, shortness of breath or fatigue during sex spoils their enjoyment and sometimes their ability to have an orgasm. If one person does enjoy the sex or has an orgasm, it can make the other person feel resentful. This situation can also make the first person feel some guilt. This is one area where communicating your fears, anxieties, frustrations and guilt is absolutely essential in maintaining a good relationship. This is something we will talk about in more detail later in this chapter.

Increasing Your Sensuality

Sensuality is helpful in relationship building. It can be good to spend more time on sensuality or foreplay and less on actual intercourse. By concentrating on ways to arouse your partner and give pleasure while in a comfortable position, your intimate time together can last longer and be very satisfying. Many people enjoy climax without intercourse; others may wish to climax with intercourse. For some, climax may not be as important as sharing the pleasure. There are many ways to enhance sensuality during sexual activity. In sex, as in most things, our minds and bodies are linked. By recognising this, we can increase the sexual pleasure we experience through both physical and mental stimulation.

Dealing with Your Emotional Concerns

Emotional concerns can also be a serious factor for someone with health problems. Someone who has had a heart attack or a stroke is often concerned that sexual activity will bring on another attack. Similarly, people with breathing difficulties worry that sex might be too strenuous and will trigger coughing, wheezing or something worse. Their partners may fear that sexual activity could cause problems or even result in death. For this, they would then feel that they have been irresponsible. Some diseases such as diabetes can make erections difficult or cause vaginal dryness. These worries can certainly test your relationship.

Coping with a Loss of Self-Esteem and a Changed Self-Image

Self-esteem and *self-image* can be subtle and create devastating sexual barriers. Many people with long-term health conditions believe that they are physically unattractive. This may be because of paralysis, shortness of breath, weight gain caused by medications, the changing shape of their joints, or the loss of a breast or other body part. Mental health problems can also damage people's sense of self, causing them to avoid sexual situations; they *try not to think about it.* Ignoring the sexual part of their relationship, or physically and emotionally distancing themselves from their partner, can cause problems.

For example, it can lead to depression, which in turn leads to further lack of interest in sex and more depression, creating a vicious cycle. However, depression can be treated, and you can feel better. For more on depression and how to help yourself overcome it, see Chapter 4. If self-management techniques are not enough then talk to your doctor or specialist nurse.

Even good sex can get better. Thankfully, there are ways you and your partner can explore sensuality and intimacy, as well as some ways to overcome fear during sex.

Overcoming Fear During Sex

Anyone who has a long term condition has without doubt at some stage experienced fear that it will worsen and that the deterioration could be life-threatening. Health problems can frequently get in the way of the activities that we want and need to do. When sex is the activity that fear invades, we have a difficult problem. At the same time as we are denying ourselves an important and pleasurable part of life, we are also feeling guilty about disappointing our partner. On the other hand, our partner may feel more fearful and guilty than we do; they may be experiencing fear that they might hurt us during sex and guilt about feeling resentful. This dynamic can cause serious relationship problems. The resulting stress and depression can produce even more symptoms. We don't have to allow this to happen.

For successful sexual relationships, the most important thing is communication. The most effective way to address the fears of both partners is to confront your fears and find ways to alleviate them through good communication and problem solving. Without effective communication, learning new positions and other ways to increase sensuality are not going to be enough. This is particularly important for people who worry about how their health problem makes them look to other people. Often they find that their partner is far less concerned about their looks than they are.

When you and your partner are comfortable with talking about sex, you can go about finding solutions. Start by sharing information about what kinds of physical stimulation you prefer

Misconceptions About Sex

Many of our sexual attitudes and beliefs are learned—they are not automatic or instinctual. We begin learning these when we are young. They come from friends, older children, parents, and other adults. We also learn them through jokes, magazines, TV, and films. Much of what we learn about sex is mixed up with our inhibitions; all those *shoulds*, *musts*, *should nots*, and *must nots*, are compounded by other misconceptions.

To maximise your sexual enjoyment, you often have to break down your misconceptions so that you are free to discover and explore your own sexuality. For example,

many people believe a number of things that simply are not true. For example:

- Older people can't enjoy sex.
- Sex is for people with beautiful bodies.
- A *real man* is always ready for sex.
- A *real woman* should be sexually available whenever her partner is interested.
- Love-making has to involve sexual intercourse.
- Sex must lead to orgasm.
- Orgasm should occur simultaneously in both partners.
- Kissing and touching should only be done when they lead to sexual intercourse.

and which positions you find most comfortable. Then, perhaps you can share the fantasies you find most arousing. It's difficult to dwell on other fears when your mind is occupied with a fantasy!

To get this process started, you and your partner may find some help with communication skills in Chapter 9 and in the problem-solving techniques dealt with in Chapter 2. Remember, if these techniques are new to you, give them time and practice. As with any new skill, it takes patience to learn.

Sensual Sex

In our society sexual attraction has become almost solely dependent on the visual experience. This leads to an emphasis on our physical image. Sight however, is only one of our five senses. Therefore, when we think about being sensual, we must also appreciate the seductive qualities of our partner's voice, scent, taste, and touch. Sensual sex is about connecting with our partner through all these senses, making love is not only achieved with the eyes, but with our ears, nose, mouth, and hands as well.

Sensual touch is particularly important because the largest sensual organ of our bodies is the skin; it is rich with sensory nerves. The right touch, on almost any area of our skin, can be very erotic. Fortunately, sexual stimulation through touch can be done in just about any position and can be enhanced with the use of oils, flavoured lotions, scents, feathers, fur gloves. Indeed, with whatever your imagination desires. Just about any part of the body is an erogenous zone. The most popular areas are the mouth, ear lobes, neck, breasts and nipples, the latter being pleasurable for both sexes. Also sensitive are the navel area and the hands, including the fingertips if you are giving pleasure and palms if you are receiving it. Your wrists, the small of your back, buttocks, toes, and the insides of the thighs and arms are all rich in sensation. Experiment with the type of touch you employ. Some people find a light touch arousing, while others prefer a firm touch. Many people also become very aroused when touched with the nose, lips, and tongue . . . or even by sex toys.

Sensuality with Fantasy

What goes on in our mind can be extremely arousing, too. If it weren't, there would be no strip clubs, sexy magazines or romance novels. Most people engage in sexual fantasy at some time or another. There are probably as many sexual fantasies as there are people. It is perfectly OK to indulge mentally in fantasy. If you discover a fantasy that you and your partner share, you can play it out in bed, even if it is as simple as a particular set of words that you or your partner like to hear during sex.

Engaging the mind during sexual activity can be every bit as arousing as physical stimulation. It is also useful when symptoms during sex interfere with your enjoyment. But you should also be careful, because fantasy can lead to unrealistic expectations. Your real partner might not compare favourably to your dream lover. You may also find decreased sexual satisfaction if you regularly fire up your imagination with explicit photos or videos of young, hard bodies.

Overcoming Symptoms During Sex

Some people are unable to find a sexual position that is completely comfortable. Others find that pain, shortness of breath, fatigue, or even negative thoughts during sex are so distracting that they interfere with the enjoyment or the ability to have an orgasm. This can pose some special problems. If you are unable to climax, you may feel resentful. On the other hand, if your partner is unable to climax, you may feel guilty about it. If you avoid sex because you are frustrated, your partner may become resentful and you may feel guilty. Your self-esteem will probably suffer. Your relationship with your partner will suffer, too. Everything suffers.

One thing you can do to deal with this situation is to time the taking of medication so that it is at peak effectiveness when you are ready to have sex. Of course, this involves planning ahead. The type of medication may be important too. If you take a narcotic-type pain reliever for example, or one containing muscle relaxants or tranquilisers, you may find that your sensory nerves are dulled along with your pain. Obviously, it would be counter-productive to dull the nerves that will give you pleasure. Your thinking may also be muddled because of your medication, making it more difficult to focus. Some medications can make it difficult for a man to achieve an erection;

others can help with an erection. Ask your doctor or pharmacist about timing or alternatives, if this is a problem for you.

Another way to deal with uncomfortable symptoms is to become an expert at fantasy. To be really good at something, you have to train for it, and this is no exception. The idea here, is to develop one or more sexual fantasies vividly in your mind, so that you can call it into use when needed. During sex, you can call up your fantasy and concentrate on it. By concentrating on the fantasy or on picturing you and your partner making love while you actually are, you are keeping your mind on your erotic thoughts rather than your symptoms or negative thoughts. However, if you have not had any experience in the visualisation and imagery techniques used for relaxation exercises, look at what has been written about this in Chapter 5. Remember that you will need to practise these techniques several times a week to learn them well. This practice need not be devoted solely to your chosen sexual fantasy. You can start with any guided imagery tape or script like those indicated in Chapter 5, and you should try to make it more vivid each time you practise.

Start with just picturing the images. When you get good at that, add and dwell on colours; then, in your mind, look down to your feet as you walk; then listen to the sounds around you;

then concentrate on the smells and tastes in the image and feel your skin being touched by the breeze or mist; finally, feel yourself touch things in the image. Work on one of your senses at a time. Become good at one of these before going on to another. Once you are proficient at imagery, you can invent your own sexual fantasy and picture it, hear it, smell it, and feel it. You can even begin your fantasy by picturing yourself setting your symptoms aside. The possibilities are limited only by your imagination.

Learning to call on this level of concentration can also help you focus on the moment. Focusing on your physical and emotional sensations during sex can be powerfully erotic. If your mind wanders, which is normal, gently bring yourself back to the here and now.

However, it is important not try to overcome chest pain or a sudden weakness on one side of the body in this way. These symptoms should not be ignored, and a doctor should be consulted straight away.

If, in the end, you decide that you wish to abstain from sexual activity because of your long-term health problem, or if it is not an important part of your life, then that's OK. However, it is very important that your partner is in agreement with your decision. Good communication skills are essential in this situation, and you may even benefit from discussing this matter with a professional therapist or counsellor.

Sexual Positions

Finding a comfortable sexual position can minimise your symptoms during sex. Doing so can also minimise the fear of pain or injury for both partners. Experimentation may be the best way

of finding the right positions for you and your partner. Everyone is different; no one position is good for everyone. We encourage you to experiment with different positions, possibly doing so before you and your partner are too aroused. Experiment with the placement of pillows or with using a sitting position on a chair. Experimentation can itself be erotic.

No matter which position you try, it is often helpful to do some warm-up exercises before sex. Look at some of the stretching exercises in Chapter 7. Exercise can help your sex life in other ways as well. Becoming fitter is an excellent way to increase comfort and endurance during sex. Thus improved fitness from exercises such as walking, swimming, cycling, and

other activities can benefit you in bed, as well as elsewhere, by reducing your shortness of breath, fatigue, and pain. They also help you to learn your limits and how to pace yourself, just as in any other physical activity.

During sexual activity, it may be advisable to change positions once in a while. This is especially true if your symptoms increase when you stay in one position too long. This can be done in a playful fashion, whereby it becomes fun for both of you. As with any exercise, stopping to rest is OK.

Special Considerations

People with certain health problems have specific concerns about sex and intimacy. For example, people who are recovering from a heart attack or stroke are often afraid to resume sexual relations for fear of not being able to perform, or of bringing on another attack. This fear is even more common in their partners. Fortunately, there is no basis for this fear, and sexual relations can be resumed as soon as you feel ready to do so. Studies show that the risk of sexual activity contributing to a heart attack is small. And this risk is even lower in individuals who do regular physical exercise. After a stroke, any remaining paralysis or weakness may require a little more attention to: finding the best positions for support and comfort; and identifying most sensitive areas of the body to caress. There may also be concerns about bowel and bladder control. The *British Heart Foundation* (www.bhf.org.uk) has some excellent guides about sex following a heart attack. The *Stroke Association* also has a leaflet that you can

find on-line at www.stroke.org.uk/factsheet/sex-after-stroke. This contains some very useful and easily understood guidance

People with diabetes sometimes report problems with sexual function. Men may have difficulty achieving or maintaining an erection, which can be caused by medication side-effects or other medical conditions associated with diabetes. Both women and men can have neuropathy, or reduced feeling, in the genital area. Women's most common complaint is not enough vaginal lubrication. For people with diabetes, the most effective ways to prevent or lessen these problems is to maintain tight management of blood glucose levels and exercise. Also, keeping a positive outlook and generally taking good care of themselves.

Lubricants can help with sensitivity for both men and women. If you are using condoms, be sure to use a water-based lubricant as petroleum-based lubricants destroy latex. The use of a vibrator can be very helpful for individuals with neuropathy. Concentrating the vibrator on the most sensual parts of the body for stimulation can help make sex pleasurable. There are new therapies for men with erectile problems. *Diabetes UK* (www.diabetes.org.uk) has considerable detailed information about sex and diabetes.

Persistent or recurring pain can dampen sexual interest. It can be difficult to feel sexy when you are hurting and are afraid that sex will make it worse. Pain is often the main symptom of arthritis, migraine headaches, bowel disease, and many other disorders. People with these conditions have the challenge of overcoming pain in order to become sexually aroused or to have an orgasm. This is one area where concentration and focus, as discussed earlier in this chapter, are helpful skills. Learning to focus on the moment, or on a sexual fantasy, can distract you from the pain and allow you to concentrate on sex and your partner. Time your pain medication in order to have favourable conditions during sex, find a comfortable position, take it slowly, be at ease with yourself, relax and enjoy extended foreplay.

People who are missing a breast, testicle, or another body part as a result of their treatment for cancer or some other medical condition; and people with surgical scars or swollen or disfigured joints from arthritis, may also have fears about sex and intimacy. In these cases, people often worry about what their partner thinks. Will their partner find them undesirable? Although this may sometimes happen, it actually occurs less often than you think. Usually when we fall in love with someone, we fall in love with who that person is, not with that

person's breast, testicle, or other body part. Here again, good communication and the sharing of your concerns and fears with your partner can help. If this is difficult to take on alone, perhaps talking with a counsellor may help. Often what you think is a problem, really isn't.

Fatigue is another symptom that can kill sexual desire. In Chapter 4 we talked a lot about how to deal with fatigue. Here we will add one more piece of advice: plan your sexual activities around your fatigue; that is, try to engage in sex during the times when you are less tired. This might mean that mornings are better than evenings.

Many mental health conditions and the medications used to treat the symptoms can interfere with sexual function and desire. Therefore, it is important to talk with your doctor about these side effects so that together you can find alternatives. Sometimes, the doctor may find another medication, change the dosage or timing of the medication. In other circumstances, the doctor may refer you to a therapist who can help you and your partner learn other coping strategies which will decrease or eliminate symptoms. In addition, individual or joint therapy can also help in dealing with other personal relationship, intimacy, and sexual problems.

No matter what your long-term health problem, your doctor should be the first person to consult for sexual problems related to your chronic condition. It's unlikely that your problem is unique; your doctor has probably heard about it many times before and may have some solutions. Remember, this is just another problem associated with your condition, just like fatigue, pain, and physical limitations. It is a problem that can be addressed because health problems need not end your sex life. Through good communication and planning, satisfying sex can prevail. By being creative and willing to experiment, taking pleasure in sex can actually improve your relationship.

Suggested Further Reading

Agravat, P. *A Guide to Sexual and Erectile Dysfunction in Men.* Leicester: Troubador, 2010.

Ford, V. *Overcoming Sexual Problems.* London: Constable & Robinson, 2010.

Hall, K. *Reclaiming Your Sexual Self: How You Can Bring Desire Back into Your Life.* Hoboken, N.J.: Wiley, 2004.

Kaufman, M., Silverburg, C. and Odette, F. *The Ultimate Guide to Sex and Disability: For All of Us Who Live with Disabilities, Chronic Pain, and Illness.* Berkeley, Calif.: Cleis Press, 2007.

McCarthy, B. W. and Metz, M. E. *Men's Sexual Health: Fitness for Satisfying Sex.* New York: Routledge, Taylor & Francis, 2008.

Schnarch, D. *Intimacy and Desire: Awaken the Passion in Your Relationship.* New York: Beaufort Books, 2009.

Other Resources

- ☐ *Arthritis Care.* www.arthritiscare.org.uk.

- ☐ *Association to aid the Sexual and Personal Relationships of People with a Disability* (SPOD).

- ☐ *British Heart Foundation.* www.bhf.org.uk.

- ☐ *Diabetes UK.* www.diabetes.org.uk.

- ☐ *Different Strokes.* This is an organisation which supports younger stroke survivors. www.differentstrokes.co.uk.

- ☐ *The Stroke Association.* www.stroke.org.uk/factsheet/sex-after-stroke.

Note: Many of the voluntary patient organisations, specific to your condition, have information. and advice on sexual relationships for people living with a long term condition.

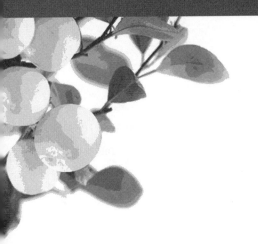

CHAPTER 11

Healthy Eating

Eating is important to all of us and eating healthily is one of the cornerstones for managing your condition. It is a central factor that influences your health. *Eating healthily* means that most of the time you make good, healthy food choices. It does not mean being rigid or perfect. It can mean finding new or different ways to prepare your meals which makes them tasty and appealing. If you have certain health conditions, you may have to be more aware of your food choices. Eating well does not usually mean that you can never eat the foods you like most. One of the few exceptions to this is where the food may interact with your medication, like eating fresh grapefruit when taking certain statins. There is more about these interactions later in this chapter on pages 189–192, where you will find more eating information for those with the most common long-term health conditions

Special thanks to Bonnie Bruce, DrPH, RD, for her help with this chapter.

173

Unfortunately, because of the Internet, new and rapidly changing research, books, other media, friends, and relatives, we can get overloaded and confused with information about what we should and should not eat. In this chapter we provide you with some simple, *science-based nutrition and diet information*. We are not going to tell you what to eat or how to eat. That is *your* decision. We will tell you what is known about nutrition for adults, and suggest some ways to help you apply this information to your specific likes and needs. We hope that this chapter will help you to make changes which will lead to healthier eating. Where appropriate we will point out any specific issues for those who are *vegetarians* or *vegans* and those whose *culture* determines some parts of their food in-take.

Why is Healthy Eating So Important?

The human body is a very complex and marvellous machine, much like a motor car. Motor cars need the proper mix of fuel in order to run well. Without it, they may not run efficiently and may even stop working. The human body is similar. It needs the proper mix of good food, or *fuel*, to keep it running well.

- You have more energy and feel less tired.

- You increase your chances of preventing or lessening further problems from health conditions such as heart disease, diabetes, and cancer.

- You feed your brain, which can help you to handle life's challenges and its emotional ups and downs.

- You can control your weight.

- You can prevent the side-effects from medication.

- You can control your blood pressure.

- You can keep your bones and kidneys functioning properly.

What is Healthy Eating?

Healthy eating is about making sensible changes, including the following:

1. *Being flexible:* At the heart of healthy eating are the long-term choices we make. Healthy eating is about being flexible, for example by allowing you to occasionally enjoy small amounts of foods that may not be too healthy. There is no such thing as a perfect eating plan. Being too strict or rigid and not allowing yourself ever to have a treat will probably cause even your best efforts to fail.

2. *Being selective and careful:* For some of us, healthy eating means being choosy about the foods we eat. For example, people with diabetes need to watch their carbohydrate intake in order to manage their

blood glucose levels. Others, who already have, or are at risk of having heart disease, will find that watching the amounts and kinds of fat they eat can help control their blood cholesterol levels. Those with high blood pressure will find that they can lower it by eating lots of fruits, vegetables, low-fat dairy foods and, for some people, cutting back on salt. Salt is an interesting case. It is made up of two components *sodium* and *chloride*. It is the sodium in salt that can lead to health problems. There are, in fact 2.4 grams of sodium in every six grams of salt. Rather confusingly, food labels sometimes use *salt* or *sodium* as though they are interchangeable, and it is important that you know the difference. By the end of 2014 only salt will be listed on food labels and sodium will not. In addition, if we are to lose or gain weight, we also need to pay attention to how many calories we eat.

3. *Changing your ideas about a good diet:* We have come a long ways since meat and potatoes were thought of as the backbone of a great diet. Today, vegetables, fruits, whole grains, low-fat milk and low-fat milk products, lean meats, poultry, and fish are at the core of a good diet. There is still a place for meat and potatoes; but it is no longer the most important place.

4. *Making healthy choices:* The real issue for most of us is not the healthy foods we choose but the less healthy ones. The less healthy choices that we sometimes make can mean that our food intake consists of too much added sugar, too much solid fat

and too much sodium. These sugars, fats, and sodium components contribute to health problems such as high blood pressure, diabetes, and obesity. In addition, we tend to eat a lot of food that is made from white flour and other refined grains.

Achieving the Right Balance

Trade-offs form a big part of healthy eating. This means learning how food affects you and then deciding when you can treat yourself and when not to do so. For instance, it may be important for you to have a very special meal on your birthday, but then you can trade off by making healthier choices when you are out for a casual lunch. *Trading off* is a tool that can help you to stay on the healthy eating path. As you get better at this, you will find it gets easier and becomes part of your everyday life.

Most dietary guidelines suggest that a good starting place is to move toward eating more plant foods: that is foods such as whole grains, fruits, vegetables, cooked dry beans and peas, lentils, nuts, and seeds. This does *not* mean giving up meats and other foods high in sugar, fat or sodium completely, but rather eating them in smaller amounts, or less often. Balancing the kinds of foods you eat and how much are the primary elements of healthy eating. We'll return to this a little later in this chapter. This all sounds very simple, but every day we are faced with hundreds of food choices. It is often easier and quicker to grab something less healthy than to *think about* what we will eat, let alone cook! So how do we put together meals that are tasty and enjoyable, yet healthy? Let's look at some key principles.

Key Principles of Healthy Eating

Choose Foods as Nature Originally Made Them

This means the less processed they are the better. By *processed* we mean foods that have been changed from their original state by having ingredients added such as sugar or fat or ingredients such as fibre or nutrients removed. The object of the manufacturer is to make them tastier, so whole grains are made into white flour for bakery products, and animal products are made into cold or sliced meats. Foods that are the least processed include: grilled chicken breast instead of fried breaded chicken nuggets; a baked potato with the skin on rather than chips; and whole-grain bread, pasta and brown rice, instead of refined grains like white bread and white rice. There are many examples of how eating unprocessed food can improve your health but one example is the reduction in your salt intake. Processed foods are usually high in salt, so a reduction in their consumption can mean a substantial reduction in your salt intake.

Get your nutrients from food rather than supplements

We know that for most people, vitamins, minerals, and other dietary supplements cannot completely take the place of food. Foods, as nature makes them, contain nutrients and other healthy compounds, such as fibre in the right combinations and amounts to make the body work properly. When we remove nutrients from their natural state in food, they may not work the way they should. They may even have harmful side-effects.

Take for example *beta carotene*, an important source of vitamin A which is found in plant foods such as carrots and winter squash. It helps our vision and enhances our immune system. However, artificial beta-carotene supplements have been shown to increase some cancer risks for some of us. This same risk does not happen when beta carotene is eaten in its natural form.

In the UK there are now a huge range of dietary supplements which makes this area a minefield for consumers.

This is a direct quotation from *NHS Choices*. Depending on how a supplement is classified, it will be subject to different regulations. Some will be considered as foods and regulated by the *Food Standards Agency* and the *Department of Health*. Others will be regulated as medicines, by the *Medicines and Healthcare Regulatory Agency* (MHRA). To further complicate the regulatory system, the European Union has a system which regulates traditional medicines. If this is an area you are particularly interested in, a good resource for clarification is the report *Supplements who needs them? A Behind the Headlines Report*, www.nhs.uk/news/2011/05May.

You might ask whether there is ever a place for dietary supplements. The answer is yes, because sometimes we cannot get enough of one or more of the nutrients we need. For example, older men and women require a large amount of calcium to help to prevent or slow osteoporosis. Although we used to get enough calcium from milk and milk products such as yoghurt or cheese, getting the amount needed can be difficult for some people.

If you are thinking of taking a supplement, talk to your GP first. They will be aware of your condition and the medications you are already taking, and most importantly they will know whether there is a need for you to take any supplements.

Eat a wide variety of colourful and minimally processed foods

The more variety in your food, the better; the more colours on your plate, the better; and the less processed your food, the better. By following these simple rules, your body will probably get all the good things it needs. This means a plate that contains minimally processed meat, fish, or poultry and a lot of colourful fruits and vegetables. Think blue and purple for grapes and blueberries; think yellow and orange for pineapple, oranges, and carrots; think red for tomatoes, strawberries, and watermelon; and think green for spinach and green beans. This colourful mix, taken along with the white and warm brown tones from mushrooms, onions, cauliflower and whole grains such as brown rice will be fine. An important benefit of eating colourful fruits and vegetables is that the different coloured fruit and vegetables contain their own combinations of vitamins and minerals. Eating a healthy diet eliminates the need for most people to take supplements.

Eat foods high in phyto-chemicals

Phyto-chemicals are compounds that are found only in plant foods such as, fruits, vegetables, whole grains, nuts, and seeds. The *phyto* part of the word means *plant*. There are hundreds of health-promoting and disease-fighting phyto-chemicals. These include the compounds that give fruits and vegetables their bright colours. Whenever a food is refined or processed, as when whole wheat is made into white flour, phyto-chemicals are lost. The more often you choose foods that are not refined, and close to how nature made them, the better. One of the benefits of eating phyto-chemicals is that there is some research which clearly indicates that naturally occurring substances in phyto-chemicals can contribute toward the reduction in certain diseases.

Eat regularly

A petrol fuelled vehicle will not run without the petrol, and a fire eventually burns out without more wood. Your body is much the same. It needs refuelling regularly to work at its best. Eating something, even a little bit, at regular intervals helps to keep your *'fire'* burning.

Eating at regular times during the day, preferably evenly spaced over time, also helps to maintain and balance your blood glucose level. Blood glucose is a key player in supplying the body, and especially the brain, with energy. If you do not eat regularly, your blood glucose drops, and depending on how low it gets, can cause weakness, sweating, shaking, and mood changes such as irritability, anxiety, and also anger, nausea, headaches, or poor coordination. Low blood glucose (*hypoglycaemia*) can be dangerous for many people.

Eating regularly means that you get the nutrients you need and also it helps your body to use those nutrients. Of course, not skipping meals, and not letting too many hours slip by between meals also helps keep you from getting overly hungry. Being *too* hungry can often lead to over-eating. This can in turn lead to such problems as indigestion, heartburn, and weight gain. One of the positive outcomes of eating regularly is that it can boost your metabolism, thereby helping your weight control.

Finally, eating regularly does not mean that you must stick to the same routine every day. Nor does it mean that you must follow the *normal* pattern of eating three meals a day. Allow yourself room for some give and take. If you have certain health conditions, such as cancer, you may find that several small meals over the day work better for you, whilst at other times fewer, bigger meals might work better. For people with diabetes, spacing meals regularly and balancing what they eat is important, but this could mean several small meals a day, or three meals mixed with a snack, or just three meals.

Which of these options is decided on depends on what suits you best.

Eat what your body needs no more and no less

This is easy to say but more difficult to put into practice. How much you should eat depends on things like the following:

- *Your age:* You need fewer calories as you get older.

- *If you are a man or woman:* Men usually need more calories than women.

- *Your body size and shape:* In general, if you are taller or have more muscle, you can eat more.

- *Your health needs:* Some conditions affect how your body uses calories.

- *Your activity level:* the more you move or exercise, the more calories you can eat.

Tips to Help You Manage Your Eating

- *Stop eating as soon as you feel full:* This helps you control the amount you eat and helps to prevent you over-eating. Pay attention to your body so you can learn what this feels like. Like all new skills, it takes some practice. If it is hard to stop eating when you *begin* to feel full, remove your plate or get up from the table and move away.

- *Eat slowly:* Eating slowly gives you more enjoyment and helps prevent over-eating. Make your meals last at least 15 to 20 minutes. It takes this much time for the brain to catch up and tell your stomach that it is getting full. If you finish quickly, wait at least 15 minutes before getting more food. If this is difficult, we have offered some more tips on pages 198–199.

- *Pay attention to what you eat:* If you are not fully aware of what you are doing, it is easy to eat an entire bag of crisps or packet of biscuits or too much of any bite-sized pieces of food, without even knowing it. This can happen easily when we are with friends, using the computer, or watching television. In these situations, portion out what you want to eat, or alternatively keep food out of reach and out of sight.

A Note About Breakfast

Breakfast is just what It says, *breaking your fast*. It refuels your body after going without eating for many hours and helps you to resist the urge to eat extra snacks or over-eat during the rest of the day.

We know that you may not want to eat breakfast. This probably not only because you don't have the time or aren't hungry, but maybe because you don't like the usual breakfast foods. There are no set rules about what you should eat in the morning. Breakfast can be anything, fruit, beans, rice, bread, broccoli, or even left-overs. The important thing is to kick-start your body each day by refuelling it with healthy foods.

■ *Know a portion size when you see one:* You need to know a little about what a portion size looks like. This is different for every food but please note the only *exact* portion size recommended by the Department of Health is the five fruits and vegetables a day. Here are some examples of food portion sizes:

- A slice of bread is one portion.

- Half a bread roll is one portion.

- A small, four-inch pancake is one portion.

- One portion of vegetables is 80 grams, or about three heaped tablespoons.

- One portion of fruit is one apple or about 80 grams.

However each person needs a certain number of calories a day to lead a healthy life. The number *you* need depends on your age, gender, and crucially, your lifestyle particularly whether you are active or sedentary. Of course, it also depends sometimes on your medical condition. Whatever the number of calories you need they should come from the *Eatwell Plate* in the portions indicated in the next section. So, if for example someone needs 2000 calories per day, approximately a third of these calories, round about 667, should come from fruit and vegetables.

It can sound a bit like a mathematical exercise to get portions right for each meal but with time and practice it will become second nature to you. You do not have to get the portions accurate for every single meal: balance them out for the day or even over a few days. In this way, you can cope if you have a special celebration meal coming up.

■ *Watch out for portion inflation:* In recent years, serving sizes have rather *beefed up*. The typical adult cheeseburger used to have about 330 calories; now it has a whopping 590 calories, almost twice the amount. Twenty years ago, an average biscuit was about 1½ inches wide and had 55 calories; now it is 3½ inches wide and has 275 calories, or *five times* the amount!

It takes an extra 3,500 calories more than we need to gain a pound of body fat. This means that over one year an extra

100 calories a day will cause you to put on 10 pounds. This is equivalent to eating an extra thick slice of white bread every day over a year. Also, watch out for plate sizes. Larger plates will encourage or deceive you about the amount of food you actually have in front of you.

■ *Whenever it's practical, select single-size portions:* Foods that come pre-packaged as single portions, sometimes labelled as *single servings*, can help you to see what a suggested portion should look like. If that portion size seems too small compared to what you usually eat, we suggest that you start slowly. Reduce how much you now eat by just a small amount gradually, over time. For example, if you usually eat four tablespoons of rice, see if you can eat three tablespoons instead.

■ *Make your food attractive:* We really do eat with our eyes! Compare the appeal of a plate with white fish, white rice, and white cauliflower with another containing golden brown chicken, baked sweet potato, and bright green spinach. Which of these two meals seems more mouth-watering to you?

An Easy Map for Healthy Eating: The *Eatwell Plate*

Eating a variety of foods is not as complicated as you might think if you use the *Eatwell Plate* method. This is something many of you will already be familiar with. The *Eatwell Plate* is a pictorial summary of the main food groups that highlights the different types of food that make up your diet and shows the proportions you should eat in *each day* in order to have a well-balanced and healthy diet. It is a method built on dietary advice from the Department of Health.

Use the *Eatwell Plate* to help your get your food balance right. There are some special circumstances where you will need to check with your doctor or a registered dietician to decide whether the *Eatwell Plate* is appropriate for your condition. Situations in which you should be careful, might include when you are trying, on medical advice, to gain weight; or perhaps you are someone who has been diagnosed with diabetes. Later in the book there is a specific chapter (Chapter 18) on self-management for people with diabetes and the subject of their nutrition needs are dealt with in more detail there.

The *Eatwell Plate* is suitable for vegetarians and meat eaters and for people of all ethnic origins.

Use the *Eatwell Plate* to help you get your food balance right. It shows how much of what you eat each day should come from each of five food groups.

The plate is divided into five sections:

1. Fruit and vegetables. Aim for at least 5 portions of a variety of fruit and vegetables a day. Remember not to include potatoes in this category as they count as starchy foods.

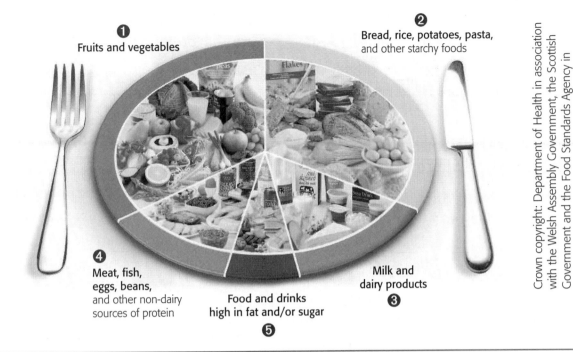

Figure 11.1 **The Eatwell Plate**

2. Bread, rice, potatoes, and pasta and other starchy foods. Choose whole-grain varieties where you can.

3. About a fifth of the plate is for milk and dairy products and/or calcium-fortified soya milk.

4. The next smaller section is for meat, fish, eggs, and other non-dairy sources of protein such as beans and pulses.

5. The smallest section is for foods or drinks high in fat and/or sugar.

Nutrients: What the Body Needs

What are nutrients? Earlier we talked about the need to get nutrients from food. The body extracts what it needs from what we eat but does not recognise the precise food it is getting. When the food goes into our mouth the digestive system takes over and breaks it down into various nutrients which it then processes, or *metabolises,* to keep us warm, alive and well. Nutrients are made up of carbohydrates, fats, protein, water, and a few vitamins and minerals.

In addition, although it is technically not a nutrient, we will also talk about *fibre.* Fortunately, it is quite easy to get all the things that we need by eating healthily.

How much: The big question for any individual is, *how much do I need to eat a day to be healthy?* An average man needs around 2500 calories a day to maintain his weight and for the average woman, it is around 2000 calories a day. As previously pointed out these values will vary depending on age, height, levels of physical activity, and the effects of some medications and certain medical conditions. Let's look at the actual nutrients involved in a bit more detail.

Carbohydrates: Your Body's Chief Energy Source

What are carbohydrates and what do they do?

Our digestive system extracts and uses carbohydrate as the major source of energy for our bodily processes. We measure the heat that any one food can produce in our body in calories. Accordingly, we need to eat a high proportion of food containing carbohydrates to keep our basic body temperature steady and generate the energy to move around.

Kinds of carbohydrates

You should note that there are two types of carbohydrate that we consume:

- *Starches, or complex carbohydrates,* are to be found in grains, rice, pasta, breads, peas and beans, root vegetables such as potatoes and carrots, and other vegetables. Complex carbohydrates take time to digest, so they help to keep blood glucose levels constant. *This is what we want.*

- *Simple carbohydrates or sugars,* are to be found in fruits and some dairy products and they are quickly absorbed. We need to watch our intake of these, especially processed foods which are made with refined or table sugar, honey, syrups and jams. These foods raise blood glucose levels quickly and then let them drop. *This is not what we need to happen.*

Which foods do we get our carbohydrates from?

Given that carbohydrates provide much of the energy we need for movement, starchy carbohydrates should form a main part of your meal. This group includes, bread, rolls, chapattis, breakfast cereals, oats, pasta, noodles, rice, potatoes, sweet potatoes, plantains and green bananas, beans and lentils. It also includes dishes made from maize and millet. However, you should avoid potato crisps because they are high in both salt and fat. Potatoes are, of course, vegetables but because they are so starchy they have been put into this group. They only continue to be included as a carbohydrate if you don't cover them in butter, salt or oil. The wholegrain varieties of starchy foods not only provide you with sustained energy over several hours but are also a good source of fibre. To summarise, about one third of what you eat should come from the carbohydrate group.

Why is fibre important?

Fibre does not quite fit into a food group, but it is nevertheless essential for healthy eating. During digestion your food moves steadily through your digestive system making use of all the nutrients. The muscular activity to keep things moving is helped by the right sort of fibrous bulk, which will then be discarded at the end of the process. If you eat very refined food with no fibrous husks or vegetables left in it, your body will have trouble moving the unusable or toxic matter. Therefore waste may stay in your system longer than is healthy and may produce uncomfortable symptoms. Fibre can also help to prevent heart disease, weight gain, diabetes and some cancers, particularly rectal and colon

Tips for Choosing Healthier Carbohydrates and Increasing Your Fibre Intake

- *Ensure that at least half of the grains you eat are whole grains,* such as brown rice, whole-grain breads and rolls, whole-grain pasta.

- *Choose foods with whole wheat or a whole grain,* like oats, listed first on the ingredients list on the food label.

- *Choose dried beans and peas, lentils, or whole-grain pasta* instead of meat, or as a side dish. Do this at least a few times each week.

- *Choose whole fruit* rather than fruit juice. Whole fruit contains fibre, takes longer to eat, fills you up better than juice and can help keep you from over-eating.

- *Choose higher-fibre breakfast cereals* such as shredded wheat or raisin bran.

- *Eat higher-fibre crisp-bread.* Choose whole rye or multi-grain crackers, especially those containing sesame, pumpkin or sunflower seeds.

- *Add fibre to your diet,* but do it gradually over a period of weeks. Drink plenty of water to process fibre and prevent constipation.

cancer. Most people in the UK do not eat sufficient fibre, a minimum of around 14 grams a day. In fact, 18 grams is the recommended amount to aim for, but you can build this up slowly if your normal intake is very low.

What foods are sources of fibre?

Fibre is found naturally in whole or minimally processed plant foods which have *skins, seeds, and strings.* Some foods have added fibre, for example when pulp is added to fruit juice. There are two types of fibre, *soluble fibre* and *insoluble fibre,* and these can help your body in different ways:

- *Insoluble fibre which does not dissolve:* This acts like nature's broom. It keeps your digestive system moving and helps to prevent constipation. Foods with insoluble fibre include fruit and vegetables with skins and pips, nuts and wholegrain cereals such as wheat, rye and rice.

- *Soluble fibre which is able to dissolve:* This type of fibre is broken down by the natural bacteria in your bowels, making your stools softer and larger. Foods that contain soluble fibre include oats, barley, pulses such as peas and beans, and fruit and vegetables. Some years ago this type of fibre was presumed not to have any calories but this has changed and it is now becoming mandatory to include the number of calories from this source in food labelling. However, the number of calories involved is very small, at approximately two calories per gram.

Fruit and vegetables usually contain a mixture of these soluble and insoluble fibres.

Oils and Solid Fats: The Good, the Bad, and the Deadly

Most of us think that *all* fat is bad for us. But we all need some fat for survival and for your body to work properly. Fat can also be used almost without limit by our bodies to store energy as body fat.

Although all fats for the same portion size have the same number of calories, some fats are healthier than others. These healthy fats we call *good* fats, and some can be harmful if we eat too much, these are the *bad* fats.

■ **The good fats** are called *unsaturated fats.* These are mostly oils that are liquid at room temperature. They help keep our cells healthy, and some can help to reduce blood cholesterol. Good fats include soybean, sweet corn, peanut, sunflower, canola, and olive oils. Nuts, seeds, and olives, and the oils they contain, are also good. Avocados too, are rich in good fats.

There is another group of good fats, the *omega-3s*, which can be helpful for some people in reducing the risk of heart disease and may help with rheumatoid arthritis symptoms. These fats are found in deep-water fish such as salmon, mackerel, trout, and tuna. Other sources of omega-3s include wheat germ, flaxseed, and walnuts. It is thought possible that the body may not use omega-3s from plants as well as it does from the fish sources.

■ **The bad fats** which are called *saturated fats*, are usually solid at room temperature as, for example in butter, lard, and bacon.

This fat can increase blood cholesterol and the risk of heart disease. Most bad fats are found in animal foods such as butter, beef fat, suet, chicken fat, and pork fat. Other foods that are high in bad fats include margarines, red meat, fatty minced meat, processed meats such as sausage, bacon, and cooked meats, poultry skin, and any cheese including cream cheese and sour cream. Palm kernel oil, coconut oil, and cocoa butter are also considered bad fats.

■ **The deadly fats** are known as *trans-fats.* They have more harmful effects on our blood cholesterol and in increasing the risk of heart disease than even the bad fats. Trans-fats are found in many processed foods, including pastries, cakes, biscuits, icing, margarine, and most microwave popcorn.

These fats are listed on food labels as *partially hydrogenated* or *hydrogenated* oils. There are no current legal requirements by food manufacturers to label trans-fats. This means that *you* must check the list of ingredients for hydrogenated fats or hydrogenated oils. If a food contains either of these it will probably contain trans-fats. Some manufacturers have stopped using hydrogenated fats or reduced the level of trans-fats in their food. They may be labelled *low in trans.*

The daily guidelines recommended by the NHS suggest that the average man should eat no more than 30 grams of saturated fat a day and the average woman no more than 20 grams and of this, trans-fats should be no more than 5 grams per day.

Tips for Choosing Good Fats and Healthier Fats

When choosing your foods:

- *Eat more poultry* such as chicken or turkey. *Eat less red meat* such as beef, lamb, venison, mutton and pork. Keep your cooked portions of meat, fish and poultry to around two or three ounces, or approximately 56–85 grams.

- *Remove the skin* on poultry, duck and turkey before cooking.

- *Eat more deep-water fish,* such as salmon, tuna, and mackerel.

- *Choose leaner cuts* of meat such as sirloin, or flank.

- *Trim off all any fat* you can see from meat before cooking it.

- *Use semi-skimmed or skimmed milk* or non-dairy products such as soya milk, and low fat or fat free dairy foods. These latter foods will include the low fat versions of cheese, sour cream, cottage cheese, yoghurt, and ice cream.

- *Use oil such as olive or sunflower oil, and soft margarines,* instead of shortening, lard, butter, or margarine in your cooking and baking

When preparing foods:

- *Measure the oil in tablespoons,* rather than pouring from the container

- *Use a non-stick pan,* or a pan requiring only small amounts of cooking oil spray.

- *Boil, grill, microwave, poach, bake or steam* when preparing meats or fish.

- *Avoid frying* or deep frying foods.

- *Skim off the fat* from stews and soups during cooking. If you refrigerate them overnight, the solid fat will lift off easily.

- *Choose low fat versions* of sausages and other meat products.

- *Use less* butter, margarine, gravies, meat-based and cream sauces, spreads, and creamy salad dressings.

- *Reduce or cut out spreads like margarine* when eating things like beans on toast.

The best recommendation is to eat very little bad and deadly fats and to replace them with the good fats, without increasing the overall amount of fat you eat.

There is one more thing you should know about fat. All fats contain twice the calories per teaspoon as protein or carbohydrate. Calories from fat add up quickly. For instance, 1 teaspoon of sugar has about 20 calories, but 1 teaspoon of oil or solid fat has about 35 calories. When we eat more calories than we need, no matter where they come from, the extra calories will be stored as body fat, and will result in weight gain.

Protein: Muscle Builder and More

How is protein used in the body?

Protein is vital for hundreds of activities that keep you lively and healthy. Protein is part of your red blood cells and of the enzymes and hormones that help to regulate your body and your muscles. It helps your immune system to fight infection and builds and repairs damaged tissues. Protein can also give you some energy. But like fat, protein is not as good a source of energy for your body as carbohydrate.

Kinds of proteins: complete and incomplete

There are two types of proteins, distinguished by how they are built.

- *Complete proteins* have all the right parts in the right amounts. Your body uses them just as they are. Complete proteins are found in animal foods for example in meat, fish, poultry, eggs, milk and other dairy products, as well as in soy foods such as soybeans, tofu, and tempeh.

- *Incomplete proteins* are low in one or more parts. They are found in plant foods such as grains, dried beans and peas, lentils, nuts, and seeds. Most fruits and vegetables contain much less protein. For your body to be able to use incomplete proteins well, you should eat them with at least one other incomplete protein or with a complete protein.

Combining complete and incomplete proteins

Over the centuries, people have learned to survive by eating protein combinations. Two of the most plentiful and commonly eaten incomplete protein pairs are *beans with rice* and *peanut butter with bread*. Although nearly all plant proteins are incomplete proteins, they are still at the heart of healthy eating. By eating a small amount of an animal protein, like chicken with a plant food such as lentils or black beans, you end up with all the benefits of a complete protein. In addition, some plant foods, such as nuts and seeds, are sources of good fats, and many plant foods are good sources of fibre. Plant foods have no cholesterol and contain little or no trans-fats.

How much protein should we eat?

The good news is that most people eat more than enough protein. Unless you have a special medical condition, there is no need to be concerned. Unfortunately, many people get most of their protein from meat, which tends to be high in bad fats. The best way to get protein is mainly from plant foods along with small amounts of lean meat, poultry and fish.

Vitamins and Minerals

Why do we need vitamins and minerals?

Vitamins help to regulate the body's inner workings. Minerals are part of many cells and cause important reactions in the body. All vitamins and minerals are essential for survival and health, and most of us can get all we need from healthy eating. But some minerals, sodium, potassium, and calcium stand out and deserve our special attention. This is because they are related to some current health problems, and many of us eat either too much or too little of these nutrients.

Sodium and salt

What is sodium? Salt is made up of two components: *sodium* and *chloride*. It is the sodium in salt that can lead to health problems. There are about 2.4 grams of sodium in six grams of salt. When looking at food labels pay particular attention to whether the word *salt* or *sodium* is used.

Why do we need sodium or salt?

We all need a little bit of salt because it helps to keep our bodily fluids at the right concentration. However the majority of us eat more salt than we need. If you do so, then your volume of bodily fluids will increase and push up your blood pressure. High blood pressure can then lead to serious problems such as heart disease or stroke.

Salt recommendations

On average, people in the UK eat about 8.1 grams of salt per day: that is equivalent to 3.2 grams of sodium. A healthy amount is no more than six grams of salt, or 2.4 grams of sodium each day.

Some tips for reducing your salt intake

Here are five tips to help you to reduce your salt intake:

■ *Salt is often a hidden ingredient in our food so it can be difficult to work out how much we are actually eating:* Some foods, like crisps or bacon, clearly taste salty so you can remove them easily from your diet. However, many ready-made foods have salt added to them. This surprisingly includes sweet foods like biscuits as well as the more obvious foods like bread.

■ *Ready-made foods are the source of approximately 75% of our salt intake:* This means

we must get into the habit of reading the food labels. As a guide, for every 100 gram serving:

◆ 1.5 grams, or 0.6 grams of sodium would be a *high* amount of salt.

◆ 0.3 grams or 0.1 grams of sodium would be a *low* amount of salt.

■ *Use less of foods which are high in salt:* For example, try to consume less bacon, cheese, gravy granules, ham, salami, smoked meat, smoked fish, soy sauce and stock cubes.

■ *Always taste your food before adding salt to it:* Food often tastes just as good without it.

■ *Don't add salt to food when cooking:* Season your food with spices, herbs, pepper, garlic, onion, or lemon, instead.

Potassium

This mineral helps to regulate your heartbeat, in addition to other important jobs it does in your body. In contrast to sodium, which raises blood pressure, potassium can help to lower it. When you follow the *Eatwell Plate*, it is easy to get enough potassium.

The main sources of Potassium are:

■ Some vegetables, such as broccoli, peas and lima beans

■ Tomatoes, potatoes and sweet potatoes

■ Winter squash fruits, including citrus fruits, cantaloupe, bananas, kiwi-fruit, prunes, apricots and nuts

■ Meat, poultry and some fish including salmon, cod and sardines

■ Milk, buttermilk, and yoghurt also contain some potassium

Calcium

You probably know that calcium helps to build bones. However, did you know that it is also needed to ensure that blood will clot normally? It is thought that calcium may help to lower high blood pressure and protect against colon and breast cancer. But for the time being, we will wait for more evidence before confirming this. The recommended amount of daily calcium consumption is 700mg for an adult. You should normally be able to get all the calcium you need from your diet but some people with certain medical conditions may not do so. People with osteoporosis or with a lifestyle confining them indoors for most of the time may need calcium supplements. Chapter 17 provides further information on this.

Calcium can be found in foods such as:

- Milk, cheese and dairy products
- Green vegetables such as broccoli and cabbage
- Nuts
- Fish such a sardines and pilchards
- Bread made with fortified flour

Vitamins

Most of us can get all the vitamins we need from eating a healthy balanced diet. However, some people choose to take supplementary vitamins, but often end up taking too much for too long which can sometimes be harmful. There is also the possibility that they might interact with your medications. So the recommendations are that you should only take additional vitamins *in consultation with a health care professional* and in specific circumstances.

For example, people who stay indoors most of the time, such as elderly residents in care homes or people who, for religious or cultural reasons, cover up their skin and are not exposed to the sun may become deficient in vitamin D. In these cases, the doctor may recommend that they take vitamin D supplements. Some vegetarians and vegans may not get all the vitamin B12 that they need from their diet and, therefore may need to take supplementary B12. There are many other vitamins which serve essential needs in our body but *supplements should always be taken under medical advice or guidance*. For more information on vitamins consult www.nhs.uk/conditions/vitamins-minerals on the NHS Website or consult the British Dietetic Association for their food facts leaflets at www.bda.uk.com/foodfacts. If you do not use a computer, why not ask your local librarian to recommend a reputable book on vitamins?

Water

The function of water

Water is your most important nutrient. Like the air you breathe, you cannot live without it. More than half of your body is made up of water, and each cell is bathed in it. Water helps to keep your kidneys working, prevents constipation, and helps you eat less by making you feel full. It also helps to prevent some medication side-effects.

Where in your diet does water comes from?

Although most people can last weeks without food, you cannot live longer than a week or so without water. Most adults lose about 2.5 litres of water each day. However, we usually have no problem getting six to eight glasses each day. This totals around 1.2 litres, which is what many experts recommend. Whilst this is less water than we lose in a day, the rest can be made up from water contained in the food we eat; this totals around one litre. Even the driest cracker contains a tiny amount of water. In addition to this the body also recovers water from chemical reactions in our body cells, providing about 0.3 of a litre.

How to check if you are drinking enough

To see if you are drinking enough, check your urine. If it is light-coloured, you are fine. When you start to get thirsty, you need more water. Milk, juice, and many fruits and vegetables are good sources of water. But be careful because drinking coffee, tea, and other drinks with caffeine, as well as alcohol, can cause you to lose water. Do not depend on these drinks for your water.

Special medical conditions

If you have kidney disease or congestive heart failure or are taking special medications, your need for water may be different. Talk to a registered dietician or your GP about your own specific needs.

Eating for Specific Long-term Conditions

The Eatwell Plate is a general plan designed to work for most of us. However, some people have different needs and different likes. These depend on your age, sex, body size, activity level, health, and even the availability and affordability of food. Here we present some information and guidelines for selected long-term health problems.

Diabetes

When you eat a meal, your body breaks down the carbohydrates into glucose, which is the basic fuel for the body's cells. The glucose is then absorbed into the bloodstream. Protein and fat usually contribute little to the body's blood glucose. The hormone insulin takes the glucose into the cells. With diabetes, the cells do not absorb or use glucose very well. The glucose builds up in the in your bloodstream which can then lead to other health problems. Managing blood glucose levels is one of the prime goals in diabetes treatment and involves many different things. These include taking medication, exercising, and keeping a careful eye on your diet. For more information on diabetes, take a look at Chapter 18. Keeping a careful eye on your diet, is really about keeping the balance of your food intake right.

People with diabetes were, for many years, told that they could not eat sweets and that they could only eat certain types of carbohydrates. As we learn more, things have changed. We now know that people with diabetes do not have to avoid any specific food. However, they do need to watch *what* and *how much* they eat. These things will vary from person to person.

Diabetes UK recommends that you use the *Eatwell Plate* as a guide for healthy eating and in helping you get the balance of your food intake right. The *Eatwell Plate* has been discussed and explained earlier in this chapter. Following the *Eatwell Plate* is especially important for preventing future problems. This is because people with diabetes are at a higher risk from heart disease and other chronic health conditions. In addition to the guidance on getting the balance of food choices right, you also need to follow other general advice about a healthy routine and how and when to eat.

General points

Here are some general points about healthy eating for people with diabetes:

- *Start each day with something to eat.* Eating something in the morning is truly *breaking the fast*. It helps fuel the body after a long night of resting and not having any food; it gives you energy to start the day's activities.

- *Space meals and snacks regularly over the day, and don't skip meals.* Spacing your meals at the usual times gives your body the chance to produce and use its insulin, and time for your medication to work to keep up your energy level. Of course, the number of meals you eat and the time between meals will vary depending on your personal health and lifestyle. Many of us eat three meals a day, when others may prefer or need to eat smaller more frequent meals.

- *Eat the same amount of food at each meal.* This helps you to maintain an even energy flow and a constant blood sugar level throughout the day. Skipping meals or mixing large meals with small meals, can throw

off your energy level. It can also lead to over-eating and to poorer, less healthy food choices. This in turn can cause swings in your blood sugar and result in symptoms such as irritability, poor concentration, shakiness, mood swings, pain, difficulty in breathing due to stomach bloating, heartburn, indigestion, and even poor sleep.

Carbohydrates

It is important that you learn to manage the carbohydrates you eat. Nearly all carbohydrates break down into glucose, so they have the greatest effect on your blood sugar. Too much carbohydrate causes blood sugar to increase; too little makes your blood sugar low. General guidelines suggest that you should eat between 45g and 60g of carbohydrates per meal, but this amount may vary widely from person to person.

For most people with diabetes, there is no such thing as a bad carbohydrate or one that is off limits. What matters most is the total amount of carbohydrate consumed, rather than the specific kind. However, it is true that some people may *feel* that certain foods affect them differently. Carbohydrates are found mostly in plant foods, milk and yoghurt being exceptions. They are also found in the form of sugars including honey, jam, table sugar, and in starches such as dried beans, winter squashes, grains like rice, and flour. You get the most benefit by getting the majority of your carbohydrates from whole grains including brown rice, oats, and wholewheat bread. Also, fruits preferably in the form of whole fruit rather than juice, vegetables, and dried beans, peas, and lentils, provide benefits. These foods are high in vitamins, minerals, fibre, and other good things that help keep your body healthy and protect it from disease. Another advantage of foods such as barley, dried beans, oats, apples, citrus fruits, carrots, and psyllium seeds are that they are absorbed by the body rather, slowly which helps you to manage your blood glucose level. They can also help to lower blood cholesterol, which will reduce your heart disease risk.

Fats, vegetables and sodium and weight

Because of the increased risk of heart disease and stroke it very important to eat fewer bad fats. As discussed on page 184, these are the saturated and trans-fats. You should replace these with good fats like olive oil. In addition, you can decide to eat more plant foods and fewer animal foods. Take in less sodium by eating fewer processed and prepared foods, and use salt sparingly, if at all. If you are carrying some extra weight, losing some of it can help lower your blood glucose. Even a small weight loss of five to ten pounds can make a big difference in your blood glucose level. Take a look at the *Tips for Healthier Eating* in the boxes on pages 183 and 185. At the same time, consult the tips for choosing healthy fats on page 184. For further more detailed information on diabetes, see Chapter 18.

Heart Disease and Stroke

Healthy eating for people with heart disease or those who have had a stroke usually involves keeping arteries from hardening or becoming clogged. Details on these issues can be found in Chapter 16. So clearly, it is important to watch the amount and kind of fat you eat. Most of your fat intake should come from the *good unsaturated fats* and very little from the *bad saturated fats*. In addition, you should eat little to no

trans-fat. By increasing the amount of fibre you eat, especially from oats, barley, dried beans, peas, lentils, apples, citrus fruits, and carrots you can manage your high blood cholesterol more effectively, and avoid a major risk factor for heart disease. Eating less salt or sodium can help you to prevent or control high blood pressure. Try to limit the total daily amount you consume to no more than six grams of table salt. If the food label refers only to the *sodium* content in the food then the maximum amount should be no more than 2.4 grams. It helps if you use herbs, spices, lemon, and vinegar for flavour. The tips provided on pages 183 and 185 also indicate how you can make healthy fat choices and increase fibre in your eating plan.

Lung Disease

For people with lung disease, especially *emphysema*, it is sometimes necessary to increase the amount of protein you eat. This helps to increase your energy, strength, and the ability to fight lung infections. When it is hard for you to eat, for example when you have little or no appetite, try eating higher-calorie foods. For example, try fruit nectars which are thick fruit juices rather than normal juice. Also try dried fruit instead of fresh fruit; or sweet potato instead of white potato; or nibbling on a small handful of nuts as another alternative during the course of the day. Our discussion of the common challenges of gaining weight in Chapter 12, on pages 216–218, gives you some tips to help you increase the amount you eat.

If you have specific concerns about what to eat, talk to your doctor or to a registered dietician. These professionals can tell you what's best for you and for your unique health needs.

Osteoporosis

Osteoporosis makes bones brittle so that they can easily be broken. It has been called a *silent disease* because its first symptom can be a bone fracture, especially in the spine, hip, or wrist. However, it is never too late to help slow down its progress. You can help by getting enough calcium and vitamin D and also by regularly doing muscle-strengthening and weight-bearing exercise like walking. We explored this earlier in Chapters 7 and 8. In addition, you should follow carefully your health care professional's recommendations, including taking your prescribed medications for bone loss.

Osteoporosis is technically not a calcium deficiency disease, and this means that after bone has been lost, simply getting more calcium will not restore it. But getting vitamin D together with your calcium intake can help your body to absorb the calcium. Everybody needs some calcium every day. The best sources are milk and foods made from milk. But some people avoid milk products because they don't like them, or they don't eat animal products, or they have problems in digesting milk sugar (lactose intolerance). You can still get enough calcium from your diet even if you have problems with milk sugar. Many people can enjoy milk products if they take them in small amounts or eat other foods with them. For example they can eat cereal with milk or use lactase tablets to help digest the lactose. Or if they can eat foods such as *kefir*, which is a fermented milk drink made with kefir grains, or yoghurt. There are also some fruits and vegetables that are high in calcium, including kale, collard greens, bok choy (also known as Chinese cabbage), and broccoli. Also you can try calcium-treated tofu; cooked dried beans; and foods with added calcium, such as soya milk, juices, cereals, and pasta. If you think you may not be getting enough calcium, talk to your doctor or to a registered dietician about your diet and ask whether calcium supplements are needed to meet your needs.

One of the main sources of vitamin D is sunshine, so getting out in daylight helps to increase your levels of vitamin D. It can also be found in reasonable amounts in oily fish such as salmon, sardines, pilchards, trout, and kippers. Eggs, milk and meat also contain small amounts of the vitamin.

For more information on Osteoporosis, you should take a look at Chapter 17.

The Importance of Food Labels

Food labels need to be taken seriously and the following notes and Charts are intended to help you to do this:

- *Consult the label:* most food packages have nutritional information food labels to help you find out what packaged foods contain. These show the suggested serving size and nutritional content which can help you make better choices. Reading and understanding the information on food labels can be overwhelming. UK food packages usually have nutritional labels on the back and may also have a colour coded label on the front of the package. Changes are underway that will make understanding and using

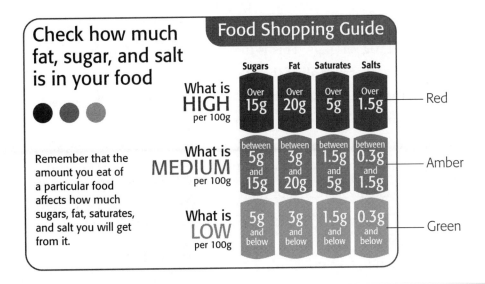

Figure 11.1 **The UK Food Standards Agency Label**

these labels easier. The labels usually provide nutritional information per 100 grams and some also give the information per serving size. We would suggest that you actively look at these when shopping and making decisions about what to buy.

■ *Make sure you understand the colour coded labels:* The label above, *Figure 11.1* is usually found on the front of the food package. It shows a table used by the *UK Food Standards Agency* that provides an easy way to see if the fat, sugar and salt content in your food is high, medium, or low. It does this by looking at food per 100 grams, and then showing the total grams of each key constituent, in a colour coded chart. The chart colour scheme is based on our traditional traffic lights. Thus, red is for stop (*top row*), amber for warning (*middle row*), and green is for go (*bottom row*). If you look at *Figure 11.1* and you want to check if the food you want to buy is low in fat, then you would look in the column headed fat for the High, Medium and Low figures. The red flag (*top*)

will tell you that the fat content is high, an amber flag (*middle*) that it has a medium content, and a green flag (*bottom*) that it is low in fat.

Some manufacturers also use a traffic-like colour code which includes information on the *total calories* present in the sugar, fat and salt in the pack. Calories are indicated in the first column in *Figure 11.2*.

■ *Investigate Food Nutritional Labels and serving size:* Not all labels give the serving size but if you look at the sample food label in

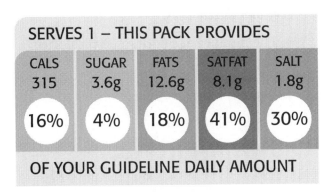

Figure 11.2 **Adding Information on Calorie Content**

Figure 11.3 you will see that this package contains three × 150g servings. This is the first thing to look at, because all of the other information on the label is based on this serving size and most packages will contain more than one serving. But the serving size on the package may not be what you usually eat. If you would usually have less or more than the stated serving size, you have to do some mental arithmetic.

This is important to take notice of, because sometimes a package that *looks like* one serving will have several, just as the label shown in *Figure 11.3* has three. A manufacturer's idea of a serving size may contain more than the recommended amounts of sugar or fat. In this situation you may need to eat *less* than one serving.

Note that our yoghurt label In *Figure 11.3* shows 409kj or100kcal. This calorie figure measures the amount of energy in the food. The recommended calories for any individual can vary depending on age, amount of physical activity done and other factors.

So let's look at our yoghurt example again, and work out how many calories there are in a serving:

Consider the calories:

- The number of calories is 100 calories for 100 grams.

- There is a total of 450 grams for three × 150 gram servings.

- Therefore, one serving is equal to 150 calories That is 450 gram divided by three.

Nutrition Information	
	Typical Values/100g
Energy	**409kj/100kcal**
Protein	**3.9g**
Carbohydrate	**13.4g**
Of which sugars	**12.8g**
Fat	**3.5g**
Of which saturates	**2.1g**
Fibre	**0.2g**
Sodium	**0.05g**
Contains 3 x 150g servings	

Figure 11.3 **Food Label for Yoghurt**

If we look at the fat content:

- There are 3.5 grams of fat in every 100 grams of yoghurt.

- If you look at Chart 1, the colour code on the shopping card, you will learn that the fat content in this yoghurt is borderline between medium and low.

Finally look at sodium:

- There is 0.05 of a gram in 100 grams of yoghurt.

- If you look at *Figure 11.1* again, you will see that the guidance is for *salt* and not for sodium. So, in order to find the amount of *salt* in the yoghurt we must multiply the amount of sodium, which is 0.05 grams by 2.5. This gives us 0.125 grams of salt. If you consult *Figure 11.3* again, you will find that the salt content in this yoghurt is low.

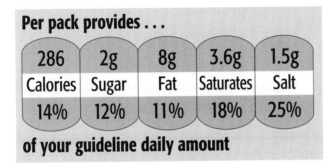

Figure 11.4 **The Guideline Daily Amount**

■ *Find out the Guideline Daily Amounts:* A final label that you will sometimes find on food packs is called the *Guideline Daily Amount* (GDA). This is illustrated in *Figure 11.4*. These guidelines are based on an average sized woman doing an average amount of physical exercise. You need to be aware of this in order that you do not over or under estimate the daily allowances that *you* will need.

From this label you can see that the food product contains eight grams of fat, which is 11% of your daily fat intake allowance. This label is probably more difficult to interpret than the traffic light system.

■ *Checking the ingredients list:* Always check a package's ingredients list. It shows you what is in the food you will be eating. Ingredients are generally listed in order by weight. If you see sugar listed first, then the food contains more sugar than anything else. Remember, too, when you see the words *partially hydrogenated* or *hydrogenated*, the product contains bad trans-fats.

A Word of Caution

At the time of writing, in 2013, the labelling of food packs still varies from manufacturer to manufacturer. There has been no overall consistency about labelling. The Government is pushing forward with proposals to make labelling more consistent but even this will be on a voluntary basis. It is hoped that an agreed system will be in place within a few years.

Eating and Your Thoughts

Do you eat when you're bored, down in the dumps, sad, or just feeling lonely? Many people find *comfort* in food and may be just eating as something to do when they need to take their minds off a problem; sometimes they eat simply because they have nothing else to do. Some people eat when they are feeling angry, or anxious, or depressed. At these times, it is easy to lose track of what and how much you eat. These are also the times when celery sticks or apples just won't do. Here are some ways to help control these understandable urges:

■ *Keep a food-mood diary:* Every day, list what, how much, and when you eat. Note how you are feeling when you have the urge to eat.

■ *Try to spot patterns so you can anticipate the problem:* You will soon know when you will want to eat without really being hungry and will be prepared.

■ *Decide whether you are really hungry:* If you catch yourself feeling bored and about to eat something, ask yourself, *"Am I really hungry?"* If the answer is no, make yourself do something else for two to three minutes, for example, go for a short walk around the house, work on a jigsaw puzzle, play a computer game or listen to the radio. Keep your mind and hands busy. Getting your hands dirty is helpful, as with gardening. Write down some *action plans* for when these situations arise. Sometimes it is easier to refer to the written word than to remember what you said you would do.

Common Challenges to Healthy Food Choices

"Healthy food doesn't taste the same as the food I am used to. When I eat, I want something with substance, like meat and potatoes or a piece of apple pie! The healthy stuff just doesn't fill me up!"

Making healthier food choices does not mean that you cannot have something that you crave for. It means *trading off* to fit in favourites while making better choices most of the time. Some of these tips are discussed in Chapter 12, and more information is available at the end of this chapter. There are also many excellent cookbooks with healthy recipes, as well as websites with plenty of healthy recipe ideas.

But what if your inner voice responds with, *"But I love to cook!"*

If you love to cook, you are in luck. Take a new cooking class: you can begin watching one on television; or treat yourself to a new cookbook on healthy cooking; or find a website featuring healthy recipes. If you have odds and ends, even left-overs, in your kitchen, do a computer search to see what recipes you can find. Play around with ways to modify your favourite recipes, particularly finding ways of making them lower in fat, sugar, and sodium.

"I'm living alone now, and I'm not used to cooking for one. I find myself over-eating so that food isn't wasted."

The first thing to do is to learn the new ways of shopping for one person. Shopping for one can be a problem when the situation is new. Make meal plans so that when you go shopping you know what to buy and can avoid buying things spontaneously that you do not need. Reduce the number of perishable foods you buy so you don't end up having to throw some away; on the other, hand buy frozen packs when they are on special offer. Buy things such as meat from your local butcher or the meat counter in the supermarket where they will weigh and cut the meat into pieces of the size you want. These are just a few tips and, as time goes on, you will learn more about your food needs and how to avoid waste. Here are some additional tips you might consider:

- *Don't eat family style by putting serving dishes on the table:* Put as much as you feel you can comfortably eat on a plate, and bring only that plate to the table.

- *As soon as you have finished eating, or even right after you have served your portion, immediately put left-overs in the refrigerator:* This strategy will give you left-overs to eat on the next day or later, whenever you don't feel like cooking a meal.

- *Have friends over for a dinner once in a while:* This means you can share food and other people's company. So, plan a pot-luck supper with neighbours, relatives, clubs, or other groups.

"Food just doesn't taste as good as before."

Many things can affect how food tastes for each of us. Having surgery, taking certain medications, being on oxygen, and even the common cold can make food taste unpleasant. When this happens, you tend to eat less. Many people try adding salt to their food to make it taste better. Unfortunately, this can also cause you to retain water or feel bloated, and these effects can increase your blood pressure.

Here are a few ideas about how you can make your food taste better:

- *Use herbs*: Put herbs such as basil, oregano, tarragon and spices such as cinnamon, cumin, curry, ginger, or nutmeg in your cooking. You can even sprinkle them on your food.

- *Squirt on some fresh lemon*: Add lemon juice to your food to your taste.

- *Use a small amount of vinegar*: Put this in, or on top of, hot or cold foods. There are dozens of different vinegars, ranging from balsamic to berry and fruit-flavoured varieties; experiment with new flavours.

- *Add healthy ingredients*: Fortify the foods you usually eat such as carrots or barley by adding them to soup, or put some dried fruits and nuts in your salads. This will give the food more texture and make them tastier.

- *Chew your food slowly and well*: This will allow the food to remain in your mouth longer and release more flavour.

If a lack of taste is keeping you from eating enough, you may need to add more calories to your meals or snacks. Tips for doing this are provided on page 217.

"It takes so long to prepare meals. By the time I'm finished, I'm too tired to eat."

This is a common problem, especially when you do not have much energy. It is a situation that calls for planning to make sure that you *do* eat. Here are some hints to help you:

- *When you do have some energy then cook extra*: Cook enough for two, three, or even more servings or meals, especially if it is something you really like.

- *Do a meal exchange*: Do this with friends or family, and freeze what you get in return in single-serving sizes for times when you feel too tired to cook.

- *Break your food preparation into steps*: You can then rest between steps.

- *Ask for help*: Do this especially for big holiday meals or family gatherings.

"Sometimes eating causes discomfort."
"I'm afraid I'll become short of breath while I'm eating."
"I really have no appetite."

People who say things like this might try the suggestions we make below. If you experience shortness of breath, or find it difficult and physically uncomfortable to eat meals you will tend to eat less. For others, eating a large meal can cause stomach problems such as indigestion, discomfort, or nausea. Indigestion, accompanied by a full stomach, reduces the space in which your breathing muscles have to expand and contract. This can aggravate breathing problems.

If these are the sort of challenges you face, then try the following:

- *Eat four to six small meals a day:* Do this rather than the usual three large meals. You will be using less energy for each meal.

- *Avoid foods that produce wind or make you feel bloated:* It's a fact that many foods can produce wind, although all foods affect people differently. Be aware that amongst the more common foods that cause discomfort are avocados, cabbage, broccoli, Brussels sprouts, onions, beans, bananas, apples, and melons.

- *Eat slowly, take small bites, and chew your food well:* Try pausing occasionally during a meal. Eating quickly in order to avoid a short breath episode can actually make it happen. Slowing down and breathing evenly reduces the amount of air you swallow while you eat.

- *Do a relaxation exercise about half an hour before mealtimes:* This relaxation and taking time out for a few deep breaths during the meal can really help.

- *Choose food that is easy to eat:* Go for foods such as yoghurt or pudding, or have a drink, like a thick fruit juice.

"I can't eat very much in one sitting."

There is no rule that says we must eat only three meals a day. In fact, many people find that four to six smaller meals work better for them. If you choose to eat more frequently, then try to include no-fuss, high-calorie snacks such as shakes, and protein or meal bars as part of these extra meals. If you still can't finish a whole meal, then eat the portion of your meal that is highest in calories, first.

Common Challenges to Healthy Eating

"I love to eat out, so how do I know if I'm eating well?"

Whether it is because you don't have time, or you hate to cook, or you just don't have the energy to shop for groceries or cook meals, eating out can often suit your needs. This is not necessarily bad, if you work out how to make the best choices possible. Here are some tips on eating out:

- *Select restaurants that have a variety of menu items:* Preferably restaurants that offer meals which have been prepared in healthy ways, for example, grilled or steamed dishes, rather than fried foods.

- *Ask what is in a dish and how it is prepared:* In this case you will know what you are eating, especially if you are eating in a restaurant where the dishes are new to you.

- *Before you go out, decide what type of food you will eat and how much:* This gives you planning time; to help, many restaurants post their menus on the Internet or at the front of the restaurant.

- *Order small plates or appetisers:* This can be an alternative to ordering main courses.

- *When you are in a group, order first:* Then you won't be tempted to change your mind after hearing what the others have selected.

- *See if you can split your main meal with a dining companion, or order a half portion:* You could also decide to eat only half of what is served, so that you can take the rest home for another meal. Ask to have the take-away container brought to you with your food, and box it up *before* you start eating.

- *Choose menu items that are low in fat, sodium, and sugar:* You can also ask if they can be prepared that way.

- *Whenever possible, order barbecued, baked, grilled, or steamed dishes:* This will be better for you than if the food is breaded, fried, sautéed, creamed, or covered in cheese.

- *Ask for your vegetables to be steamed or raw:* Also you can insist that they are also without butter, sauces, or dips.

- *Eat bread without butter:* You can ask that no butter or dips are served with your bread.

- *Request salad with dressing on the side:* This gives you more control. Also, try dipping your fork into the dressing before spearing each mouthful.

- *For dessert, select fruit, non-fat yoghurt or sorbet:* This will mean that you can avoid temptation!

"I snack while I am doing other things—watching TV, working on the computer, or reading."

If this is a problem for you, plan ahead by keeping a list of healthier snacks that you can grab.

Here are some examples:

- *Choose your snacks:* Avoid eating crackers, crisps, and biscuits, by choosing to munch on fresh fruit and raw vegetables. Have some ready and prepared in the fridge.

- *Measure out your snack in a single-portion size* so that you won't be tempted to eat more.

- *Make specific places at home and work eating areas* and don't eat anywhere else.

"I just can't afford to buy the healthier foods having a young family and on low income"

- *There is a special government scheme for families on very low incomes:* This also applies to those with children under four years old or pregnant mothers. It is called *Healthy Start* and it will help you to buy healthier foods through a voucher scheme. Leaflets with application forms are sometimes available in surgeries, libraries and job centres.

- *There are many recipe books or on-line suggestions on preparing healthy meals:* These are often based on inexpensive ingredients. For more details look at the end of this chapter.

"I follow a vegan diet, so what can I do about the Eatwell Plate?"

A healthy vegan diet should consist of plenty of fruit and vegetables and starchy foods, together with some non-dairy sources of protein such as beans and pulses. It should also contain some dairy alternatives such as fortified soya milk and just a small amount of fatty and sugary foods. The *Eatwell Plate* accommodates these needs as well as those who follow a vegetarian diet.

Summing Up the Basic Principles of Healthy Eating

Healthy eating is about the food choices you make *most* of the time. It is not about *never* being able to eat certain foods. There is no such thing as a perfect food. Healthy eating means enjoying a moderate amount of a wide variety of minimally processed foods, consumed in the proper amounts for your body. It should also allow for occasional treats.

Eating this way can help you maintain your health, prevent future health problems, and let you manage your condition and symptoms in the best way possible. Eating healthily, however, may mean making some changes to what you are now doing. These could include making food choices that are higher in good fats and fibre and fewer food choices that are high in bad and trans-fats, sugar, and sodium. Healthy eating is just as important when it comes to losing weight, keeping it constant, or gaining weight. Take a look at Chapter 12, on this issue.

If you choose to make some of the changes suggested in this chapter, then think of it as doing something positive and wonderful for yourself, not as a punishment! As a good self-manager, it's up to you to find the changes that are best. And, if you experience set-backs, try to identify the problems and work at resolving them. You can do it!

Suggested Further Reading

Chan, W. *Counter, G.I. and G.L.* London: Hamlyn, 2006. This is a small reference book to hundreds of foods with information on their Glycaemic Index, calories, average portion sizes and nutrition.

Pinnock, D. *The Medicinal Chef: Eat Your Way to Better Health*. London: Quadrille Publishing, 2013.

Warshaw, H. *Eat Out, Eat Right: The Guide to Healthier Restaurant Eating*, 3rd ed. Chicago: Surrey Books, 2008.

Woodruff, S. and Gilbert-Henderson, L. *Soft Foods for Easier Eating Cookbook: Easy-to-Follow Recipes for People Who Have Chewing and Swallowing Problems*. Garden City Park, N.Y.: Square One, 2010.

Other Resources

☐ BBC: A website with interesting food suggestions. www.bbc.co.uk/food/diets/healthy

☐ Healthy Eating: Food fact sheets can be found on the *British Dietetic Association* website. www.bda.uk.com/foodfacts

☐ Heart Health: Although this is a heart charity website, a lot of the advice given which is applicable to all of us. www.bhf.org.uk/heart-health/prevention/healthy-eating

☐ Live Well: This site gives you ideas on healthy meal preparation. www.nhs.uk/Livewell/healthy-recipes

☐ Mayo Clinic, "Nutrition and Healthy Eating." www.mayoclinic.com/health/nutrition-and-healthy-eating/MY00431

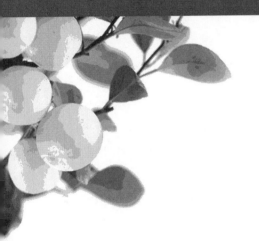

CHAPTER 12

Maintaining a Healthy Weight

WEIGHT AFFECTS OUR HEALTH, how we look, and our ability to move; and it can affect how we feel about ourselves. *Too much weight* contributes to arthritis, because of excessive joint stress, diabetes because of high blood glucose, and high blood pressure. *Being underweight* can weaken our immune system and make us less able to fight infection. Being underweight can also increase our likelihood of developing osteoporosis, sometimes called *thin bones*, and in younger women it can affect fertility and result in menstrual problems. Therefore being either overweight or underweight can have major effects on your life and health.

Special thanks to Bonnie Bruce, DrPH, RD, for her help with this chapter.

Why Is Body Weight Important?

Being at a healthy weight can help us to achieve better health and a better quality of life. It can help us manage symptoms such as lack of energy, joint pain, and shortness of breath. It can help us by preventing or holding off related health problems such as diabetes and high blood pressure. In addition, maintaining a healthy weight can help you to be more active and to sleep better. In general, it can increase your ability to do the things you want and need to do. In this chapter we clarify what we mean by a healthy weight, suggest how you might make changes, how to decide whether you should seek to lose or gain weight, and how you can maintain any changes you make.

What Is a Healthy Weight?

Most people's weight tends to shift up and down over time. This can happen even over the course of a few days. So, a healthy weight is not just one specific number on a scale, or a mysterious *ideal* number. There is no such thing as an ideal weight. A healthy weight tends to cover a range that is unique and personal to you. Keeping within this range will help you to lower your risk of developing or further worsening health problems and help you feel better in both body and mind. There is a chart used by your doctor to determine whether your current weight is considered healthy for someone of your sex and height which we will now look at in more detail. You can see this in *Chart 12.1*.

Using Charts to Work Out Your Healthy Weight

To get a sense of a healthy weight range for you, look at the chart in *Chart 12.1* on page 203. This may be very familiar to you, because it is used frequently by GPs in their surgeries. You can check if you are approximately the right weight for your height. The chart will give you some idea of whether you fall into a category where you are classified as underweight, a healthy weight, over-weight, fat or obese or very obese. For example, a healthy weight for someone who is 5 foot 5 inches tall lies between eight stone (50.8kg) and 10 stone 10 pounds (69.8kg).

However, you should remember that pinpointing your healthy weight range and deciding whether you need to change your weight depends on several things. These include: your age, your health, how much and where your body fat is located, and your family history of weight-related health problems, such as high blood pressure or diabetes.

People who are very active and exercise regularly may have built up a lot of muscle in their body. Muscle weighs heavier than fat and *Chart 12.1* does not allow for someone who is very muscular. In a similar way there may be an

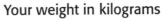

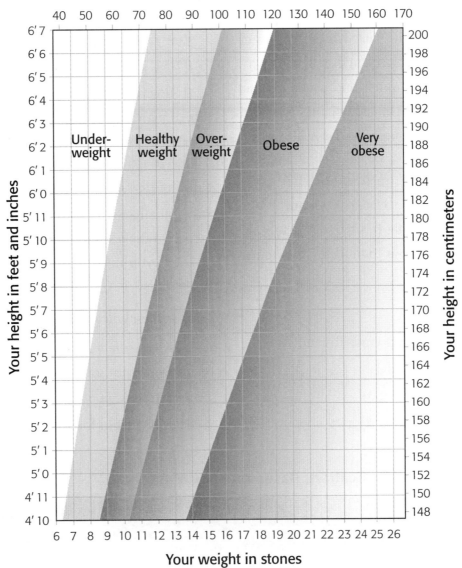

Chart 12.1 **Height and Weight Chart for Men and Women (BMI Chart)**

underestimation of body fat in older people who have lost muscle.

Take some time thinking about where you fit on this chart. There can be several reasons why you might be *under-weight* such as a medical condition such as an overactive thyroid gland, a chronic respiratory disease or simply because your diet is not providing you with enough calories. If you fall into the under-weight group it is advisable to see your doctor to ascertain the reasons.

If you fall into the group where your weight is *a healthy weight* for you it is still important to eat a balanced diet. Take *The Eatwell Plate* (see pages 180–181) seriously and include physical activity as part of your lifestyle.

If you are *over-weight*, obese or very obese: it means your weight is too much for your height and it is time to address the situation for the sake of good health.

Using the bmi chart: the body mass index

You can use the *BMI Chart (Chart 12.1)* to determine your healthy weight. This will give you your Body Mass Index (BMI). Although it is not a perfect tool, it is a useful, quick, and general guide for adults based on weight and height. For many people it relates to total body fat and health risks.

How to calculate your body mass index

The formula used is to measure your body weight in pounds, divide this by your height in inches squared, and then to multiply the figure you get by 703.

Here is an example:

1. Your body weight is pounds lbs and your height is 60 inches.

2. 153 divided by (60 × 60).

3. 153 divided by 3600 = 0.0425

4. 0.0425 × 703 = 29.87

5. Your Body Mass Index is 29.87. This means that you are just below the BMI level for obese.

If you hate maths or find the calculations difficult, you can find an easy calculator on NHS website at www.nhs.uk/tools/pages/healthy-weightcalculator.aspx. Then, all *you* have to do is type in the measurements and it will automatically calculate your BMI.

Now take a quick look at *Table 12.1*. *Table 12.1* tells you in BMI units where your current weight falls.

What do these calculations tell us?

■ *A BMI less than 18.5 means*: That you are under-weight for your height.

■ *A BMI 18.5–24.9 means*: That you are a healthy weight for your height.

Table 12.1 **Weight Classifications Based on Body Mass Index**

Body Mass Index	Weight Classification	What It Means
Less than 18.5	Underweight	Unless you have other health problems, being in this weight class may not be an issue if you are small or petite.
18.5 to 24.9	Normal weight	This is the healthy range to aim for.
25 to 29.9	Overweight	This range suggests that you are carrying extra pounds. But it may not be of much concern if you are healthy, have few or no other health problems or risk factors, and are physically active or have a lot of muscle.
30 to 39.9	Obese	This range signals that it is likely you have a large amount of body fat. This puts you at increased risk for weight-related health problems.
40 and over	Extremely, or morbidly, obese	This weight class pinpoints that a high proportion of your body weight is fat. It puts you at very high risk of developing and complicating serious health problems.

- *A BMI 25–29.9 means:* That you are over-weight for your height.

- *A BMI 30–39.9 or more means:* That you are obese and this puts you in a category where you are at risk of health problems like heart disease, stroke or diabetes.

- *A BMI 40 and over means:* That you are extremely obese and puts you in a category where there is a very high risk of developing serious health problems.

Other ways of calculating a healthy weight for your height

Another way to judge your weight is to use a rough rule of thumb: Give or take 10%, women should weigh about 105 pounds for the first five feet of height and another five pounds per inch after that; men should weigh about 106 pounds for the first five feet and then an added six pounds per inch. For example, for a woman who is 5 foot 5 inches tall a healthy weight would be 125 pounds, and her healthy weight range would be roughly 112–138 pounds. Note: this weight range places her in the BMI *normal weight* class.

An alternative way to judge your weight is to measure the distance around your waist: If you are overweight and most of your body fat is around your waist rather than on your hips and thighs, you are at higher risk for heart disease, high blood pressure, and Type 2 Diabetes. For non-pregnant women, health risks go up with a waist size that is more than 35 inches (88 cm). For men, this risk level is associated with a waist circumference that is greater than 40 inches (100 cm). To measure your waist correctly, stand and place a tape measure, using one that is not too old and stretched, around your bare middle, just above your hipbone. Measure your waist just after you breathe out.

Taking the Decision to Change Your Weight

Reaching and maintaining a healthy weight may mean that you will need to make some changes in your eating habits and lifestyle. This is true whether you want to gain or lose weight. Make changes that you believe you can stick with for a long time. If you decide to make changes for someone other than yourself, or want to plan for only short-term changes, you probably won't succeed.

So, an important piece of advice is this: you must decide to make these changes for yourself and not simply to please your friends or family.

To get started, review the information about *action planning* which you will find in Chapter 2. If you think that you seriously want to change your weight, then you should consider asking your doctor to refer you to a registered dietician for help. This is not something you need to do alone.

When making this decision, you must ask yourself two important questions:

1. *Why do I want to change my weight?* The reasons for losing or gaining weight will be personal and different for each of us. The most important reason for some may be physical health, but for others there may be personal or emotional reasons for wanting to change.

To help you to begin and to increase your chances of success, think about the reasons that make you want to gain or lose weight. Here are some examples:

- *To improve my symptoms* such as reducing pain, fatigue and shortness of breath.

- *To manage my blood glucose.*

- *To have more energy* so that I can do the things I want to do.

- *To feel better about myself.*

- *To change the way others think about me.*

- *To enable me to feel more in control of my life.*

Jot down some of your own important reasons here:

_____

_____

_____

_____

_____

_____

_____

2. *Am I ready to make lifelong changes?* You need to work out whether this is a good time for you to start making changes in your eating and exercise. If you are not ready, you may be setting yourself up to fail. However, the truth is that there may never be a *perfect* time. So take a look at your situation to see how things can work for you. Even if you aim for a small change or weight loss this may give you an incentive to go on and achieve a more significant loss later on, which will contribute significantly to better health.

Consider the following:

- Is there someone, or something, that can be supportive and make it easier for you to begin and continue with your changes?

- Are there problems or obstacles that will keep you from becoming more active or changing the way you eat?

- Will worries or concerns about family, friends, work, or other commitments alter your ability to carry out your plans successfully?

Use *Table 12.2* help you identify some of these factors. If you find barriers, use some of the problem-solving tools you will find in Chapter 2.

After you have thought about these issues, you may find that now is not the best, or right, time to start. If it is not, then set a future date to review the situation. In the meantime, accept that this is the right decision for you at this moment. You can then focus your attention on other goals. If you do decide that now *is* the right time, start by changing the things that are simplest, easiest, and most comfortable for you by taking *baby steps*. This means working on only one or two things at a time; do not try to do too much, too quickly. Remember, slow and steady wins the race. Use the steps involved in *action planning* to make progress.

Table 12.2 **Factors Affecting the Decision to Gain or Lose Weight *Now***

Things That Will Enable Me to Make My Desired Changes	Things That Will Make It Difficult for Me to Change
Example: I have the support of family and friends.	*Example:* The holidays are coming up and it will be too difficult to start to make changes when away from home.

Where to Start

A good starting point is to keep a diary of what you eat now and how much physical activity or exercise you currently do. Do this for a week. It will help you learn where you need to make changes. In doing so, write down:

- What are you currently eating.

- Where you are eating.

- Why you are eating; are you hungry or just eating because you are bored?

- How you feel when eating; describe your mood and emotions.

- What you are doing now in terms of exercise or physical activity; and what are you not doing?

You might also have a section in your diary for ideas about what you would like to do differently. There is no need to worry if all your ideas don't work out right away, you can always go back to them. Our sample lifestyle tracking diary, which is shown in *Table 12.2*, may be useful to you.

How to Make Changes

Two important ingredients for successfully changing your weight are to start small by taking *baby steps*, and then only making changes that you know will work. Whether you want to lose or gain weight, there is no easy way to achieve it; most people will need to change the amount and perhaps the way they eat. This may seem scary or even impossible, but by starting with things that are do-able, you can be successful. This could mean that if you want to lose weight you will need to eat a little less, or if you want to gain weight eat a little more. For instance, instead of eating three ounces of rice, eat one ounce less or one ounce more. To help you eat less, try eating more slowly; to help you increase your calories, spread out your eating over several small meals a day. You might find it useful to refer back to Chapter 11 on *Healthy Eating*.

- *When you find things you want to change, start by choosing only one or two things at a time.* It is really important, so allow yourself time to get used to these changes and then slowly add further changes later on. If you tell yourself you are going to walk five miles a day every day of the week and never eat potatoes or bread again, you won't be able to stick with that for very long. It is likely you won't lose weight, and will become frustrated and discouraged. But if you make a plan to have only one piece of toast at breakfast instead of two pieces and take two ten-minute walks four times a week and stick to it, you will be making good, long-term changes that will lead you to success.

- *When you change your weight slowly over time, you have a better chance of maintaining*

Table 12.3 **Lifestyle Tracking Diary**

Date	Time	What I Ate	Where I Ate	Why I Ate	My Mood or Emotions	My Exercise

that change. This is partly because your brain begins to recognise the changes you are slowly making as part of your regular routine and It's not just a temporary thing. The *goal-setting* and *action-planning* skills discussed in Chapter 2 will help with this. Remember, the best plan combines both healthy eating and exercise and is a slow, steady plan that feels right to you.

A Way to Get You Started Using the 200 Plan

What is the 200 Plan?

The *200 Plan* is a simple and practical plan to get you started. It involves making small daily changes in what you eat and in the amount of physical activity you do. You have to change what you do by only 200 calories a day. This can add up to a 20-pound weight change over a year. The *200 Plan* is a good way to balance eating and exercise and helps you make a long-term change in your weight management.

Therefore, to *lose weight*, you must eat 100 fewer calories a day than you do now and, in addition burn off 100 calories a day more with extra exercise. If you would like to *gain weight*, then add 100 calories while keeping your exercise at the recommended level of 20 to 40 minutes for most days of the week. Sticking to this kind of plan on a daily basis will bring success.

■ *But how can I change what I eat by 100 calories a day?* Start by checking out one of the food guides recommended in the previous chapter. These provide you with estimated serving sizes and calories. For example, you will find that a one-ounce slice of bread has close to 100 calories. So, by not eating one of the slices of bread on your sandwich, instantly cuts out close to 100 calories. To easily eat 100 calories more, you could add about two tablespoons of nuts to your food intake over the day. Of course, if you have a nut allergy then you will have to find an alternative extra input.

■ *What must I do to burn off an extra 100 calories a day?* If you add 20 to 30 minutes to your regular exercise routine, which could be walking, cycling, dancing, or gardening, then you have done it. In addition, you could also use the stairs more and park further away from the shops. If time is an issue for you, doing your exercise in three five to ten-minute chunks of time over the day works just as well as doing it all at once.

Exercise and Weight Loss

Exercise can help you to lose weight and keep it off

However, it is very difficult to exercise enough to lose weight without also changing what you eat. Adding aerobic or cardio-vascular exercise is the best for weight loss. This is the kind of exercise that gets your heart pumping: walking, jogging, cycling, swimming, and dancing all do the trick. These kinds of exercises help you lose weight because they use the large muscles in the body that burn the most calories. The guideline suggestions in Chapter 8, recommending that you get 150 minutes of moderate or brisk aerobic activity a week are the same for general health, weight loss, and for keeping the weight off. Exercising in ten-minute bouts works as well as longer workouts. If you can add more minutes, then that is even better.

It is true that the more calories you burn with exercise, the more weight you can lose. However, that is only one part of the story. It is important to understand that most success comes from making exercise and eating changes together. And making changes *that become part of your daily life.*

When you add more exercise to your routine, be honest with yourself about what you can do and what is safe and enjoyable for you. If you exercise too hard or too long for your body, you are more likely to have to stop because of injury, fatigue, frustration, or loss of interest. The truth is that whatever you do to increase your physical activity will be helpful only if you do it regularly and at a pace that is good for you.

Some people become discouraged after a while

The pounds may not melt off straight away, or your weight loss may grind to a halt. This may be true even if you are still exercising and being careful about what you eat. There are many reasons why weight loss slows down. For example, your exercise may be building muscle and reducing fat. Muscle weighs more than fat, so you could be losing fat but the scales are not showing it. If you keep track of your body measurements such as waist and hips, or notice that your clothes fit better or are looser, this can also be a signal that your exercise is working. And remember, when you exercise regularly, even if you don't lose weight, you are doing good things for your body. Regular aerobic exercise can help give you more energy and help anyone who might be *pre-diabetic* to avoid diabetes. It can also: reduce blood glucose and blood fat levels; increase good cholesterol; reduce risk of heart disease; and help with depression and anxiety.

Pointers for Losing Weight

Many studies show that eating fewer calories and being physically active are both important for successful weight loss. Just eating less is usually not enough. Being active will not only help you burn calories, but it will also help to build up your muscle which burns more calories than fat. In addition, activity and greater muscular development will give you more strength and energy. You will be able to move and breathe better. You will find more information about exercise and tips for choosing the particular activities that suit your needs and lifestyle in Chapters 6, 7, and 8. For now consider the following suggestions:

■ *Set small, gradual weight loss goals:* Break the total amount of weight you want to lose into small, reachable goals. For example, think in terms of a loss of one to two pounds each week or five to seven pounds each month. This is much less daunting than looking at the total weight you would like to lose, especially if this is a considerable amount. For most people, aiming to lose one to two pounds a week is realistic and do-able. When you set small goals rather than large ones, your goals become more possible and practical.

■ *Identify the exact steps you will take to lose your weight.* For example you could decide to walk 20 minutes a day for five days each week, not to eat between meals, and to eat more slowly.

■ *Keep on top of what is happening.* Keep track of your weight on a schedule that works for you. Some people decide that when their weight rises again by say, three pounds, it is a signal to get back into action.

■ *Think long-term.* Instead of saying *"I really need to lose ten pounds right away,"* tell yourself, *"Losing this weight gradually will help me keep it off for good."*

■ *Be in the present when you eat.* By focusing on what you are eating and not what you are doing, like watching television, you will be more likely to enjoy your food, become satisfied sooner, and eat less.

■ *Eat more slowly.* If you take less than 15 or 20 minutes to eat a meal, you are probably eating too fast and not allowing yourself to feel the enjoyment of eating. You may be surprised to learn that many of us can both enjoy food more and eat less, simply by eating more slowly. If you find it hard to slow down, try putting your fork down on the table between bites, and pick it up only after you have swallowed the previous mouthful.

■ *Become keenly aware of your stomach.* Learn to become aware of when your stomach is starting to feel full. Stop eating as soon as you get that signal. This will take attention and practice. When you do recognise the feeling of becoming full, remove your plate immediately or leave the table, if you can.

■ *Portion out your food.* Especially when first starting to make changes, measure out your portions. Do this frequently over time. It is amazing just how easily three ounces of rice can *grow* to a four ounce serving! Try to use food products that are already in single-sized portions. But take note of the difference between a portion and a serving size. This issue is considered in Chapter 11.

■ *Choose smaller portions.* When eating away from home, you can select appetisers or first courses rather than main meals, or order a child's meal. This will help you eat fewer calories. Over a year, it takes only an extra 100 calories a day to put on ten pounds. This is like eating one extra slice of bread a day. There are many published serving sizes recommended for different foods. The reference books listed at the end of Chapter 11 list some common serving sizes for a variety of foods, along with information on selected nutrients.

■ *Use a smaller plate.* If you do this, you won't be able to put as much food on it as you would on a standard plate.

■ *Clock yourself.* Make it a habit to wait about 15 minutes before either consuming another portion or starting to eat a dessert or a snack. You'll often find that this is enough time for the urge to eat or continue eating, to evaporate.

Common Challenges Around Losing Weight

"I need to lose ten pounds in the next two weeks. I want to look good for a special event."

Does this sound familiar? Almost everyone who has tried to lose weight wants to lose it fast. There are hundreds of weight-loss diets promising fast and easy ways to lose weight. However, these promises are false. There is no *magic bullet*. Remember, if it sounds too good to be true, it probably is.

During the first few days of almost any weight-loss plan, your body will lose mostly water, along with some muscle. This can amount to five or even ten pounds. Because of this, those fad and fast-weight-loss diets are able to claim that they are successful! But these pounds will come right back just as soon as you return to your old ways. Also, when you use fad diets, you may experience light-headedness, headaches, constipation, fatigue, and poor sleep. This is because such diets are often badly imbalanced in the kinds and amounts of foods which they allow. With fat loss, the amount you really want to lose will typically happen after a few weeks of eating fewer calories.

So, rather than wasting time with fad diets, do it properly. Set small, realistic goals; do action planning; and use positive thinking and self-talk. All these activities are discussed in greater detail in Chapters 2 and 5. Remember, the weight didn't go on overnight and it won't go away overnight.

"I just can't seem to lose those last few pounds."

Almost everyone reaches a time, sometimes called a plateau when their weight loss stops, despite their continued efforts. This is frustrating and can make us want to give up. Plateaus are usually temporary. They can mean that your body now needs fewer calories and has adapted to its lower calorie intake and higher activity level. Although your first impulse may be to cut your calories even further, this could actually be counter-productive and make your body burn fewer calories, making more weight loss even harder.

This is a good time to ask yourself how much of a difference those last few pounds really make to you. If you are feeling good and doing well with your blood glucose or cholesterol or other health issues, you may not need to lose more weight. If you are relatively healthy, staying active, and eating a good diet, it is usually not bad to carry a few extra pounds. Also, you may have replaced some of your body fat with muscle, which will weigh more than fat. This is a type of weight gain that is good. However, if you decide that those pounds *must* go, then consider the following tactics:

- *Instead of focusing on weight loss, focus on staying at the same weight.* Do this for at least a few weeks and then go back to your weight loss plan.

- *Increase your physical activity.* Your body may have adjusted to your lower weight and therefore require fewer calories, so you may need to exercise more to burn off more calories. Adding more exercise will help to kick-start your body into doing this. There are tips for safely increasing your exercise in Chapter 6.

- *Keep thinking positively.* Remind yourself of how much you have achieved. Here's a tip: write words that will encourage you on sticky notes and post them where you will see them.

"I always feel so deprived of the foods I love when I try to lose weight."

You are a special person. This means that the changes you decide to make must meet your special likes, dislikes, and needs. Unfortunately, our brains can get channelled into thinking about what we don't want to do or what we should not be doing. Think instead in a supportive or encouraging way, when you are considering losing weight.

Thinking uses both pictures and words. This means that you must teach yourself to see things in a better light, telling your brain to stop thinking about certain things, and to replace negative thoughts with positive ones that work for you. You'll find more on positive thinking in Chapter 5. Here are a couple of examples:

- *Replace any thoughts that include the words never, always, and avoid;* instead, tell yourself that you can enjoy things occasionally *"but a healthier choice is better for me most of the time."*

- *Tell yourself that you are retraining your taste buds.* Reflect on the fact that making healthier choices can help you to manage your weight and feel better.

"I eat too fast or I finish eating before everyone else and find myself reaching for seconds."

If you are finishing meals in just a few minutes or before everyone else at the table, you are probably eating too fast. You may be doing this for a number of reasons. You may be letting yourself get too hungry by allowing too much time pass between meals and then you *wolf down* your food when you finally get to eat. Or, you may be hurried, anxious, or stressed when you sit down. Slowing down your eating can help you eat less and enjoy your food more. Here are some tips for cutting down your eating speed:

- *Do not skip meals*; you will then avoid becoming overly hungry.

- *Make it a challenge*; try not to be the first person to finish eating at the table.

- *Work on thinking about what you are eating and how you are enjoying it*; practise doing this without diversions that demand your attention, such as friends, video games, or television.

- *Take small bites and chew slowly*; be careful to swallow each bite before you take another. Chewing your food well before swallowing also helps you enjoy your food more and feel better after the meal by reducing heartburn and other digestive upsets.

- *Put your cutlery down between mouthfuls*; this slows you down mechanically!

■ *Use a relaxation method about a half hour before you eat.* Remember that several methods were discussed in Chapter 5.

"I can't do it on my own."

Losing weight is challenging, and sometimes you just need some outside support and guidance. For help, you can contact any of the following resources:

■ *Registered Dieticians:* You can find out about the local services provided by dieticians in various ways:

◆ Contact your local hospital or GP surgery for dietary advice.

◆ Search for a freelance dietician on the *Dietician Unlimited* website. This is run by the *British Dietetic Association* (BDA). Contact them at info@bda.uk.com or by telephone on 0121 200 8080.

◆ You can also get details from the *Health and Care Professional Council* (HCPC). Dieticians must be qualified and registered with the HCPC. Nutritionists are qualified to give advice about food and nutrition but, unlike registered dieticians, they are not qualified to give advice about special diets for medical conditions. They too must be qualified as Registered Nutritionists with their professional Organisation. You can contact them by telephone on 0845 300 6184 or at www.hcpc.org.uk.

■ *Your surgery:* Some surgeries run a special weight clinic, but even if they don't, they can still offer advice on losing or gaining weight.

■ *Support groups like Weight Watchers:* This is where you can meet other people who are also trying to lose or maintain a healthy weight.

■ *Weight loss programmes*: These are offered by your local NHS providers, hospitals, private health insurance companies, community schools, and some employers.

Common Challenges in Retaining Your Weight Loss

"I've been on a lot of diets before and lost a lot of weight. But I've always gained it back, and even some more. It's so frustrating, and I just don't understand why this happens!"

This happens to many people. In fact, it is the down-side of quick weight-loss diets, because they typically involve drastic changes. They do not focus on a long term change in eating habits, exercise, and lifestyle. Typically, once you have tired of the diet or have reached your goal weight, you return to your old ways, and the weight comes back on with a vengeance, and sometimes even more on top!

The key to maintaining a healthy weight is to develop healthy eating and exercise habits that you enjoy, that fit into your lifestyle, and that become part of a new lifestyle that you can stick to. We have already given you many tips earlier in this chapter. Here are a few more:

■ *Set a personal weight gain alarm*; this can be a specific number of pounds gained, say three pounds. If you hit this mark, then return to your regular programme. The sooner you start, the faster the added pounds will come off.

■ *Monitor your activity level*; once you have lost some weight and are exercising three to five times a week you will dramatically improve your chances of keeping weight off. Research suggests that to maintain weight loss, some people should be exercising for nearly an hour a day. But don't worry, this time includes normal activities *and* planned physical exercise. Also remember that increasing activity does not just mean exercising for longer. It can mean going faster or doing something that is harder to do. For example, you might eventually be walking uphill or swimming with paddles attached to your hands.

"I can manage to keep weight off for a short time. Then something happens beyond my control, and I stop caring about what I eat. Before I know it, I've slipped back into my old eating habits."

Everyone is going to slip up at one time or another; no one is perfect. If it was only a little slip, don't worry about it. Just continue as if nothing has happened and get back on your plan. If the slip is bigger, try to work out why it happened. If there is something that is taking a lot of your attention at a particular time, then weight management may need to take a back seat. That's perfectly OK. The sooner you realise this, the better. Just try to set a date when you will re-start your weight management programme. You may, for extra support, want to join a weight support group and stay with it for at least four to six months. If so, look for a support group that does the following:

■ Lays emphasis on healthy eating.

■ Advocates lifelong changes in eating habits and lifestyle patterns.

■ Gives support in the form of on-going meetings and long-term follow-up.

■ Avoids making miraculous claims or providing guarantees. Remember, if something sounds too good to be true, it probably is.

■ Doesn't rely on special meals or supplements.

Common Challenges of Gaining Weight

Sometimes long-term health problems make it difficult to gain weight or keep it on. This could be because your condition or its treatment makes it hard for you to eat. Perhaps it is because you aren't hungry or or you are sad and depressed. Perhaps your body is unable to use the food you take in, or is burning up the calories faster than you can replace them.

When you aren't hungry or are having trouble eating, few foods sound appealing. At this time it is more important to eat something rather than to worry about whether the food is *healthy* or not. You need to eat for energy and strength and to meet your body's nutrition needs. That must over-ride being sure that what you eat is *healthy*. During difficult times like this, try to feel comfortable about eating whatever you can; it will probably only be temporary and then you can return to healthy eating.

Here, too, slow and steady wins the race. Use the 200 Plan which is described on page 210, making sure that you eat an extra 100 calories a day, every day. This alone can result in a ten-pound weight gain over a year. Also be sure to choose foods that you really enjoy, focusing on your favourites. Keep easy-to-cook or ready-prepared foods handy so that you don't need to spend too much time cooking.

If you experience a continual or extreme weight loss or have trouble keeping weight on, you're not alone. *However, it is wise to check out this kind of weight loss with your doctor if only for reassurance.* Let's look at some common challenges and some ideas for dealing with them.

"I don't know how to add calories to my current diet."

Here are some ways to increase the calories and nutrients you take in without increasing the quantity of food you need to eat:

- *Choose foods that are higher in fat;* but try to stick with foods that contain good fats, these are explained on page 184. Increasing your intake of fat is necessary because fat will give you many more calories than carbohydrate or protein, For example, you can snack on calorie-rich foods such as avocados, nuts, seeds, or peanut butter.

- *Eat dried fruit or thick fruit juices;* eat these rather than fresh fruit or regular juice.

- *Choose sweet potatoes* instead of normal white potatoes.

- *Use whole milk* instead of lower-fat dairy products, and use it instead of stock or water in soups and sauces.

- *Take liquid supplement drinks;* you can have these with or between meals.

- *Drink high-calorie beverages* such as shakes, malts and fruit whips.

- *Top salads, soups, and casseroles;* you can use grated cheese, nuts, dried fruits, or seeds.

"I just don't have much of an appetite."

Check with your doctor or a registered dietician to see if the following suggestions are appropriate for you:

- *Eat tiny meals;* or at least smaller meals several times a day.

- *Keep some nuts or dried fruit close by;* eat a few pieces every time you walk past the bowl.

- *Eat the highest-calorie foods on your plate first;* saving lower-calorie foods for later, for example, eat buttered bread before cooked spinach.

- *Add extra whole milk or milk powder;* put it in sauces, gravies, cereals, soups, and casseroles.

- *Add melted cheese;* tasty when added to vegetables and other dishes.

- *Use butter, margarine, or sour cream;* add these as toppings.

- *Consider keeping a snack at your bedside;* then you can eat something if you wake in the middle of the night.

Other common problems related to making changes in your eating habits are discussed in Chapter 11. More information on body weight can also be found in the resources listed below.

Conclusion

People come in many shapes and sizes and this fact can affect their health and their symptoms, whether they carry too much weight or too little. There is no such thing as a perfect or *ideal* weight. Rather there is a range of weight that will be good for us. Being in a healthy weight range helps you to achieve overall health and well-being, in body and mind. The most effective approach to achieving a healthy weight range involves both healthy eating and activity. Once you get to your healthy weight, keeping it within this good range is most important. Tailoring what you do to meet your needs and match your lifestyle is the best way. Choose realistic lifelong strategies that you can stick with. Avoid trying quick fixes, which usually do not work. Set your sights on success by building on small changes over time.

Suggested Further Reading

Ferguson, J. M., and Ferguson C. *Habits, Not Diets,* 4th ed. Boulder, Colo.: Bull Publishing, 2003.

Hensrud, D. D., ed. *Mayo Clinic Healthy Weight for Everybody.* Rochester, Minn.: Mayo Clinic Health Foundation, 2005.

Nash, J. D. *Maximize Your Body Potential,* 3rd ed. Boulder, Colo.: Bull Publishing, 2003.

Schoonen, J. C. *Losing Weight Permanently with the Bull's-Eye Food Guide.* Boulder, Colo.: Bull Publishing, 2004.

Thompson, A. W., Gorindi, A. and Suthering, J. *The Diabetes Weight Loss Diet.* Lanaham, Ma: Kyle Books, 2008. Printed in association with *Diabetes UK*, this book is relevant to not only to those with diabetes but to others as well.

Other Resources

Because weight control is an integral part of healthy living nearly all of the patient websites listed in previous chapters are a source of information for achieving or maintaining a healthy weight. In particular *Diabetes UK* and the *British Heart Foundation* have published pamphlets relevant to all of us. The *NHS* websites also offer a lot of advice and information. In addition, your local GP surgery will have information and will be able to point you in the direction of other resources.

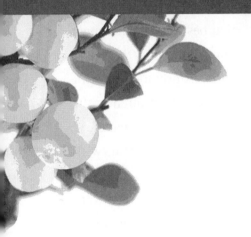

CHAPTER 13

Managing Your Medicines

HAVING A LONG-TERM CONDITION usually involves taking one or more medications. It is therefore a very important management task to understand the nature of your medications and how to use them appropriately. This chapter will help you do just that.

General Words about Medications

Regulation and Advertising of Medicines in the UK

In the United Kingdom the classification of medicines determines how they can be obtained. There are three major classifications:

1. *Prescription only medications (POM):* these are prescribed by a qualified medical doctor and dispensed by a qualified pharmacist. Recently some nurse practitioners have been allowed to prescribe any medicine for any medical condition, including some controlled medicines, with the exception of diamorphine, cocaine and dipipanone for the treatment of addiction. POM medicines cannot be advertised to the general public.

2. *Pharmacy Medicines (P):* these can be sold over the counter, but only by a qualified pharmacist who will askthe purchaser some questions in order to clarify the appropriateness and safety of the sale. These medications can be advertised.

3. *General Sales List (GSL):* These are available off the shelf and do not require a trained pharmacist to sell them; for example, they can be bought at a supermarket or garage. These can be advertised.

The advertising of prescription only medicines in the UK is strictly controlled by the *Medicines and Healthcare products Regulatory Agency (MHRA)*. This agency routinely scrutinises magazines, medical journals and the Internet for the promotion of licensed medicines and checking on advertising to the general public where this is prohibited. If you would like more details about medicine regulation then look at *The Blue Guide: Advertising and Promotion of Medicines in the UK*. This can be viewed on-line at www.mhra.gov.uk

What is the Function of Medicines?

Your body is often its own best healer, and given time, many common symptoms and disorders will improve. The *prescriptions* provided by your body's own *internal pharmacy* are frequently the safest and most effective treatments. So, patience, careful self-observation, and monitoring with your doctor are often excellent choices to make.

It is also true that medications can be a very important part of managing a long-term condition. However, these medications do not cure the condition. They generally have one or more of the following purposes:

- *To relieve symptoms*: For example, an inhaler delivers medications that help expand the bronchial tubes and make it easier to breathe. Similarly, a nitro-glycerine tablet expands the blood vessels, allowing more blood to reach the heart, thus alleviating angina. Paracetamol can be used to relieve pain.

- *To prevent further problems*: For example, medications that thin the blood (or extend it's clotting time) help to prevent blood clots, which cause strokes and heart and lung problems.

- *To improve or slow the progress of disease*: For example, non-steroidal anti-inflammatory drugs (NSAIDS) can help arthritis by alleviating the inflammatory process. Likewise, antihypertensive medications can lower blood pressure.

■ *To replace substances that the body is no longer producing adequately*: This is how insulin is used to manage diabetes and thyroid medication assists an under-active thyroid.

Thus the purpose of medication is to lessen the consequences of disease or to slow its course. You may not be *aware* that the medication is doing anything. But it is, in fact, slowing the course of your disease, thereby keeping you from getting worse or helping you get worse more slowly. Because you don't feel anything, you may think that the drug isn't working. It is important to continue taking your medications, even when you cannot see how they are helping. If this concerns you, ask your doctor.

Side Effects

We pay a price for having such powerful tools. Besides being helpful, all medications have undesirable side effects. Some of these effects are predictable and minor, and some are unexpected and life-threatening. Adverse drug reactions account for a significant number of hospital admissions in the UK. At the same time, not taking your medications as prescribed is also a major cause of hospitalisation. There is a system in place to report the side effects of your medications called the *Yellow Card Scheme*. To report a side effect, complete the Yellow Card which you can get from your surgery or pharmacy; then return it to the address on the card. Alternatively you can use the Yellow Card free phone number to report the side effects, by telephoning 0808 100 3352.

Mind Power: Expect the Best

Medication affects your body in two ways. The *first* is determined by the chemical nature of the medication. The *second* is triggered by your beliefs and expectations. What you believe and have confidence in, can change your body chemistry and your symptoms. This reaction is called the *placebo* effect. It is an example of how closely the mind and body are connected.

Many studies have shown the power of the placebo, the power of mind over body. When people are given a placebo, which means a pill containing no medication, some of them improve anyway. Placebos can relieve many symptoms such as back pain and chronic pain, fatigue, arthritis, headache, allergies, hypertension, insomnia, asthma, irritable bowel syndrome, chronic digestive disorders, depression, anxiety, and pain after surgery. The *placebo effect* clearly demonstrates that our positive beliefs and expectations can *turn on* our self-healing mechanisms. You can learn to take advantage of your powerful internal pharmacy.

Every time you take a medication, you are swallowing your expectations and beliefs as well as the pill. So expect the best!

Let's look at some ways to do that:

■ *Examine your beliefs about the treatment*: If you tell yourself, *I'm not a pill taker,* or perhaps *medications always give me bad side effects*, then how do you think your body is likely to respond? If you don't think the prescribed treatment is likely to help your symptoms or condition, these negative beliefs will undermine the ability of the pill to help you. You can change these negative images into more positive ones. If you take a few moments to review the discussion of positive thinking in Chapter 5 this will help you with this.

- *Think of your medications in the way you think about vitamins*: Many people associate healthy images with vitamins, often more so than with medications. Taking a vitamin makes you think that you are doing something positive to prevent disease and promote health. So, if you regard your medications as health-restoring and health-promoting, like vitamins, you may obtain more powerful benefits.

- *Imagine how the medicine is helping you*: Develop a mental picture of how the medication is supporting your body. For example, if you are taking thyroid hormone replacement medication, tell yourself it is filling a missing link in your body's chemical chains, which will be able to help balance and regulate your metabolism. For some people, forming a vivid mental image can be very helpful. An antibiotic, for example, might be seen as a brush sweeping germs out of the body. Don't worry if your image of what's happening inside of you is not physiologically correct. It's your belief in a clear and positive image that counts.

- *Keep in mind why you are taking the medication*: You are not taking your medication just because your doctor told you to. You are taking your medication to help you live your life. It is therefore important to understand how the medicine is helping. You can use this information to help the medicine do its job. Suppose a woman with cancer is given chemotherapy. She has been told that it will make her feel like she has the flu, she will vomit, and her hair will fall out. So of course, that is what she thinks about and that is what happens. But suppose she is also told that the symptoms will last only a few days and that hair falling out is a good sign because it means that cells that grow fast, like cancer *and* hair, are being destroyed. Also reinforcing the positive message by reassuring her is the clear promise that her hair will grow again after chemotherapy finishes. In that case, she may regard her hair loss, flu-like symptoms, and vomiting as signs that the drugs are working. She can then take actions to counter these effects and will have an easier time tolerating them. The presence of side effects can sometimes be your proof that the medicine is working.

Taking Multiple Medications

People with multiple problems often take many medications: medication to lower blood pressure, anti-inflammatory drugs for arthritis, a pill for angina, a bronchodilator for asthma, antacids for heartburn, a tranquiliser for anxiety, plus a handful of over-the-counter (OTC) remedies and herbs. The more medications you are taking, including vitamins and OTC remedies, the greater the risk of unpleasant reactions. Also, not all drugs like each other, and when they get together, they sometimes cause problems. Fortunately, it is often possible to take fewer medications and lower the risks. However, you should not do this without the help of your doctor. Most people would not change the ingredients in a complicated cooking recipe or throw away a few parts when repairing a car. It is not that changing your medications can't be done. It is just that if you want the best and safest results, you will need expert help.

How you respond to any one medication depends on many factors: your age, metabolism, daily activity, the waxing and waning of your symptoms, your long-term condition, your genetics, and your frame of mind. To get the most from your medications, your doctor will depend on you. Report what effects the drug has had on your symptoms and any side effects. Based on this critical information, your medications may be continued, increased, discontinued, or otherwise changed. In a good doctor-patient partnership, there is a continuing flow of information in both directions. Unfortunately, this vital interchange is often rather underdone. Studies indicate that often patients getting new prescriptions don't ask any questions about them. Doctors tend to interpret patient silence as understanding and satisfaction. Problems often occur because patients fail to receive enough information about medications or do not understand how to take them. In addition, all too often people do not follow instructions carefully enough. Safe, effective drug use depends on your doctor's expertise and equally, on your understanding of when and how to take the drug, and any necessary precautions you need to take.

You must ask questions. Our discussion of communication in Chapter 9 can help with this. Some people are reluctant to ask their doctor questions. They are afraid that they will seem foolish, or stupid, or that they might be perceived as challenging the doctor's authority. But asking questions is a necessary part of a healthy doctor-patient relationship. It has been recognised, in the last few years in the NHS, that doctors working *in partnership* with patients is the most effective way of achieving good outcomes.

The goal of treatment is to maximise the benefits and minimise the risks. This means taking the fewest possible medications, in the lowest effective doses, for the shortest period of time. Whether the medications you take are helpful or harmful often depends on how much you know about them and how well you communicate with your doctor. Another important way to be informed is to read the leaflet that always comes with the medication, or is on the attached label. This gives you a comprehensive summary of practically all you need to know about the medication which has been prescribed for you.

What You Need to Tell Your Doctor

Even if your doctor doesn't ask, there is certain vital information about medications that should be mentioned during every consultation. Here are some of the important matters to consider:

1. Are you taking any other medications?

Report to your doctor and your dentist about all the prescription and non-prescription medications you are taking, including birth control pills, vitamins, aspirin, antacids, laxatives, alcohol, and herbal remedies. An easy way to do this is to carry with you a list of all medications you take and the dosage. Alternatively, you can bring all your medications to the doctor's appointment. Simply saying that you are taking *the little green pills* is not very helpful!

This is especially important if you are seeing more than one doctor. Each doctor may not know what the others have prescribed. Thankfully, this situation should improve when the new *Summary Care Record* system is fully established. Knowing all your medications and supplements is essential for correct diagnosis and treatment. For example, if you have symptoms such as nausea or diarrhoea, sleeplessness or drowsiness, dizziness or memory loss, impotence or fatigue, they may be caused by a drug side-effect rather than the disease. Also, if your doctor does not know about all your medications, he or she cannot protect you from drug interactions.

2. Medication reviews with your GP

Patients in receipt of repeat prescriptions have their medicines reviewed on a regular basis. The date of the next review should be indicated at the bottom of each prescription. The review enables your doctor to make sure that you are taking what you need. At the same time it is an opportunity to review your various medical conditions. The review involves checking that the medication you are taking matches the medication in your records in terms of both dose and frequency. It is also a very good opportunity to discuss any side-effects or interactions between your drugs. However, any allergic reactions should be communicated urgently to your doctor and not withheld until your review. From a wider perspective, the introduction of *Summary Care Records* should improve some situations in managing your drugs, because all the doctors involved in your health care will have access electronically to your personal Care Record which will list all your medications. You can consult pages 160-161 in Chapter 9 on *Communication* for a detailed explanation and rationale for Summary Care Records.

3. Have you had allergic or unusual reactions to any medications?

Describe any symptoms or unusual reactions caused by your medications. Be specific: which medication and exactly what type of reaction? A rash, fever, or wheezing that develops after taking a medication is often a true allergic reaction. If any of these develop, call your doctor at once. Nausea, diarrhoea, ringing in the ears, light-headedness, sleeplessness, and frequent urination are likely to be side-effects rather than true drug allergies.

4. What are your chronic diseases and other medical conditions?

Many diseases can interfere with the action of a drug, or may increase the risk of using certain medications. Diseases involving the kidneys or liver are especially important to mention because these diseases can slow the metabolism of many drugs and increase their toxic effects. Your doctor may also avoid certain medications if, now or in the past, you have had such diseases as high blood pressure, peptic ulcer, asthma, heart disease, diabetes, or prostate problems. Be sure to let your doctor know if you may be pregnant or are breastfeeding. Many drugs cannot be safely used when this is the case.

5. What medications were tried in the past to treat your disease?

It is a good idea to keep your own records. What medications have you used in the past to manage your condition, and what were the effects? Knowing what has been tried and how you reacted will help to guide the doctor's recommendations for any new medications. However, the fact that a medication did not work in the past does not necessarily mean that it can't be tried again. Diseases change and sometimes the same medication can work the second time round.

What to Ask Your Doctor or Pharmacist

There is also important information that you need to know about your medications. Be sure you ask the following nine questions:

1. Do I really need this medication?

Some doctors prescribe medications not because they are really necessary but because they think their patients want and expect drugs. Doctors often feel under pressure to do something for the patient, so they prescribe a new drug. So, don't pressure your doctor into prescribing medications. If your doctor doesn't offer a medication, consider that good news. Also, ask about non-drug alternatives. In some cases, lifestyle changes such as exercise, diet, and stress management should also be considered. When any treatment is recommended, ask what is likely to happen if you postpone it. Sometimes the best

medicine is none at all, but on other occasions taking a powerful medication early can help you avoid permanent damage or complications.

2. What is the name of the medication, and what dosage do I take?

Keep a record of each medication you take, noting:

■ Its *brand name*, for example it might be *Crestor* which is one of the statins;

■ The *generic, or the chemical name*, which for Crestor is *Rosuvastatin*;

■ The *dosage* your doctor has prescribed.

If the medication you get from the pharmacy doesn't match this information, ask the pharmacist to explain the difference. This is your best protection against mix-ups with your medication.

Note that many medications have *two names* because more than one version of the medicine may be available. We provide a detailed explanation of medication names later in this chapter.

3. What is your medication supposed to do?

Your doctor should tell you *why* the medication is being prescribed and *how* it might help you. For example is the medication intended to prolong your life, completely or partially relieve your symptoms, or improve your ability to function? So, if you are given a medicine for high blood pressure, the medication is given primarily to prevent later complications, such as stroke or heart disease, rather than to stop a headache. On the other hand, if you are given a pain reliever such as ibuprofen, the purpose is to help ease the headache. You should also know how soon you might expect results from the medication. Drugs that treat infections or inflammation may take several days or up to a week to show improvement. Antidepressant medications and some arthritis drugs typically take several weeks to start providing relief.

4. How and when do I take my medication, and for how long?

If medications are going to work then you must take them *when* you are supposed to, *in the amounts* you are prescribed, for *as long as* you are supposed to take them and *at the correct intervals*. Following this advice is crucial for safe and effective use. If you are puzzled, then ask. Does *every six hours* mean every six hours while you are awake or every six hours around the clock? Should the medication be taken before meals, with meals, or between meals? What should you do if you accidentally miss a dose? Should

you skip it, take a double dose next time, or take it as soon as you remember? Should you continue taking the medication until you have fewer symptoms or until you finish the current medication? Some medications are prescribed on a *PRN* basis. The acronym PRN comes from the Latin phrase *pro re nata* meaning *as needed*. So, you need to know when to begin and end your treatment and how much medication to take. It's important to work out a plan with your doctor to suit your individual needs.

Taking your medication properly is vital, and if you are still not sure exactly how to take the medication contact your doctor or pharmacist.

5. What foods, drinks, and other medications or activities should I avoid while I'm taking this medication?

Food in your stomach may help protect it from some medications but may render other drugs ineffective. For example, milk products or antacids block the absorption of the antibiotic tetracycline. This drug is best taken on an *empty* stomach. Some medications may make you more sensitive to the sun, putting you at increased risk from sunburn. It is very important to ask questions. For example, will the medication prescribed interfere with driving safely? Other drugs you may be taking, even over-the-counter drugs and alcohol, can amplify or lessen the effects of the prescribed medication. Taking aspirin along with an anticoagulant medication can result in bleeding. On some occasions both of these may be prescribed for patients by their doctor. However, in that situation the aspirin is not an simply an over-the-counter drug, it is a considered part of the treatment and these patients will be closely monitored by the

GP. The more medications you are taking, the greater the chance of an undesirable drug interaction. So ask your doctor about possible *drug-drug* and *drug-food* interactions. Take great care to make sure you are aware of exactly which pill is which. Sometimes you may be prescribed two lots of medication and the shape and colour of the pills are very similar. If you mix them up this will lead to you missing a dose of one medication and taking too much of the other. Using a pill organiser box can help to make sure you get the right pills and the right dose at the right time and on the right day.

6. What are the most common side-effects, and what should I do if they happen to me?

All medications will have side-effects. Sometimes, your doctor may try several medications before hitting on the one that is best for you. You need to know what symptoms to be on the look-out for and what action to take if they develop. If you have an adverse reaction, should you seek immediate medical care, discontinue the medication, or call your doctor? Of course the doctor cannot be expected to tell you every possible reaction to the drug, but the most common and important ones should be discussed. So it may be up to you to ask your doctor or pharmacist if there are any likely adverse reactions. The *National Institute for Health and Clinical Excellence* (NICE) has produced a pamphlet giving guidelines on medication prescribing. The pamphlet is easy to read and jargon free. It is entitled: *You and your prescribed medicines: enabling and supporting patients to make informed decisions*. It is available on-line at www.nice.org.uk/nicemedia. It is referenced as pamphlet *CG76*. One of the recommendations

is that professionals should ask patients if they have any concerns about their medications.

7. Are there any tests necessary to monitor the use of my medication?

Most medications are monitored according to the improvement or worsening of symptoms. However, some medications can disrupt body chemistry before any noticeable symptoms develop. In some cases these *invisible* adverse reactions can be detected by laboratory tests such as blood counts or liver function tests. In addition, the level of some medications in the blood needs to be measured on a regular basis to make sure you are getting the right amounts. Ask your doctor if the medication being prescribed has any of these special requirements.

8. Can a less expensive alternative or generic medication be prescribed?

Every drug has at least two names, a *generic name* and a *brand name*. The generic name or scientific name is the name for the active ingredient in the medicine which is identified by an expert committee and is understood internationally. The brand name is given to a medicine by the pharmaceutical company that makes it. For example *Sildenafil* is the generic name of a medicine to treat erectile dysfunction. Pfizer, the company that makes Sildenafil, sells it under the brand name *Viagra*. When a drug company develops a new drug in the United Kingdom, it is granted exclusive rights to produce that drug for 20 years. In some cases the license can be extended. After this 20 year period, other companies may market chemical equivalents of the drug. These generic medications are considered to be as safe and effective as the original brand-name drug but often cost much less. In some cases, your doctor may have a good reason for preferring a particular brand.

9. Is there any written information about the medication?

Your doctor may not have time to answer all of your questions. In addition, you many not remember everything that was said. Fortunately, there are many other good sources of information, including pharmacists, nurses, package inserts, pamphlets, books and websites. Several useful sources are listed at the end of this chapter. The *package inserts* mentioned earlier are a very important way of finding a lot of information about your particular prescription. It tells you what your medication is, how it works, how you should take it and when. It warns you when you should not take this medication, for example if you have certain conditions, and it also provides information about other medicines which will react with it. Indeed, the package insert is a thorough and reliable source of information about your medication.

How to Read the Prescription Label

One important safeguard in dealing with your medication is the prescription label. The illustration in *Figure 13.1* will help you to learn how to read these labels. The label will repeat the instructions for using the medication that your doctor will have given you verbally. You should note that Aspirin should not be given to children under the age of 16 years. For you the label provides all the information you need to ensure you take the medication safely:

- The pharmacy details.

- Your name, date of birth and address: this ensures it is *your* prescription.

- What the medication is and the dosage.

- Specific instructions on how and when to take it.

- Any additional warnings.

Green Lake Pharmacy, 600 London Road, Utopia

Date: 15-06-2013 tel. 01119 777777

Aspirin 75mg.

James Scott 16.07.1991. 3, King's Castle, Roundhead Hill, Utopia.

Do not take more than eight in 24 hours.

Do not take indigestion remedies two hours before or after you take this medicine.

Swallow this medicine whole, do not chew or crush. Contains aspirin. Do not take anything else containing aspirin while taking this medicine.

Figure 13.1 **The Label on Your Medication**

A Special Word about Pharmacists

Pharmacists are an under-used resource. They have gone to university for many years to learn about medications, how they act in your body, and how they interact with each other. Your pharmacist is an expert on medications who will readily answer questions face-to-face, over the phone, or even via e-mail. Pharmacists can be based in, or near, your local surgery, in local chemists and hospital pharmacies. As a self-manager, don't forget pharmacists. They are potentially important and helpful consultants.

Medications may be prescribed to be taken in forms other than tablets

This includes taking injections of insulin for diabetes or betaferon for multiple sclerosis. Also your medications can be taken by using a patch, nasal spray, cream or syrup.

The same rule applies to all medications in that you must follow the instructions given to you on how to take them. It is also important that you follow the exact instructions on *storing* the medications. For example, some medications will require refrigeration and others must be kept out of direct sunlight.

Healthy Living Pharmacies

The importance and ability of pharmacists to contribute toward helping people live a healthy lifestyle has been recognised much more in the in recent years. The evaluation of a pilot study, where certain community pharmacies were set up specifically as *Healthy Living Pharmacies*, concluded that they had much to offer. The idea of a Healthy Living Pharmacy is aimed at achieving the consistent delivery of a broad range of high quality services to improve health and wellbeing and to reduce health inequalities. These pharmacies have a lead professional trained in healthy lifestyles and offer a range of services above and beyond that of merely dispensing your prescriptions. For example, consider the following services:

- *Medicine MOT:* If you have a long-term health condition and take medicines prescribed by your doctor, your pharmacist can meet with you. He or she will discuss the best time to take your medicines and their side effects, and also talk about how your drugs may interact with over-the-counter medicines, or with food or alcohol. People with asthma or COPD can be invited back after six months to check their progress with inhaler technique.

- *Stop smoking:* This is a service which supports, monitors and advises people on stopping smoking.

- *Weight management:* The pharmacy can offer a personalised weight loss support service to help motivate you to lose weight. If you have a Body Mass Index of over 30 the service is free. For more detail on BMI take a look at Chapter 12.

- *Rethink your drink:* After a simple assessment, if you find that the amount of alcohol you drink is putting your health at risk, the pharmacy can offer quick and effective solutions to help you cut down.

- *Minor Ailments Service:* The scheme can include treatment for a wide variety of common conditions and help in obtaining the relevant medicine from the NHS.

- *Emergency Contraception:* The pharmacy can provide the *morning-after pill* and offer objective advice.

At the time of writing, Healthy Living Pharmacies have not been set up nationally so accessing them currently will depend on where you live. The standard of service, as in every organisation, will vary and depend on the individuals involved.

Taking Your Medicine

No matter what the medication, it won't do you any good if you don't take it. Nearly half of all medicines are not taken as prescribed. This has been called *the other drug problem.* There are many reasons why people don't take their prescribed medication: forgetfulness, lack of clear instructions, complicated dosing schedules, bothersome side-effects and sometimes the cost of the medications. Whatever the reason, if you are having trouble taking your medications as prescribed, discuss this with your doctor. Often simple adjustments can make things easier. For example, if you are taking many different medications, perhaps one or more can be eliminated. If you are taking one medication three times a day and another four times a day, your doctor may be able to simplify this regimen, perhaps even prescribing medications that you need to take only once or twice a day. Understanding more about your medications, including how they can help you, may also help in motivating you to take them regularly.

If you recognise these problems, ask yourself the following questions and discuss your answers with your doctor or pharmacist:

- Do you tend to be forgetful?

- Are you confused about the instructions about how and when to use the medications?

- Is the schedule for taking them too complicated?

- Do your medications have unacceptable side effects?

- Is your medicine too expensive? Certainly, those who need to take several medicines and are not eligible for free prescriptions can find that the costs can mount up alarmingly.

- Do you feel that your disease is not serious or unpleasant enough to need regular medications? It is a fact that with some diseases such as high blood pressure, high cholesterol, and early diabetes, you may not have any obvious symptoms.

■ Do you feel that the treatment you are getting is unlikely to help?

■ Are you really denying that you have a disease that needs treatment?

■ Have you had a bad experience with the medicine you are supposed to be taking, or with another medication?

■ Do you know someone who has had a bad experience with the same medication?

Perhaps you are you afraid that something similar will happen with you.

■ Are you afraid of becoming addicted to the medication?

■ Are you embarrassed about taking it, or view it as a sign of weakness or failure?

■ Maybe you fear you'll be judged negatively if other people know about it?

■ Ask yourself about some of the benefits you might expect if you take the medication as prescribed.

Remembering to Take Your Medicines

If forgetting to take your medication is a problem, here are some suggestions to help you remember:

■ *Make it obvious:* Place the medication, or a reminder, next to your toothbrush, on the breakfast table, in your lunch box, or in some other place where you're highly likely to stumble over it. At the same time, be careful where you put the medication if there are children around. Alternatively, you might put a reminder note on the bathroom mirror, the refrigerator door, the kettle, the television, or in some other conspicuous place. If you link taking the medication with some well-established habit, such as meal times or watching your favourite television programme, then you'll be more likely to remember.

■ *Use a checklist or an organiser pillbox:* Make a medication chart listing each medication you are taking and the time when you

take it, or you can check off each medication on a calendar as you take it. You might also buy a pillbox at the chemist. This container separates pills according to the day, and time of day, they should be taken. You can fill the pillbox once a week so that all of your pills are ready to take at the proper time. A quick glance at the pillbox lets you know if you have missed any doses and prevents you double-dosing.

■ *Use an electronic reminder:* Get a watch or mobile phone that can be set to beep at pill-taking time. There are also *high-tech* containers that beep at pre-set times, to remind you to take your medication. If you have a smart phone, you can also download *apps* that can track and remind you to take your medication.

■ *Enlist the support of others to remind you:* Ask members of your household to remind you to take your medications at the appropriate times.

- *Don't run out of supplies:* Avoid waiting until you reach your last pill. When you get a new prescription, mark on your calendar the date a week before your medications will run out. This will serve as a reminder to re-order your prescription. Also be careful that you don't forget to pick up your repeat prescriptions when the time comes.

Travelling

Plan in good time before you travel. There are many things you need to be aware of if you plan to travel, some relating to short trips others to much longer ones:

- Talk to your GP at least two months ahead of your trip so you will be aware of any special arrangements you will need to make.

- Check the rules for taking your medication out of the UK and into the country you are going to. Some countries have rules about the types and quantities of medication that you are allowed to bring in.

- Be aware that some medicines you may have bought over-the-counter in the UK may be controlled in other countries and vice versa.

- Countries such as India, Pakistan and Turkey have a list of medicines that they will not allow in.

- Always carry your medication in a correctly labelled container.

- Carry your medication in your *hand luggage* but also take spare medication in your luggage in case one or the other is lost.

- It's a good idea to carry a copy of your prescription with you and a letter from your GP explaining the details of your medicine and the conditions for which you are taking them.

- Make sure you have taken out medical insurance for non-EU countries you may be travelling to, for example when visiting the USA.

- Carry your *European Health Insurance Card* (EHIC): This card is entirely free and for detailed information about its use you can phone the *Overseas Health Care Team* on 0191 218 1999. If you need to call from abroad then telephone +44 191218 1999.

Self-Medication : A Practical Management Guide

Here are some pointers for self-medication:

- *Over-the-counter medications (OTC):* These are medications that you buy for yourself and it is important that you find out exactly what it is that you are taking, why, and how to use the medication wisely.

- *Consult your doctor before self-medicating:* Especially if you are pregnant, nursing, have a long-term condition, or are already taking multiple medications.

- *Read the labels:* Follow the directions carefully.

■ *Check with the pharmacist before you buy:* Let the pharmacist know which prescription medicines you are taking because OTC medicines can interact with prescription drugs causing a variety of problems. These can range from mild to life-threatening. Quite simple things such as herbal remedies or vitamins can react with some prescription medications.

■ *Never be tempted to use medicine from an unlabelled container.*

■ *Do not take medicines left over or prescribed for someone else:* We sometimes retain medications from a previous illness or are tempted to use medicines which were prescribed for someone else.

■ *Pills can sometimes get stuck in your throat:*
  ◆ Your pill may go down more easily with well chewed food.
  ◆ Drink at least half a glass of water with your pills.
  ◆ Remain standing or sitting upright for a few minutes after you taking pills.

◆ Some medicines are better taken on an empty stomach while others should be taken with food.

◆ Check with your pharmacist the best way to swallow your particular tablets.

■ *Do not exceed the recommended dose or the length of the treatment period:* Unless you have discussed this with your doctor.

■ *Store your medicines in a safe place:* Well out of the reach of inquisitive children.

■ *Make sure you read the instructions on how to store your medicines:* For example, in a cool place or away from sunlight.

■ *Many medicines have an expiry date of two to three years:* Get rid of all out-of-date medicines by taking them to your pharmacy. Don't flush them away in the lavatory.

Medications can help or harm. What often makes the difference is the care you exercise and the partnership you develop with your doctor.

Prescriptions and Prescription Charges

The prescription charges quoted here are correct for June 2013 and apply to England. This is because prescription charges have been abolished in Scotland, Northern Ireland, and Wales.

Charges

■ The current prescription charge is £7.85p per item. You can save money by purchasing a *prescription prepayment certificate* which is £29.10p for three months or £104 per annum. These prepayment certificates can save you money if you need four or more items over three months, or if you need 14 or more items in any one year.

■ For wigs and fabric supports charges increased in 2013 by an overall 2.5%. One pair of elastic hosiery support now costs £15.70

A Special Word about Alcohol and Recreational Drugs

The use of alcohol and recreational drugs, the illegal use of prescription medications used for non-medicinal purposes, has been increasing in recent years, particularly amongst people over the age of 60. These drugs, whether legal or illegal, can cause problems. They can interact with prescription medications, making them less effective or even causing harm. They can blur your judgment and cause problems with balance. In turn, this can cause accidents and injure both you and others. In some cases, alcohol or recreational drugs can make existing long-term conditions worse. Alcohol use is associated with an increased risk of hypertension, diabetes, gastrointestinal bleeding, sleep disorders, depression, erectile dysfunction, breast and other cancers, and injury.

Current NHS guidelines say:

Women should not drink more than two or three units a day: that is, no more than a standard 1.75ml glass of wine.

Men should drink no more than three or four units per day: that is, no more than one strong pint of beer.

In practical terms what does a unit mean?

The size of the glass determines the number of units. Where the strength of the alcohol is 13% then for red, white or rosé wine

A small glass is 1.25ml = 1.6 units.

A standard glass is 1.75ml = 2.3 units.

A large glass is 2.5ml = 3.3 units.

For Beer

One pint of beer 4% alcohol = 2.3 units.

One pint of beer 5.2% alcohol = 3 units.

One pint of beer 8% alcohol = 4.5 units.

If you are at the *at risk* level for alcohol or are regularly using recreational drugs, you should seriously consider cutting down or stopping their use.

Talk to your doctor about your use of these drugs. Doctors are often hesitant to raise the issue because they don't want to embarrass you. So, it is up to you to introduce the subject. Doctors will be very willing to talk about it. They have heard it all, and they will not think less of you because of it. An honest conversation now might save your life.

Free prescriptions

Some groups of people are eligible for free prescriptions including:

- Those aged under 16.
- Those aged under 19 and in full-time education.
- Those who are aged 60 and over.
- Those who are pregnant or have had a baby in the previous 12 months.

- Those with a continuing physical disability that prevents them from going out without help from another person.

- War Service Pensioners needing treatment for accepted disabilities.

- Those who are NHS in-patients.

- Those who have certain specified medical conditions; for example Type 1 Diabetes or

Type 2 when medication is required to treat the disease, or anti-convulsive medication for epilepsy.

■ Those on low incomes. This is a more complicated group and individual patients may need advice to see if they qualify. Currently, it includes people on income support or income-based job seeker's allowance.

Cancer as a special case

■ Prescription charges for cancer patients were abolished in 2009. Your doctor can authorise a certificate for this exemption.

■ The abolition covers current treatment for cancer, the effects of cancer and the effects of current or previous cancers.

■ Other medications, not relating to your cancer, are also prescribed free of charge.

■ This exemption is not intended for those patients who have been treated and are apparently clear of cancer and where no further treatment is planned. In these cases, treatment is carefully defined and does *not* include routine follow up with planned discharge at a later date.

The situation in Wales, Northern Ireland, and Scotland

Prescriptions in Wales, Northern Ireland, and Scotland are free. This is because the devolved government powers in these countries have legislated to abolish prescription charges.

Suggested Further Reading

Publishing and Royal Pharmaceutical Society. *British National Formulary* (BNF). BMJ London: Pharmaceutical Press: 2013

This book is a comprehensive reference book used by the medical profession including your own GP. It is published every six months to include all recommended changes in prescribing medicines. It has 1100 pages and costs approximately £25. It is not a browsing book.

Baxter, K. *Stockley's Drug Interaction Pocket Companion.* London: Pharmaceutical Press: 2013

Martin, E., ed. *A–Z of Medicinal Drugs: a family guide to over-the-counter and prescription drugs.* Oxford: Oxford University Press, 2010

Williamson, E., ed. *Stockley's Herbal Medicines Interactions.* (2nd Edition) London: Pharmaceutical Press: 2013

Other Resources

☐ www.nhs.uk/medicine-guide/pages
This is an NHS site on side effects, interactions and dosages.

☐ www.herbsociety.org.uk/mh-legislation
This site provides a guide to the EU traditional Herbal Medicines Directive and its possible implications.

☐ www.mhra.gov/safety-information
This is the official body for regulating medicines in the UK and the link concerns using medicines safely.

☐ www.anxiety.org.uk.
This organisation has a section on herbal medicine.

☐ MedlinePlus: *Drugs, Supplements, and Herbal Information*, a service of the U.S. National Library of Medicine and National Institutes of Health.
www.nlm.nih.gov/medlineplus/druginformation.html.

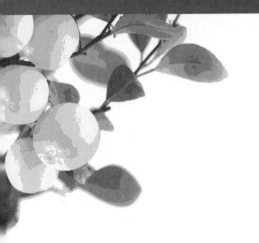

CHAPTER 14

Making Informed Treatment Decisions

IN THE UK, ADVERTISING FOR PRESCRIPTION MEDICINES is closely regulated so we are protected, to some degree, from being overwhelmed by pressures to use these drugs. Nevertheless we still hear about new drugs, nutritional supplements, and alternative treatments on a regular basis, particularly those classified as over-the-counter medicines. Hardly a week goes by without a new treatment or research of some kind being reported in the news. What can we believe from what we read and hear? How can we decide what might be worth trying and find out if it is available and suitable for us?

Treatment Options

For lots of long-term conditions, there is no single, universal treatment. We are faced by a whole range of possible treatments to consider, and it's not just the medical factors that we must take notice of. Our own personal preferences are very important too. It may be that the risks involved in an operation must be balanced against living in discomfort. It could mean deciding if the possible side effects are worth the possible treatment benefits. We must weigh effects such as hair loss, erectile dysfunction, or weight gain against the benefits deriving from a more controlled condition. We are more likely to make the best personal decisions if we consider all the risks and options available, and our preferences. Most people want more information and a greater say in what treatments they are given. Indeed, not being properly informed about our illness and the treatment options is the most common cause of patient dissatisfaction. Your health care professional can provide you with information about treatment choices available to you. Then, there are tools which can help you to consider these options, tools like the *NHS Right Care Patient Decision Aids*.

Ask Three Questions

There are really three simple questions you can ask your health care professionals when you are considering treatments:

- Firstly, what are my options?

- Secondly, what are the pros and cons of each treatment option for me?

- Thirdly, how do I get support in making a decision that is right for me?

An important part of managing your own care is being able to evaluate the myriads of claims and recommendations we hear, so that we can make an informed decision about whether to try something new, or not. In doing this, there are some other important questions that you should ask yourself when you are coming to a decision about treatment, whether it is a mainstream, complementary or alternative treatment. Here is some guidance on *nine* of these questions:

1. Where did I learn about this treatment option?

Was it reported in a scientific journal, a newspaper, a magazine, a TV advertisement, a website, or a flyer you picked up somewhere? Or, did your doctor suggest it?

The source of the information is important. Results that are reported in a respected scientific journal are more believable than those you find in a tabloid newspaper or in advertising. Results reported in scientific journals, such as the *Lancet, New England Journal of Medicine,* or *Nature* are usually based on research studies. These studies are carefully reviewed for scientific integrity by other scientists, who are very careful about what they approve for publication. However, many alternative treatments and nutritional supplements have not been studied scientifically, so they are not as well represented in the scientific literature as medical treatments are. As this is the case, you need to be vigilant and critical when evaluating what you read or hear.

2. Were the people who showed improvements from this treatment like me?

In the past, many studies were done with *easy-to-reach* people. So older studies were often carried out on students, nurses, and white men! This has changed, but it is still important to find out if the people that improved or got better were like you. Were they from the same age group? Did they have similar lifestyles? Did they have the same health problems as you do? Were they the same gender and race? If the people *aren't* like you, then the results may not be the same for you.

3. Could anything, other than the treatment, have caused the positive changes noted?

For example, a woman who returns from a two-week stay at a spa in the Mediterranean reports that her arthritis has improved dramatically. She gives thanks for the special diet and supplements she received. But ask yourself whether her improvement was all to do with the special diet and supplements, when warm weather, relaxation, and pampering may have had even more to do with her improvement?

It is important to look at everything that has changed since you started a particular treatment. It is common to adopt a generally healthier lifestyle when starting a new treatment; could that be playing a part in any improvement? Did you start another medication or treatment at the same time? Has the weather improved? Are you under less stress than you were before you started the treatment? Can you think of anything else that could have affected and improved your health?

4. Does the new treatment involve stopping other medications or treatments?

Does it require that you stop taking another basic medication because of possible dangerous interactions? If the other medication is important, this will require a discussion with your doctor before making such an important change.

5. Does treatment involve not eating a well-balanced diet?

Does it eliminate any important foods or concentrate on only a few foods that might be harmful to you? Maintaining a balanced diet is important for your overall health. Be sure that you're not sacrificing important vitamins. Alternatively, make certain that you're getting them from another source, perhaps by consulting your doctor or dietician. Also be sure to avoid putting excessive stress on your organs by concentrating on only a few food groups to the exclusion of others.

6. Can I think of any possible dangers or harm in this treatment?

Some treatments take a toll on your body. All treatments have side-effects and possible risks. Discuss these matters thoroughly with your health care professionals. Only you can decide if the potential problems are worth the possible benefits. But you must have all the information in order to make that decision.

Many people think that if something is natural, it must be good for you. This is not always true. *Natural* isn't necessarily better just because a treatment ingredient comes from a plant or animal. Take the case of the powerful heart medication *digitalis*, which comes from the foxglove plant. It is *natural*, but the dosage must be exact or it could be very dangerous. Hemlock comes from a plant, but it is a deadly poison. Some treatments may be safe in small doses but dangerous in larger doses. Be careful.

7. Are nutritional supplements regulated?

Nutritional supplements and traditional herbal medicines are regulated in the UK according to whether they are classified as foods or medicines. If they are classified as food, they are regulated by the *Food Standards Agency* and the *Department of Health*. If they are classified as medicines then they will be regulated by the *Medicines and Healthcare Regulatory Agency* (MHRA). Some traditional herbal remedies come under the *EU Regulations* for herbal medicines. If you are particularly interested in the subject of nutritional supplements, you should read the very user-friendly pamphlet *Supplements: Who needs*

them? A Behind the Headlines Report. This can be found on-line at www.nhs.uk

8. Is the new treatment available to me?

Is your health strong enough to maintain this new treatment regime in the timeframe it seems to need to produce an improvement? Will you be able to handle it emotionally? Will this put a strain on your relationships at home or at work? Is it currently available in your area?

9. Am I willing to go to the additional trouble or expense?

Do you have the necessary support in place? Would you be able to attend clinics regularly for treatment, perhaps for hours or even days, if this is required? Would you accept the possible side-effects of the treatment, such as erectile dysfunction, hair loss or weight gain, when measured against the benefits?

Deciding to Try a New Treatment

If you ask yourself all these questions and more and then decide to try a new treatment, it is important to inform your health care professional of your decision. After all, you are partners, and you will need to keep your partner informed about your progress during the time you are taking the treatment.

The Internet can provide information about new treatments very quickly and is therefore a resource for up-to-date information about them. But be cautious, not every piece of information on the Internet is correct or even safe. Seek out the most reliable sources by noting the author or sponsor and the Internet address. Addresses ending in *.edu*, *.org*, and *.gov* are generally more

objective and reliable; they originate from universities, non-profit organisations, and governmental agencies, respectively. Some *.com* sites can also be good, but because they are maintained by commercial, profit generating organisations, their information may be biased in favour of their own products. For more information on finding resources on the Internet and elsewhere, take a look at Chapter 3.

Making decisions about new treatments can be difficult, but a good health self-manager uses the questions presented in this chapter and the decision making steps dealt with in Chapter 2 to achieve the best personal results.

Suggested Further Reading

Chapman, G. B. and Sonneberg, F. A. (Eds). *Decision Making In Health Care.* Cambridge: Cambridge University Press, 2003.

Edwards, A. and. Elwyn, G. *Shared Decision Making in Health Care: Achieving Evidenced Based Patient Choice,* 2nd edition. Oxford: Oxford University Press, 2009.

Other Resources

- ☐ For patient decision aids look at www.sdm.rightcare.nhs.uk/pda

- ☐ "Ask 3 Questions" has been adapted with kind permission from the MAGIC programme, supported by The Health Foundation. "Ask 3 Questions" is based on Shepherd H.L., et al. "Three questions that patients can ask to improve the quality of information physicians give about treatment options. A cross-over trial." *Patient Education and Counselling,* 2011;84:379–85.

- ☐ Patient Empowerment at About.com. This website has useful information about making decisions as a patient. www.patients.about.com

- ☐ *Quackwatch.* This site helps you to distinguish between trusted and not so trusted websites. www.quackwatch.org

- ☐ *Supplements: Who needs them? A Behind the Headlines Report.* www.nhs.uk/news/2011/05May/Pages/supplements-special-report.aspx.

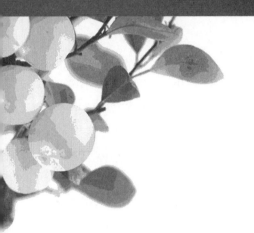

CHAPTER **15**

Managing Chronic Lung Disease

SHORTNESS OF BREATH, TIGHTNESS IN THE CHEST, wheezing, persistent coughing, and thick mucus: if you have chronic lung disease, these symptoms may be all too familiar. When your lungs aren't working well, you may have trouble getting enough oxygen to your organs, and you may not be able to get rid of unhealthy waste air containing carbon dioxide. There are many types of lung disease; the most common are asthma, chronic bronchitis, and emphysema. In each of these diseases there is something getting in the way (an obstruction) of the airflow in and out of the lungs. Chronic bronchitis and emphysema are often referred to as chronic obstructive pulmonary disease (COPD). Although asthma, chronic bronchitis, and emphysema can all be described separately, many people have a mixture of these diseases. Self-management and treatment of these conditions are similar and often overlap.

Special thanks to Cheryl Owen, RN, Karen Freimark, and Roberto Benzo, MD, for help with this chapter.

Understanding Asthma

Asthma is caused in two ways: firstly, by a tightening of the muscles in the walls of the airways that is known as *bronchospasm;* secondly, by the inflammation and swelling of the airways. Take a look at the normal lungs as shown in *Figure 15.1.* The airways (*bronchioles*) are very sensitive, and when exposed to irritants such as smoke, pollens, dust, or cold air, the muscle will contract, and the airway narrows. As the airway narrows, the flow of air is obstructed or blocked. This causes an *asthma attack* or a *flare-up* characterised by shortness of breath, coughing, chest tightness, and wheezing. Wheezing is a high-pitched whistling sound as air pushes through narrowed airways. Treatment is aimed at relaxing the temporarily tightened airway muscles.

The irritants, sometimes called *triggers*, also cause inflammation of the airways. When this happens, the airways swell and produce mucus. To make things worse, chemicals are released from the lining of the airways that make them even more sensitive. This sets up a vicious cycle leading to more bronchospasm and more inflammation.

An acute flare-up of asthma can be treated with medications that relax the muscles in the airways. These medications are called *bronchodilators*, but that may not be enough. Effective treatment also includes avoiding irritants and the use of anti-inflammatory medications such as corticosteroids or intal. These medications reduce the swelling, inflammation; and excessive sensitivity of the airways. To prevent these attacks, you

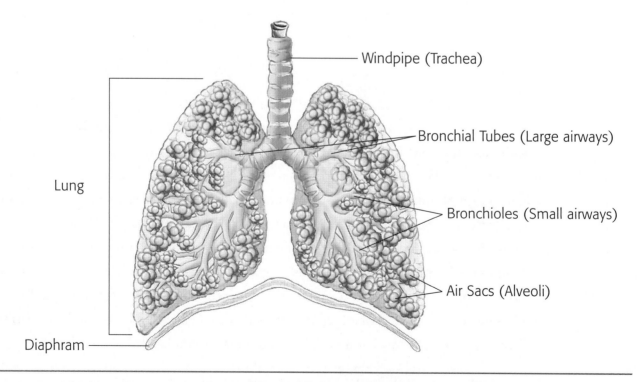

Windpipe (Trachea)

Bronchial Tubes (Large airways)

Bronchioles (Small airways)

Air Sacs (Alveoli)

Lung

Diaphram

Figure 15.1 **Normal Lungs**

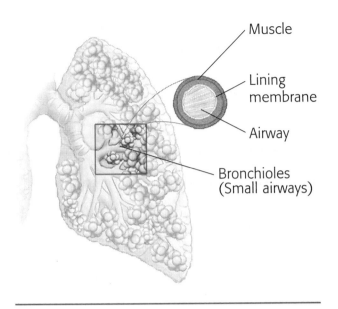

Figure 15.2 **The Bronchiole or Small Airway**

should avoid irritants and you should not smoke. You should also avoid second-hand smoke. If the cold brings on your symptoms, then you should cover your nose with a scarf in cold weather and not exercise outside. In addition, you may need to take anti-inflammatory medications *even when you have no symptoms.*

Asthma varies greatly from person to person. Symptoms may consist of mild wheezing or shortness of breath at night. Indeed, asthma symptoms tend to be worse during sleep. The attacks may be mild and infrequent, or severe and life-threatening. Asthma can usually be managed, but you must be an active partner in the management process. Learn your triggers and avoid them. Take action to prevent symptoms and acute attacks. Your specialist nurse may also teach you to monitor your lung function. Develop a plan with your doctor to recognise and treat your symptoms. Learn how to breathe effectively and exercise properly. Although these measures cannot completely cure or reverse the disease, they can help you to reduce symptoms and to live a full, active life. By taking an active self-management role, you should be able to participate fully in work and leisure activities, sleep through the night without coughing or wheezing, and avoid urgent visits to the doctor or the A&E department.

Understanding Chronic Bronchitis

In chronic bronchitis, the walls inside your airways become swollen and thick. This inflammation narrows the airways and interferes with your breathing. The inflammation also causes the glands that line the airways to produce large amounts of thick mucus. The results are often a chronic cough that produces mucus or sputum, and shortness of breath.

Chronic bronchitis (meaning a long-term bronchitis) is primarily caused by smoking or inhaling second-hand smoke. Air pollutants, dust, and toxic fumes can also be causes. These irritants keep the airways inflamed and swollen. The key to management is to stop smoking, stay away from smokers and avoid other irritants. If this is done, especially early in the disease, you can often prevent it from becoming worse. If you have chronic bronchitis, you should get an *influenza jab* every year and a one-time *pneumococcal pneumonia vaccine* as well. If you have a respiratory condition or are over 65, you may need a second pneumonia vaccination. You should also avoid exposure to anyone with a cold or flu because these infections can make your bronchitis much worse. If symptoms get worse with an increased cough, yellow brown sputum coupled with increased shortness of breath and a fever, consult your doctor. The doctor may decide to recommend the use of medications to thin and liquefy the mucus and provide an occasional treatment with antibiotics.

Understanding Emphysema

In emphysema, the tiny air sacs, called *alveoli* at the very ends of the airways become damaged. Take another look at *Figure 15.1*. As a consequence of this, the air sacs lose their natural elasticity, become overstretched, and often break. When the air sacs are damaged, it is harder for your blood to get oxygen and rid itself of carbon dioxide. The tiniest airways also become narrow, lose their elasticity, and tend to collapse when you breathe out. As a result stale air is trapped in the air sacs and prevents fresh air from coming in.

A large amount of lung tissue can be destroyed before there are any symptoms. This is because most of us have more lung capacity than we normally need. However, eventually the lung capacity is reduced to the point where you begin to notice shortness of breath with activity or exercise. As the disease progresses, the shortness of breath becomes worse with less activity. Later, it may be present even when you are at rest. You may also develop a cough that produces mucus.

Smoking and second-hand smoke are the major causes of emphysema. Cigarette smoking is the most common and most dangerous cause, but cigar and pipe smoking are also damaging. Even if you do not smoke, daily exposure to second-hand smoke is almost as bad. It is important that your home, car, and workplace stay smoke-free. There is also a rare hereditary type of emphysema caused by not having enough of a particular enzyme that protects the elastic tissue in the lungs.

Emphysema tends to get worse over time, especially if you continue smoking. The key to prevention and treatment is avoiding all smoking. Of course, it is better to stop smoking sooner rather than later, but *stopping at any stage* of the disease can help preserve your remaining lung function. People with emphysema can learn a variety of self-management skills, ranging from proper breathing to exercise. These will help them to lead an active life. Medications and oxygen can sometimes be helpful in emphysema. We describe the use of these later in this chapter.

Asthma, Chronic Bronchitis and Emphysema

Asthma, chronic bronchitis, and emphysema most often overlap, so you could have one or more of these conditions. You may have to undergo Pulmonary Function Tests (PFTs) like a spirometry tests where you will be asked to breathe into a machine called a spirometer. This measures the amount and speed of the air you can blow out in order to evaluate how well your lungs are working and the types of treatment that might help you. Although the treatment varies somewhat depending on your specific symptoms and disease, some of the principles and strategies for management are similar. Now take some time to look at some self-management tools that are specific for chronic lung disease.

Avoiding Irritants and Triggers

The best way to manage chronic lung disease is to avoid the things that make it worse. Several irritants can trigger the symptoms of asthma and worsen the symptoms of other chronic lung disease. Fortunately, you can avoid most of these.

Smoking

Smoking is the main cause of chronic bronchitis and emphysema and a major trigger for asthma. Whether you smoke yourself or are around people who smoke, smoking will irritates and damage your lungs. The hot smoke dries, inflames, and narrows the airways. The poisonous gases which are present will paralyse the cilia, the tiny hair-like *sweepers* in your airways that help clean out dirt and mucus. The carbon monoxide in cigarette smoke robs your blood of oxygen and makes you feel tired and short of breath. The irritation from smoking makes infections more likely and can irreversibly damage the air sacs in your lungs. Unfortunately, once air sacs are destroyed, they cannot be repaired. The good news is that most of these harmful effects can be eliminated by stopping smoking and by avoiding second-hand smoke.

If you have tried to stop and failed, do not give up. This is a common experience and you can get help. The NHS runs *Quit Smoking Programmes* which are both free and easily accessible. This is not something you have to do on your own.

Air Pollution

Car exhaust fumes, industrial wastes, household products, aerosol sprays, and wood smoke can all irritate sensitive airways. On particularly smoggy days, check your radio and TV for air pollution alerts, and stay indoors as much as possible.

Cold Weather or Steam

For some people, very cold air can irritate the airways. If you can't avoid the cold air, because of your daily obligations, try breathing through a cold-weather mask. These masks are available at most chemists, or as an alternative you can wear a scarf. For some people even steam in the shower, can be a trigger.

Allergens

An allergen is anything that triggers an allergic reaction. If you have asthma, an attack may be triggered by almost anything, indoors or out. Avoiding your allergens completely can become a full-time job. But, if you are careful a few sensible measures can significantly reduce your exposure. Try some of the following suggestions:

- *Avoid outdoor allergens:* by closing the windows and using an air conditioner when pollen and mould spore counts are at high levels.

- *For some people the major allergic triggers are found indoors:* these come in the form of dust mites, animal detritus from skin flakes and fur and moulds. Often pets, including dogs, cats, and birds, must be banished from the house altogether, or at least from bedrooms.

- *Bath dogs and cats weekly:* this will reduce the allergens present.

- *House dust mites tend to live in mattresses, pillows, carpets, upholstered furniture, and clothing:* if this is a problem, vacuum your mattress and pillows and then cover them with an airtight cover. Wash your bedding, including blankets and bedspreads, weekly in hot water; avoid sleeping or lying on upholstered furniture; and remove carpets from your bedroom. It is often better to avoid dry dusting and vacuuming by using a damp cloth or mop instead.

- *Change the heating and air-conditioning filters every month.*

- *Avoid air fresheners that produce ozone:* these can make asthma worse. All of this takes time, but in the long run the effort will pay off.

- *Be aware that asthma symptoms can easily be triggered:* by perfumes, room deodorisers, fresh paint, and some cleaning products.

Sometimes, indoor air cleaners can be helpful in reducing allergens in the air.

- *Particular foods can be triggers for some people:* the worst offenders are peanuts, beans, nuts, eggs, shellfish, and milk products. Food additives, like sulphite in wine and dried apricots, can also sometimes trigger asthma symptoms.

If you cannot identify your triggers, allergy testing may help you. *Immunotherapy* or allergy injections may also help to de-sensitise some people to certain allergens.

In addition to breathing problems, some people with respiratory conditions also have *gastric reflux*. This happens when acid from the stomach backs up and irritates your gullet and your airways. This may sometimes cause heartburn symptoms. The irritation of the airways may lead to coughing or breathing trouble. Treatment of gastric reflux includes keeping your head and chest elevated when sleeping; avoiding smoking, caffeine, and foods that irritate the stomach; and when necessary, taking antacids and acid-blocking medications.

Medications

Some medications, including anti-inflammatories such as aspirin, ibuprofen, and naproxen, and beta-blockers such as propranolol (*Inderal*), can result in wheezing, shortness of breath, and coughing. ACE-inhibitor medications like lisinopril, which are often used to treat hypertension and congestive heart failure and protect the kidneys in diabetes, can cause problems. For example, by causing a dry, tickling, chronic cough. If you suspect that you have symptoms related to a medication, do not stop your medication, but talk to your health professional or doctor about it soon.

Infections

Individuals with lung problems can experience difficulties with infection. For example, colds, flu, sinus infections, and infections of the airways and lungs can make breathing more difficult. Even though you can't prevent all infections, you can reduce the risks. Be sure to get your flu and pneumonia vaccinations. Try to avoid people with colds, wash your hands frequently, and don't rub your nose and eyes. Talk with your doctor about how to adjust your medications if you get an infection. Early treatment can often prevent serious illness and hospitalisation.

Exercise

Exercise can be a problem *or* a benefit for people with chronic lung disease. On the one hand, physical activity can improve strength and enhance the capacity of your heart and lungs. On the other hand, vigorous physical exercise can trigger asthma symptoms and cause uncomfortable shortness of breath if you have chronic lung disease. Read through pages 257–259 for ways to choose exercise routines. Also you will learn how to adjust your medications before exercising, so that you can prevent exercise-induced asthma. If being able to exercise comfortably is a problem, discuss this with your doctor.

Emotional Stress

Stress does not cause chronic lung disease. However, it can make the symptoms worse by causing the airways to tighten and breathing to become rapid and shallow. Many of the breathing and relaxation exercises in this book can help to prevent the worsening of your symptoms. Also, learning how to manage your condition helps you feel more in control and less stressed.

Note that all these *triggers* can add up. For example, your cat may not trigger an attack on its own, but if you add in a cold, or cleaning chemicals, or stress, then an attack may happen.

Monitoring Your Lung Condition

Lung conditions change over time. Sometimes it will be under better control than at other times. By monitoring your symptoms, you can often predict when a flare-up is coming and do something to keep things from getting worse.

There are two ways to monitor your lung condition. It is important to use at least one of them. For best results, use both. The first is *symptom monitoring* for asthma, COPD, bronchitis, and emphysema. The second, is *peak flow monitoring* which is for asthma.

Symptom Monitoring: for Asthma, COPD, Bronchitis, Emphysema

This monitoring requires that you pay attention to your symptoms and how they change. Here's how you can tell that a flare-up is coming:

■ You experience worsening symptoms, worse coughing, wheezing, shortness of breath, chest tightness, fatigue, increased or thickened sputum, or a new fever. Or perhaps the symptoms occur more often, or more of them are present than is usual.

- You find that you need more puffs than usual of your quick-relief medicine, like your salbutamol inhaler, or the medicine is required more often than twice a week, even though you are not engaging in much physical activity.

- You find that your symptoms cause you to wake up more frequently or are interfering with your work, school, or home activities.

If you experience any of these changes in symptoms, then discuss the situation with your doctor or other health professional.

Using a Peak Flow Monitoring Meter for Asthma

Take a look at the Peak Flow Monitoring Meter illustrated in *Figure 15.3*

Peak Flow monitoring uses a tool called a peak flow meter to measure if the breathing tubes are open enough for normal breathing. These measurements can warn you when a flare-up is starting even before your symptoms increase, and can help you to work out how bad the flare-up might be.

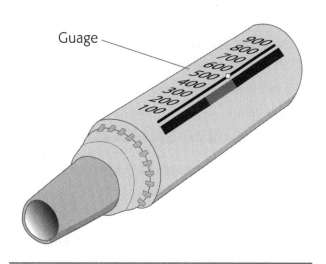

Figure 15.3 **The Peak Flow Monitoring Meter**

If you have moderate or severe asthma, the peak flow meter can become a best friend. It can alert you to problems before they become severe. It can help you and your doctor to know when your medications need to be increased and when they can be safely tapered off. It can help you to distinguish between worsening asthma and breathlessness caused by anxiety or hyperventilation. Best of all, it can help you manage your asthma better.

When the peak flow reading is close to your *personal best benchmark*, which we will describe shortly, the breathing tubes are more open, and the asthma is under control. When the peak flow reading is further away from your personal best, the breathing tubes are less open. Even if you feel OK, a lower peak flow reading can warn you that a flare-up is starting. So you are warned in advance of the need to take action and adjust your medications. Asthma self-management planning is worked through on pages 251–253, so you could take a look now.

If you do not have a peak flow meter or are not sure how to use it, ask your specialist nurse or doctor. You will need to measure your personal best peak flow when you are feeling well and in good control. This means that you are well prepared to take quick action when your peak flow begins to drop. Because different meters can give slightly different readings, *use the same meter all the time.*

You can keep track of your symptoms and peak flow measurements by writing them in an *Asthma Diary*. Your medical professional can give you one, or you can easily make your own. Keeping a diary can help you work out what triggers the asthma, whether the medicines are working and also allows you to spot when flare-ups are about to begin.

You'll need to work out an individual action plan with your doctor. We've provided a sample *asthma self-management* plan for you to study, in the next section. If you wait until your symptoms get worse, they will be more difficult to treat. Early action and adjustment of your medications can make a critical difference.

An Asthma Self-Management Plan

Work out a personal plan with your doctor about what specific actions you should take, and when.

The following guide is an example of a workable plan. These plans will vary depending on you and your doctor or consultant.

Managing Your Asthma: A Day-to-Day Self-Management Plan

GREEN ZONE: GO AHEAD
Your asthma is under good control.

No Symptoms

- You can sleep without waking.
- You have no cough, wheezing, chest tightness, or shortness of breath.
- *Quick-relief* medicines are needed no more than two days per week – except when exercising.
- You are able to participate in most activities without asthma symptoms.
- You have not missed any work or school time.
- You rarely, if ever, need emergency care.
- Your peak flow is scoring 80%–100% of your personal best.

GO AHEAD: Take your medicine daily as prescribed, and avoid triggers .

YELLOW ZONE: BE AWARE

You are having a mild asthma attack.
Possible Symptoms

- You are experiencing some coughing.
- You have some mild wheezing.
- You have a slight chest congestion or tightness.

- Breathing when resting is slightly faster than normal.
- You need to use quick-relief medications more than two days a week (except when exercising).
- Your peak flow is between 50%–80% of your personal best.

BE AWARE:

1. Take quick-relief medicine every four hours as needed to relieve your symptoms.
2. Increase the dose of your inhaled *preventer* medicine until you no longer need quick-relief medicine and are back in the Green Zone. Do not take extra *Seretide, Serevent,* or *Foradil.*
3. If symptoms continue for more than two days or if quick-relief medicine is needed more than every four hours, see *Red Zone*. Call for advice if you need to.

RED ZONE: STOP AND TAKE ACTION
You are having a severe asthma attack.

Possible Symptoms

- You have difficulty breathing when at rest.
- You are experiencing persistent coughing or wheezing.

continues on page 252 ▼

- Your coughing, wheezing, or shortness of breath is waking you up.

- Your breathing is faster than usual.

- Your symptoms are not getting better after two days in the Yellow Zone.

- Your peak flow is less than 50% of your personal best.

TAKE ACTION:

If you need quick-relief medicine every two to four hours and you still have Red Zone symptoms, take the following steps:

1. Take your quick-relief medications immediately. If symptoms do not improve after 20 minutes, take the medications again. If symptoms do not improve after another 20 minutes, take the medications for a third time and, at the same time, *contact your doctor.*

2. Start your *burst* medicine, if prescribed. Keep in mind that it may take four to six hours for burst medicine to work.

3. If you have taken steps 1 and 2 and there is still no relief, you are having a severe asthma attack. Go to the nearest **A&E Department** or **dial 999** now. As you wait, continue to take your quick-relief medicine as needed.

Understanding Your Medications

Medications cannot cure chronic lung conditions, but they can help you to breathe easier. Effective management often involves more than one medication, so don't worry if you are prescribed several medications. Here are some likely issues to take into account:

- *Bronchodilators* will relax the muscles surrounding the airways, open up the airways, and relieve wheezing and shortness of breath. Most inhaled bronchodilators can be used frequently and work in minutes. There are some exceptions to this, but your doctor will have advised you how to use them if they are prescribed for you. It is very important that you follow the advice given to you by your doctor on all your medications and also that you follow what is written in your personal plan.

- *Anti-inflammatory medications* may be prescribed to reduce the inflammation, swelling, and the reactivity of the airways. Medications to loosen mucus, such as mucolytics and expectorants, as well as antibiotics may also be helpful if you have chronic bronchitis or emphysema.

- *Some of the medications provided may be used as symptom relievers.* These will help you with symptoms like wheezing, while others may be used to prevent *and* treat other symptoms. When the medications are being used to prevent symptoms, they must be taken regularly, *even when symptoms are not present.*

- *Don't stop taking your medication prematurely.* Too often people stop their medications because they feel better. Discuss with your doctor which medications to continue and which may be stopped as your symptoms improve.

■ *Some people worry that they will become addicted to the medication or that they may become immune and no longer respond to it.* None of the medications used to treat lung disease are addictive. Nor do patients become immune to them. If your medications are not working effectively in controlling your symptoms, discuss this with your doctor so that adjustments can be made.

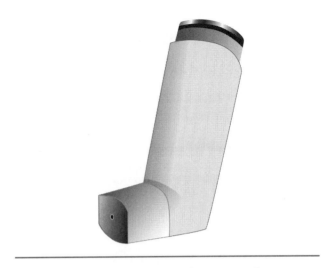

Figure 15.4 **One type of Metered-Dose Inhaler**

Using Metered-Dose Inhalers

Some lung medications, including bronchodilators and corticosteroids can be taken by inhalation. They come in a special canister called a *Metered-Dose Inhaler* (MDI). When used properly, these inhalers are a highly effective way of quickly delivering medication to your lungs. By breathing medicine directly into the lungs instead of swallowing it in pill form, you take less medication into the bloodstream, causing fewer side-effects. Inhaling medication also allows more to reach the lungs. The key to using a metered-dose inhaler is to do it effectively:

1. Exhale gently to empty your lungs.

2. Inhale slowly through your mouth at the same time as you press down on the top of the MDI canister to release the medication.

3. Hold your breath for ten seconds and wait a minute or so before taking any additional puffs to let the previous puff get to work.

Learning to use an inhaler properly is more difficult than swallowing a pill. It takes proper instruction and some practice. One study revealed that whereas 98% of patients said they knew how to use their inhalers properly, fully 94% made errors when using them. So, even if you think you are an expert, it is a good idea to have a health professional check out your technique every so often. Pharmacists are very willing to help you learn the most effective and the safest techniques.

If you have *never* been taught how to use an inhaler, ask your health professional for instructions. It is a fact that the improper use of inhalers is one of the most important reasons for difficulty in controlling symptoms. So if you are prescribed an inhaler, be certain to get help in using it properly. Look on www.asthma.org.uk which is the *Asthma UK* website. There, you will find well illustrated step-by-step instructions on how to use different types of inhaler.

Using your Medications to Best Effect

Use the quick-acting, symptom-relieving *bronchodilator*, medication *first*. Then, wait several minutes for it to open up your breathing tubes

Common Errors to Avoid When Using an Inhaler

- You forget to shake the canister.

- You hold the inhaler upside down. Remember that the mouthpiece should be on the bottom.

- You don't exhale properly before inhaling from the inhaler.

- You breathe through your nose.

- You try to inhale too fast.

- You fail to hold your breath for ten seconds after inhaling

- You don't realise that you are using an empty inhaler.

so that your next step, the use of the preventive controller, an *inhaled anti-inflammatory medication* can get into your lungs better.

Using Spacers or Holding Chambers

Take a look at the Spacer illustrated in *Figure 15.5*

To make using an inhaler easier, safer, and more effective, many doctors strongly recommend using a *spacer device* or *holding chamber*. This is a chamber, usually in the form of a specially designed tube or bag. Into this chamber, you spray the medication from the inhaler. You

then inhale the medication *from the spacer*. The spacer makes it more likely that you can inhale the smaller, lighter droplets of medication, now inside the spacer, further into your airways. The spacer also collects on its walls some of the larger, heavier droplets of medication that would otherwise settle in your mouth or throat. This can reduce side-effects like yeast infections when using inhaled steroids. Some spacer devices have a whistle that sounds only when you are inhaling too rapidly. This reminds you not to take a fast breath because this will deposit more of the medication in your mouth and less in your lungs.

Inhalers with spacers are *easier to use* than metered-dose inhalers without spacers. You don't have to worry about pointing the spray in the right direction and your inhalation doesn't have to be as carefully timed and co-ordinated with the spray. And, because more of the medication reaches your lungs and less is left in your mouth, the medication tends to be safer and more effective. This is especially important if you are using a steroid inhaler.

If you are using a corticosteroid inhaler, rinse your mouth out with water after use. Do not swallow the water. Swallowing the water will increase the chance that the medication will

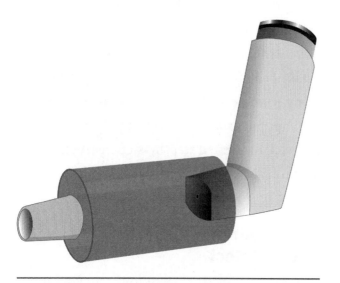

Figure 15.5 **A Spacer for your Inhaler**

get into your bloodstream. This may increase the side-effects of the medication. Some powder may build up on the inhaler over time. Whilst it is not necessary to clean the inhaler every day, you should occasionally rinse the mouthpiece, cap, and case.

How do I determine how many puffs are left in the metered-dose inhaler?

An inhaler may still seem to release puffs of medicine even when there is no medicine left. The best way to tell how many puffs of medicine are left is to keep a note of the number of puffs you have used already. There are two ways you can do this:

- *Read the label on a new canister to find out how many puffs it contains.* Write down one number for each puff on a sheet of paper. For example, if your canister has 100 puffs in it, you could write each number from 1 to 100 on a sheet of paper. Each time you take a puff of the medicine, cross off one number. When all the numbers are crossed off, the canister doesn't have any more medicine left.

- *Divide the number of puffs of medicine in the inhaler by the number of puffs you use each day.* This gives you a clear idea of how many days the medicine will last and therefore you know when you will need to start using a new canister. For example, if the inhaler has 100 puffs and you take 2 puffs a day, the inhaler will last for 50 days. That is100 puffs divided by two puffs a day makes 50 days. Count off the days on a calendar, and mark the day when the inhaler will be empty. Be

sure to renew your prescription before you run out of the medicine.

If you cannot find the number of puffs on the label of the inhaler, simply ask your doctor or pharmacist what it is.

It's best to be cautious. In the past some people have tried floating their MDI canister in water to figure out how many puffs were left. This method certainly does *not* work. We recommend that you use one of the two methods we have described.

Using Dry Powder Inhalers

Dry powder inhalers (DPIs) deliver the medicine as a powder. They are a bit different and are used without a spacer. When using a dry powder inhaler, you need to exhale first and then inhale *rapidly and deeply*. Note that, quite unlike the *slow inhalation* necessary for metered-dose inhalers, with dry powder inhalers the *inhalation needs to be rapid*.

Using Nebulisers

Now take a look at the Nebuliser in use in *Figure 15.6 on page 256*.

Nebulisers are machines that deliver quick-relief medicine as a fine mist. They are often used in the *clinic* or the *emergency room* to give a five to ten-minute *breathing treatment*. Sometimes they are used at home for people who cannot use an inhaler with a spacer. However, nebulisers are bulky and are less convenient than inhalers. Taking four to six puffs of quick-relief medicine from an inhaler with a spacer, when done correctly, works just as well as a breathing treatment with a nebuliser.

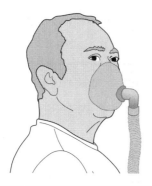

Figure 15.6 **A Nebuliser with a mask that goes over your nose and mouth**

Using Oxygen Therapy

Some people with chronic lung disease cannot get enough oxygen from ordinary air because their lungs are damaged. If you are tired and short of breath because there is too little oxygen in your blood, your doctor may order oxygen for you. Oxygen is a medicine. It is not addictive. Yet some people try not to use it for fear of becoming dependent on it. Other people don't like to be seen with oxygen equipment.

Supplemental oxygen can provide that extra boost your body needs to remain comfortable and it can enable you do the things you want to do without extreme shortness of breath. Most important, it may slow down your disease and make your brain function better. Some people may require the continuous use of oxygen, while others may require it only to help them with certain activities such as exercise or sleep.

Oxygen either comes in large tanks of compressed gas or in small portable tanks of oxygen in the form of a gas or a liquid. If you are using oxygen, be sure that you know the proper dose. This means knowing about the flow rate, when to use it and for how long. You also need to know how to use the equipment, and when to order more oxygen. And don't worry, your oxygen tank will *not* explode or burn! However, oxygen can help other things to burn, so keep your tank at least ten feet away from any open flame, including cigarettes.

How to Breathe Better

In addition to medications, there are other things you can do to improve your breathing. Here are some important examples:

Improving Your Breathing through Exercise

We breathe in and out nearly 18,000 times a day. It is not surprising that breathing is a central concern of people with lung conditions. Yet many people find it surprising that proper breathing is a skill that has to be learned. This is especially important for people with lung conditions. You can learn some ways to breathe that

will enhance the functioning of your respiratory system.

Diaphragmatic or *abdominal breathing* helps strengthen respiratory muscles, especially so in the diaphragm. It also helps to rid the lungs of stale, trapped air. One of the primary reasons why people with lung conditions feel short of breath and can't seem to get enough air, is that they don't get the old air out very effectively. Breathing exercises can help you empty your lungs more completely and take advantage of your full lung capacity. Read pages 47–49 for full instructions on how to do the necessary breathing exercises.

Improving Your Posture

If you are slouched over, it may be very difficult to breathe in and out. Certain body postures make it easier to fill and empty your lungs. For example, if you are sitting now, try leaning forward from the hips with a straight back. You can then rest your forearms on your thighs or rest your head, shoulders, and arms on a pillow placed on a table. Or you can use several pillows at night to make breathing easier. For more on this see page 50.

Clearing Your Lungs

Sometimes excess mucus blocks the airways, making it difficult to breathe. Your doctor or respiratory therapist may recommend certain positions for *postural drainage*. For example, by lying on your left side on a slant with your feet higher than your head, you may be able to help the mucus from certain areas of the lung drain more effectively. Why not ask your doctor, respiratory nurse, or physiotherapist which, if any, postures they think might be helpful for you? Also remember that drinking at least six glasses of water a day may help to liquefy and loosen unpleasant mucus. However, don't drink like this, if you have ankle swelling or have been told by your doctor to limit your fluid intake. For more information and guidance on clearing your lungs look on page 46.

Using Controlled Coughing

A deep cough, one that produces a strong jet of air, is a good way of clearing mucus from the airways. By contrast, a weak, hacking, tickle-in-the-throat, sort of cough can be exhausting, irritating, and frustrating. You *can* learn to cough better. Cough from deep in your lungs and put air power into the cough to clear the mucus. Start by sitting in a chair or on the edge of the bed with your feet planted on the floor. Grasp a pillow firmly against your abdomen with your forearms. Take in several slow, deep *belly breaths* through your nose, and as you exhale fully with pursed lips, bend forward slightly and press the pillow into your stomach. On the fourth or fifth breath, slowly bend forward while producing two or three strong coughs without taking any quick breaths between coughs. Repeat the whole sequence several times to clear the mucus. There's more on this on page 49.

Exercising with Chronic Lung Conditions

Exercise is among the simplest and best ways to improve your ability to live a full life with a chronic lung condition. Physical activity strengthens the muscles, improves your mood, increases energy levels and enhances the efficiency of your heart and lungs. Although exercise does not reverse the damage to the lungs, it can improve your ability to function within whatever limits you now have.

One of the most important things to remember when you start to exercise is to begin at a low intensity. For example, take a slow walk rather than a fast one and exercise for relatively short periods of time. You can gradually increase what you do as you find that you can do more without becoming too breathless. Good communication with your health care providers to manage your symptoms and adjust your medications will let you get the most benefit and enjoyment from an exercise programme.

Exercising with Asthma

Some people with asthma may cough or wheeze when they exercise. If you do, you may wish to start using two puffs of salbutamol (*Ventolin*) or Intal 15 to 30 minutes before starting. Ask your doctor about this. Wearing a scarf or a mask over your face in cold weather may help to prevent the cold air from triggering your asthma. Swimming usually does not trigger asthma.

Here are a few tips for exercising with a chronic lung condition:

Use your medicine, particularly your inhaler, before you exercise. This will help you to exercise longer and with less shortness of breath.

- *If you become severely short of breath with only a little effort,* your doctor may want to change your medicines or even have you use supplemental oxygen before you begin your exercise regime. Mild shortness of breath is normal during exercise, but it may take you some time to find the right balance of *exertion* and *time* for you to stay in your comfort zone.

- *Take plenty of time to warm up and cool down during your exercise activities.* This should include exercises such as pursed-lip breathing and diaphragmatic or abdominal breathing. You will find information about this on pages 47–49.

- *Everyone experiences a normal anticipatory increase in heart and breathing rate even before exercise begins.* This can be worrisome if you are afraid of getting too short of breath. Pursed-lip and diaphragmatic breathing will help you relax and stay calm.

- *Pay attention to your breathing.* Make sure you breathe in deeply and slowly and use pursed-lip breathing when you breathe out. There's more about this on pages 47–49. Learn to take two or three times longer breathing out as when you are breathing in. For example, if you are walking briskly and notice that you can take two steps while you're breathing in, you should breathe out through pursed lips every four to six steps. Breathing out slowly will help you exchange air in your lungs better and will probably increase your endurance.

- *Remember that arm exercises may cause shortness of breath and a faster heart rate sooner than leg exercises.*

- *Cold and dry air can make breathing and exercise more difficult.* This is why swimming in a warm, moist pool is an especially good activity for people with a chronic lung condition.

- *Strengthening exercises such as callisthenics, gymnastic exercises, light weightlifting, and rowing may be helpful.* This is particularly so for people who have become weakened or de-conditioned.

Exercising with Severe Lung Disease

If you can get out of bed, you can exercise for ten minutes a day. Here is how you do it. Every hour, get up and walk slowly across the room or around your chair for one minute. Doing this, ten times a day adds up to ten minutes of exercise. Then you can increase this gradually to a daily exercise routine that will help you feel stronger and more comfortable when moving about. Here are some things to remember as you start to get more active:

■ *Don't hurry.* Many people with lung disease can sometimes hurry up to get there before their breath runs out! It is much better to slow down. Move slowly, breathing as you go. At first, this will take a real effort. With practice, you will find that you can go further more comfortably. If you are afraid to try this alone, have someone walk with you, carrying a chair or a shooting stick, or use a walker with a seat so that whenever necessary, you can sit down.

■ *As you begin to feel stronger and more confident, walk for two minutes every hour.* You have just doubled your exercise and are now up to 20 minutes a day. When this feels comfortable, change your pattern to walking three to four minutes *every other* hour. Wait another week or two, and then try five minutes three or four times a day. Next, try six to seven minutes two or three times a day. You now have the basic idea. Most people with severe lung conditions can build up to walking for ten to 20 minutes, once or twice a day, within a couple of months.

■ *If being up on your feet is a problem, try using a restorator, it's like a portable bicycle crank and pedals.* This is especially helpful if you have a low level of endurance, or do not have stand-by help, or are afraid of exertion. The restorator lets you sit where you are and use your legs to pedal. It's a good device for building confidence and for getting accustomed to exertion in a secure atmosphere.

Sleep Apnoea

If you snore and you tend to feel sleepy during the day, you may have a special type of breathing problem called *sleep apnoea*. If you have this, your throat becomes blocked during sleep. Then for short periods of time, maybe ten seconds or more, you may stop breathing. If you have sleep apnoea, you probably don't know it until someone says something to you about your snoring. This condition is one of the most common undiagnosed serious health problems today.

Sleep apnoea may cause you to wake up feeling tired or with a headache. You may then feel sleepy or have trouble with concentration throughout the day. Sleep apnoea can also lead to more serious problems such as high blood pressure, heart disease, and stroke. It can even mimic the memory problems seen in dementia and Alzheimer's disease. Sleep apnoea is diagnosed by doing a sleep study. This can be done in a laboratory or by wearing a small monitor at home.

You can treat sleep apnoea at home by making lifestyle changes. These include losing weight, if appropriate; sleeping on your side and avoiding alcohol. You should not smoke and and you should start using medication to relieve nasal congestion and allergies. You can also use a breathing device that uses gentle air pressure to keep tissues in the throat from blocking your airway. This process is known as *Continuous Positive Air Pressure* (CPAP). Alternatively, your doctor may recommend using a dental device (oral breathing device) to help in keeping your airway open.

Conclusion

Asthma, chronic bronchitis, and emphysema are not curable. But you can, in partnership with your health care team, work to reduce the symptoms and improve your ability to live a rich, rewarding life. The goal is to control your symptoms so that you can undertake daily activities, exercise and sleep comfortably. They also help you to avoid situations where you have to go to the hospital or A&E departments.

Suggested Further Reading

Ayres, J. *Understanding Asthma.* Poole, Dorset: Family Doctor Publications Ltd, 2008

Haas, F. and Spencer Haas, S. *The Chronic Bronchitis and Emphysema Handbook.* New York: Wiley, 2000.

Lee, D.. *COPD: Chronic Obstructive Pulmonary Disease.* Poole, Dorset: Family Doctor Publications Ltd, 2008

Shimberg, E. F. *Coping with COPD: Understanding, Treating, and Living with Chronic Obstructive Pulmonary Disease.* New York: St. Martin's Griffin, 2003.

Other Resources

☐ *Allergy UK* (The British Allergy Foundation): Provides information, advice and support network. Helpline 01322 619898. www.allergyuk.org.

☐ *Asthma UK*: This is a Specialist Helpline staffed by asthma nurses. Telephone Helpline are as follows: England: 020 7786 4900; Scotland 0131 226 2544; Northern Ireland 028 9073 7290; Wales 029 2043 5400. www.asthma.org.uk.

☐ *British Lung Foundation*: The Foundation offers information and advice. The *Breathe Easy Club* is run predominately by patients. Helpline 03000 030 555. www.blf.org.uk.

☐ *NHS Smoking Helpline*: This is funded by the Department of Health. It offers advice and support to those who want to stop smoking or to those needing continuing support. Helpline 0800 022 4 332. www.smokefree.nhs.uk.

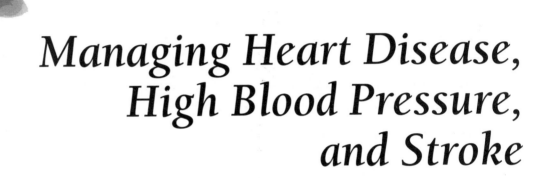

CHAPTER 16

Managing Heart Disease, High Blood Pressure, and Stroke

WE KNOW A LOT ABOUT THE TREATMENT of heart disease, high blood pressure, and stroke and have many ways of preventing and treating these life-threatening diseases. We can save lives and keep people out of hospitals. People with heart disease and even those who have had strokes can look forward to long, healthy, and enjoyable lives.

There are many forms of heart disease. The arteries that supply the heart muscle can be blocked, as in *atherosclerosis*. When a person has heart failure, the heart muscle is damaged and is unable to push blood effectively to the lungs and the rest of the body. If the valves inside the heart are damaged, the result is *valvular heart disease*. Again, blood may not reach the rest of the body. The electrical system that controls the beating of the heart can also be disrupted. This causes the heart to beat too fast, or too slow, or irregularly. This irregularity is called *arrhythmia*. In this chapter, we will talk about all of these as well as other problems with the circulatory system, including strokes and high blood pressure.

261

Coronary Artery Disease

Coronary artery disease, the most common form of heart disease, causes most heart attacks and heart failures. Coronary arteries are blood vessels like *pipelines* that wrap around the heart. The coronary arteries deliver the oxygen and nutrients that the heart needs to perform its job. Healthy arteries are elastic, flexible, and strong. The inside lining of a healthy artery is smooth, so the blood flows easily. Arteries narrow as they become clogged with cholesterol and other substances. This is called *atherosclerosis*, also known as *Coronary Artery Disease* (CAD). The blocked or narrowed area is called a *stenosis*.

Atherosclerosis is the result of a gradual process that occurs over many years. The first stage is damage to the wall of the artery. This damage can be caused by high cholesterol, high triglycerides, diabetes, smoking, or high blood pressure. Triglycerides are the fats you use for energy and come from the fatty foods you eat. Any excess can be stored in the blood. This first stage damage, allows the low-density *lipoprotein cholesterol* or LDL cholesterol which is the bad cholesterol, to enter your artery wall and cause inflammation. Some people have this damage as early as their teens.

Over time, more cholesterol is deposited and the fatty areas grow larger. These fatty areas are called *plaques* and they can completely block off blood flow in an artery. Plaques can also crack open, causing a blood clot to form at the injured site. In both cases, blood flow to the heart is blocked, and the person may experience angina, a temporary chest pain, or a heart attack.

Heart Attacks and Angina

A heart attack is also known as a *myocardial infarction* (MI) and, if not treated immediately, can cause permanent damage to the heart muscle. When a part of the heart muscle has been damaged, that part can no longer help the heart to pump blood.

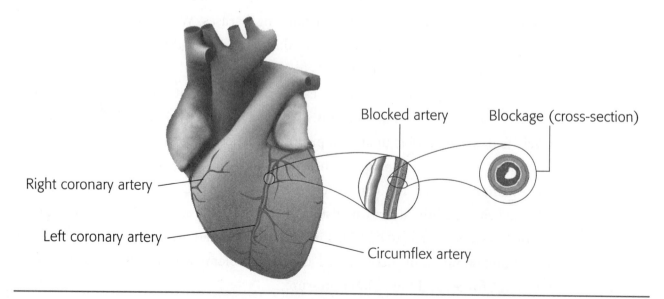

Figure 16.1 **The Arteries of the Heart**

The pain of angina or a heart attack may be on the left side of the chest over the heart but may also radiate into the shoulders, arms, neck, and jaw. Some people with angina or a heart attack may also experience nausea, sweating, shortness of breath, and fatigue.

Female Response to Heart Disease

Symptoms of heart disease in women may be different from those just described, which are more typical for men. Women may be unusually tired and experience sleep disturbances, shortness of breath, nausea, cold sweats, dizziness, and anxiety. These symptoms are more subtle than the crushing chest pain that is often associated with heart attacks. This may be because women tend to have blockages not only in their main arteries but also in the smaller arteries that supply blood to the heart. This condition is called *small vessel heart disease*. Many women turn up in A&E after heart damage has already occurred. This is because their symptoms are not the ones that most people think of as symptoms of a heart attack. Check this out by reading the section *Seek Emergency Care Immediately* on page 267.

Arrhythmias

People with heart disease may notice irregular heartbeats or *palpitations*. This is caused by irregularities in the conduction system or electrical wiring of the heart. Damage to this system can result in irregular heartbeats, skipped beats, or racing beats. Doctors refer to all these patterns as *arrhythmias* or *dysrhythmias*.

Most irregular heartbeats are minor and not dangerous. However, some types of arrhythmias can cause problems. Dangerous occurrences are sometimes accompanied by episodes of fainting, dizziness, shortness of breath, or irregular heartbeats lasting for some minutes. Such arrhythmias may be more dangerous for people with severely weakened hearts and for those with heart failure.

Sometimes the heart can beat irregularly and you may not even notice the difference. However, if you notice irregular heartbeats, take note of how frequently they occur, how long they last and how fast your heart is beating, by checking your pulse, and also how you feel during the episode. This information will help your doctor decide whether or not your arrhythmias are dangerous. Remember that infrequent, short bouts of irregular beats are common for people both with and without heart disease. They are generally not a cause for concern and should not require any change in activity or treatment.

Peripheral Vascular Disease

Peripheral Vascular Disease (PVD), which is also called *Peripheral Arterial Disease* (PAD) or *Peripheral Artery Occlusive Disease* (PAOD), occurs when the arteries in the legs harden, form plaque deposits and become narrow. This is called *atherosclerosis*. Atherosclerosis in the legs is usually the result of the same disease process that happens with atherosclerosis in heart disease.

The main symptom of PVD is leg pain when walking, referred to as *claudication*. Some people may experience leg sores that don't heal or heal slowly. Some of the treatments and medication are similar to those for heart disease: stopping smoking is the most important action, but exercise, medications, and sometimes surgery can help to restore blood flow to the legs.

Heart Failure

Heart failure does not mean that your heart has stopped working or is going to stop. It means that your heart's pumping ability is weaker than normal; your heart still beats, but with less force. This condition is sometimes called *congestive heart failure* because fluid tends to collect in the lungs and legs. Heart failure can be treated and its symptoms managed, even when the heart cannot be returned to normal.

So, What Are the Signs and Symptoms of Heart Failure?

Here are some symptoms you need to consider:

- *Excessive tiredness, fatigue, and weakness:* When your heart is not pumping with enough force, your muscles do not get enough oxygen. You may be more tired than usual and not have enough energy for your normal activities.

- *Shortness of breath:* Sometimes breathing becomes more difficult due to excess fluid in your lungs. You may have trouble catching your breath, a frequent or hacking cough, difficulty breathing when you are lying flat, or wake up at night because you are having difficulty breathing. If you need to prop yourself up with many pillows or sleep in a recliner, this may be a sign of heart failure.

- *Weight gain and swelling:* These are common signs of heart failure. The weight gain is due to fluid retention. When your body is holding on to extra fluid, your weight will go up. Sometimes, this weight gain happens rapidly, in a matter of days, and sometimes it happens more slowly. You may develop *oedema, a* swelling in your feet and ankles, your shoes and socks may be too tight, rings on your fingers may become immoveable, your stomach may feel bloated, and there may be tightness at your waistline.

- *Changes in how often you urinate:* When you pass water, your kidneys are helping your body to get rid of extra fluid. At night more blood is pumped to your kidneys because your brain and muscles are resting and need less blood. This allows your kidneys to *catch up.* You may experience more frequent urination at night or at all times.

Although heart failure is a serious condition, keeping daily track of your weight and eating a low-sodium (low-salt) diet can relieve symptoms and prevent unnecessary trips to the hospital.

Track Your Weight

It is important that you weigh yourself properly and frequently if you are to catch trends that may indicate that you have health problems. Here's how to do it:

- *Weigh yourself at about the same time every day*: We suggest weighing every morning, just after waking up, after urinating and before eating.

- *Weigh yourself with the same amount of clothing on each time*: Or without clothing at all.

- *Use the same scales*: Check to be sure the scales are set to zero before weighing yourself. Make sure your scales are on a hard surface.

- *Write your weight on a daily weight chart*: Also keep some other record, a calendar works well.

- *Repeat weighing if you have doubts*: Doubts about the scales, your procedures, or about your weight.

- *Bring your daily weight chart to all your medical appointments.*

- *Speak to your doctor if you put on more than four to six pounds in one week*: This is especially important if you are also becoming short of breath or have increased swelling in your ankles.

Eat Healthy Foods Low in Sodium

Sodium is an important mineral that helps to regulate the fluid levels in your body. Excessive sodium makes your body hold on to too much fluid. People with heart failure need to eat less sodium in order to avoid retaining excess fluid. This is because the fluid can back up in your lungs and cause shortness of breath. To learn more about healthy eating, how to keep you sodium intake low and discover the difference between sodium and salt, read page 187 in the *Healthy Eating* section of Chapter 11.

Stroke

Strokes happen when a blood vessel in the brain is either blocked or bursts. Without blood and the oxygen it carries, part of the brain will start to die. So, the part of your body controlled by the damaged area of the brain will be unable to work properly.

There are two types of stroke:

1. *An ischemic stroke*: This is the most common stroke and it happens when a blood clot blocks a blood vessel in the brain. The clot may form in the blood vessel or travel from somewhere else in the blood system, perhaps from the heart valves or the arteries in the neck.

2. *A haemorrhagic stroke*: This happens when an artery in the brain leaks or bursts causing bleeding inside the brain.

The symptoms of a stroke will depend on the area of the brain that is damaged. You may experience any of the following:

- Sudden numbness, tingling, weakness, or paralysis in your face, arm, or leg, mostly on one side of your body.

- Sudden vision changes, rather like a curtain coming down.

- Sudden trouble in speaking.

- Sudden confusion or difficulty in understanding simple statements.
- Sudden problems with your walking or balance.

Brain damage from a stroke can begin in minutes. Most of us will be aware of the Department of Health's very successful *FAST* campaign. This is designed to make us all aware of the symptoms of stroke and the need to act quickly if we suspect someone is experiencing this.

Facial weakness: Can the person smile? Has their mouth or eye dropped?

Arm weakness: Can the person raise both arms?

Speech problems: Can the person speak clearly and understand what you say?

Time: If you see anyone with any of these three signs, it's time to dial 999 and call an ambulance.

A speedy response can help to reduce the damage to the person's brain and improve their chance of a full recovery. A delay in getting help can result in death or long-term disability.

Sometimes the symptoms of a stroke develop and then go away within minutes. This is called a *Transient Ischemic Attack* (TIA), sometimes referred to as a *mini-stroke*. Do not ignore these symptoms. They may be a warning sign that a stroke may soon happen. See your doctor if you have symptoms that seem like a stroke, even if they go away quickly. Getting early treatment for a TIA can help prevent a stroke.

If you have had a stroke, you may notice improvements for several months. Stroke rehabilitation programmes can be especially helpful in recovery, as well as in preventing future strokes. They are most helpful if started as soon after a stroke as your doctor considers it is safe. This is usually days, not weeks later. You can help prevent future strokes by not smoking; getting regular exercise; keeping your blood pressure, cholesterol, and diabetes under control; and taking certain medications designed to improve recovery.

High Blood Pressure

What is High Blood Pressure?

Heightened blood pressure, or *hypertension* increases the risk of heart disease, stroke, and kidney and eye damage. Blood pressure is a measurement of the amount of pressure in an artery, expressed as two numbers. The *systolic* pressure, which is the higher first number, is the pressure in the artery when the heart contracts and pushes out a wave of blood. The *diastolic* pressure, the lower second number, is the pressure when the heart relaxes between contractions.

The two pressures are recorded in *millimetres of mercury* expressed as *mm Hg*. So a blood pressure of 120/80 often referred to as *120 over 80* means that the systolic pressure is 120 mm Hg and the diastolic pressure is 80 mm Hg. Both numbers are important because a high reading for either type of pressure can cause damage.

Symptoms of High Blood Pressure

High blood pressure is often called the *silent disease* because most people who have it have no symptoms and cannot really tell whether their blood

Seek Emergency Care Immediately

If you are having symptoms that might indicate a heart attack or stroke, *you must seek medical care immediately*. New treatments are available that can dissolve blood clots in the blood vessels of the heart and brain. These restore blood flow and prevent heart or brain damage. However, these treatments *must be given within hours of the heart attack or stroke.* The sooner you act the better. **Do not wait!** Dial 999 and ask for an ambulance if you have any of the following symptoms:

Heart attack warning signs include:

- Having a severe, crushing, or squeezing chest pain.

- Pain or discomfort in one or both of your arms, back, neck, jaw, or stomach.

- Chest pain which lasts longer than five minutes when there is no apparent cause. Also, if the pain is not relieved by rest, or by heart medications like nitroglycerin.

- Chest pain occurring with any of the following characteristics: rapid or irregular heartbeat, sweating, nausea, vomiting, shortness of breath, light-headedness, passing out, or a state of unusual weakness. For women, chest pain may not be present with these symptoms.

If you think you are having a heart attack:

1. Stop what you are doing.

2. Sit down.

3. Dial 999 and ask for an ambulance. It Is important *not* to try to drive yourself.

4. If you are not allergic to aspirin, take one adult (300mg) or four baby (75mg) aspirin tablets.

Stroke warning signs include:

- A sudden numbness or weakness of the face, arm, or leg, especially on one side of the body.

- A sudden confusion, accompanied by difficulty in speaking and understanding.

- Sudden trouble seeing in one or both eyes, which does not clear when you blink.

- Sudden trouble in walking, dizziness, and a loss of balance or co-ordination.

- Sudden severe headache with no obvious cause.

Remember that minutes matter! Fast action can save lives, maybe your own. Don't wait more than five minutes to dial 999 or your local emergency response number.

---

pressure is high, or not. The only way to find out is to measure it. But because people whose blood pressure is high may feel perfectly well, they find it hard to believe that anything is wrong with them, and so may not consider treatment. However, the silent disease may not stay silent. Over the years, untreated high blood pressure can damage blood vessels throughout the body. In some people this damage can cause strokes, heart attacks, heart failure, or damage to the eyes or kidneys. The reason for treating high blood pressure is to prevent these serious complications. That's why it is extremely important to control your blood pressure even when you feel perfectly well.

Blood Pressure Measurements

Over 90% of hypertension is called *primary* or *essential*. This really means that the exact cause is not known.

So, what is normal blood pressure? A healthy blood pressure is at rest around 120 systolic and 80 diastolic, or 120 over 80. *Prehypertension* is higher than normal but below 140/90. *Hypertension* will be considered when you have a readings of 140/90 or higher. For most people, having a lower blood pressure usually means less risk of complications. And for some people, for example, those with diabetes or chronic kidney disease, it may be important to keep their blood pressure in a lower range.

In fact, your blood pressure varies from minute to minute. Hypertension is diagnosed only when blood pressure measurements on separate occasions consistently show your blood pressure to be at 140/90mmHg or higher. Except in severe cases, the diagnosis is never based on a single measurement. That's one reason it is important to have repeated measurements of your blood pressure.

The White Coat Hypertension Phenomenon

Some people's blood pressure tends to go up only in the doctor's surgery. This is a stress reaction called *white-coat hypertension*. So, it is very helpful to have additional measurements for diagnosing hypertension and monitoring blood pressure treatment. There are many ways to get your blood pressure checked. Ask at your doctor's surgery. You can even get a machine and take your own blood pressure at home. Collect three or four blood pressure readings, and see how these can change, depending on what you are doing. Take these with you to the doctor. Sometimes your doctor can arrange for a 24-hour *ambulatory blood pressure* monitoring. A blood pressure monitor is attached to your arm and records your blood pressure at regular intervals over the 24 hours. This gives your doctor more detailed information about your blood pressure.

Can Blood Pressure be Lowered?

Your blood pressure can often be lowered by a combination of a low-sodium diet, exercise, maintaining a healthy weight, limiting alcohol, and using your prescribed medications. Understandably, some people are reluctant to use these medications due to fear of side-effects. The surprising news is that many people with high blood pressure actually feel better with less fatigue and fewer headaches, when they take the medications.

Diagnosing Heart Disease

Sometimes the symptoms of heart disease are clear and *classic*, such as chest pain following physical activity. Fortunately, there are now many tests available to determine whether heart disease is present and how severe it is.

The following are the most common tests and treatments:

■ *Blood Tests*: Blood tests to measure fat-like substances (cholesterol and triglycerides) can estimate your risk of heart disease. They are also used to monitor the effects of cholesterol-lowering medications. If you are having chest pains, your physician may order tests of cardiac enzymes such as troponin, to confirm the diagnosis of a heart attack. With heart failure, your blood levels of a hormone called *Brain Natriuretic Peptide* (BNP) may rise.

■ *Electrocardiogram:* An electrocardiogram (ECG) measures your heart's electrical activity. It can show a lack of oxygen to the heart, identify a heart attack or heart enlargement, and assess an irregular heart rhythm. It is a *snapshot* of your heart's activity. Sometimes, ECGs need to be repeated to see whether a heart attack is occurring. However, an ECG cannot predict your risk for a future heart attack. On some occasions a portable *Holter* or ambulatory monitor is worn for several hours or days to detect abnormal heart rhythms that come and go.

■ *Echocardiogram:* In this procedure, painless ultrasound waves are bounced off the heart. This produces detailed images which a computer converts into echoes which can be displayed on a TV screen. The pictures are recorded and can show your heart size, heart motion, valve function, and certain types of heart damage. This test may also be done with exercise, called *stress testing*, to see how the heart responds to stress.

■ *Stress Test:* Sometimes the problems appear only when the heart is under increased *stress*. In this case, stress refers to something that makes the heart work harder, rather than emotional stress. The test takes place while you are exercising on a treadmill or stationary bicycle, or after the injection of a chemical to stimulate the heart without exercising. An ECG is also attached to the chest. The ECG, blood pressure, and symptoms are all monitored during the test and for a few minutes after the test. A stress test is done for the following reasons:

♦ To evaluate the symptoms associated with exercise or exertion.

♦ To confirm a suspicion of heart disease.

♦ To evaluate your treatment.

♦ To assess your progress after a heart attack.

♦ To determine any irregularities in your heart rhythm.

A positive test result suggests the presence of coronary artery disease.

■ *Nuclear scan:* In this case, a weak radioactive substance such as thallium is injected into a vein. A scanner or special camera is used to take two sets of pictures, with and without stress, which are then compared. The stress is induced by exercise or medication. This test shows the blood distribution to the heart muscle and how well the heart is pumping.

■ *Cardiac catheterisation and coronary angiography:* A long plastic tube called a catheter is inserted through a major blood vessel, usually in the groin but sometimes in the radial artery in the arm. It is then gently guided into the heart. A dye is injected into the catheter and this allows the coronary arteries to show up on X-rays. This test helps your doctor to decide the best treatment if the arteries are clogged. It can also give information about the function of the heart muscle and the valves.

Prevention and Treatment of Heart Disease, High Blood Pressure, and Stroke

There are three general approaches to help prevent and treat heart disease: lifestyle changes, medications and other medical procedures including surgery. Most people will benefit from one or more of these.

Lifestyle Changes and Non-drug Treatments

Heart attacks, strokes, and high blood pressure can often be prevented or controlled by taking the following actions:

- *Not smoking:* Smoking damages the inner lining of the blood vessels and raises blood pressure. Giving up smoking is the best thing you can do for your health. Fortunately, there are now a variety of support programmes available, ranging from telephone counselling to online and group sessions. In addition, there are medications available, ranging from nicotine gum and patches to calming medications. These can help you to quit and stay smoke free. The NHS is one of the major organisations offering programmes to help you stop smoking and these *Quit Smoking* programmes will be advertised in your local surgery and in hospitals.

- *Exercising:* Exercise strengthens your heart. It can also lower your cholesterol and blood pressure and helps you to control your weight. Inactive people double their risk

for heart disease. Even small amounts of daily physical activity can lower your risk of heart disease and help you to feel better and have more energy. Check out the suggestions made in Chapters 6, 7, and 8.

- *Healthy eating:* Cholesterol is a fat-like substance in the blood. It can cause fatty deposits called plaque to build up and narrow your blood vessels. The higher your cholesterol level, the greater your risk for heart disease. Chapter 11 indicates ways to lower your cholesterol. Unfortunately, not all cholesterol can be controlled by what you eat. The body also *makes* cholesterol which means that some people have a genetic tendency to produce too much cholesterol and consequently medications may be necessary. No matter how it is done, through lifestyle changes or medications or both, lowering cholesterol considerably reduces the risk of heart attacks and strokes.

- *Maintaining a healthy weight:* Being overweight makes your heart work harder and can raise your unhealthy cholesterol and blood pressure levels, and increase your chances of developing diabetes. The highest risk is excess weight around your midsection. Regular exercise and healthy eating are the most important steps to prevent weight gain, maintain your weight, or lose weight. For information about this have a look at Chapters 11 and 12.

■ *Managing emotional stress:* Stress increases your blood pressure and your heart rate. This can damage the lining of the blood vessels and lead to heart disease, as described in Chapter 5.

■ *Limiting alcohol:* The NHS guidance is that you should drink only in moderation which means that:

  ♦ Men should not regularly drink more than three to four units a day.

  ♦ Women should not regularly drink more than two to three units a day.

  ♦ In this context *regularly* means every day or most days.

For more information on healthy eating see Chapter 11 and for the definition of *units* see Chapter 13

■ *Controlling diabetes:* If you have diabetes your risk for heart disease more than doubles. This is because high blood glucose damages the blood vessels. By controlling your blood glucose and taking certain heart-protective medications, you can greatly lower the risk of heart attack and stroke. This is discussed further beginning on page 291.

■ *Controlling high blood pressure:* You should recognise the contribution of foods high in cholesterol and this is fully considered in Chapter 11.

Medications for a Healthy Heart

A variety of medications are available to treat heart disease and high blood pressure. Some of these are also very useful in preventing future heart attacks, stroke, and kidney damage. We used to think that medication should only be used if lifestyle changes such as healthy eating and exercise had failed. Newer research suggests that the way to get the greatest benefit is to *combine* certain medications with beneficial lifestyle changes.

If you have heart disease, diabetes, stroke, peripheral arterial disease, chronic kidney disease, or an abdominal aortic aneurysm you will already have received some advice. Your doctor will have discussed with you which of the heart-protective medications are right for you. If one medication is not working or is causing you unpleasant side-effects, discuss this with your doctor. Usually an alternative medication can be found that will work just as well. Most heart medications are taken for a lifetime, continuing to reduce your risk of heart disease, heart failure, and stroke. These are not addictive and usually can be used safely over many years. Do not start or stop these medications without discussing it with your doctor. Look at *Table 16.1* which shows some of the main drugs your doctor may prescribe for heart and related problems.

Heart Procedures and Surgery

With certain heart problems, or in cases when using medications on their own is insufficient, several types of heart procedure and surgery may be helpful.

■ *Coronary or balloon angioplasty:* Coronary angioplasty relieves the symptoms of coronary artery disease by improving the blood flow to the heart by opening up the blockages. A *catheter*, a long narrow tube with a balloon at the tip, is inserted into a narrowed

Table 16.1 **Medications for Heart Disease or High Blood Pressure**

Class of Drug	Example of Generic Names	Type of Heart or Related Problem	What it Does
Statins	Simvastatin, Atorvastatin	High Cholesterol	Reduces cholesterol
Anti-coagulants	Heparin, Warfarin	Atrial fibrillation , artificial heart valve	Prevents blood clots forming
Anti-platelet drugs	Aspirin, Clopidogrel	Reduce risks of heart attacks strokes	Prevent blood clots developing
ACE inhibitors	Ramipril, Lisinopril	Protect against heart failure, heart attacks high blood pressure	Relaxes blood vessels, improves blood flow to the heart
Angiotensin 11 receptor antagonists	Valsartan, Candesartan	High Blood Pressure	Relaxes blood vessels, improves blood flow to the heart
Beta Blockers	Bisoprolol, Atenolol	Slows heart rate, protects against heart attacks. Reduces blood pressure.	Slows heat rate thus reducing the amount work the heart has to do. Increases amount of blood that heart pumps with each beat
Diuretics (Water tablets)	Bumetanide, Furosemide	Heart failure, high blood pressure, heart valve disease	Removes excess water from the body thus reduces workload on heart
Nitrates	Glyceryl trinitrate (nitroglycerin) spray under the tongue, tablets or patch Oral Nitrates Isosorbide dinitrate (tablets or capsules)	Relieves angina	Relaxes walls of arteries and veins allowing blood to flow more easily
Potassium channel activators	Nicorandil	Prevent or treat angina	Relaxes the walls of arteries

artery to widen it. Your surgeon may choose to insert a tiny mesh tube called a *stent* to help keep the narrowed vessel open. Many stents, termed *drug-eluting stents*, contain medications that may help to prevent the artery from clogging up again.

- *Coronary artery bypass surgery:* Bypass surgery creates a *new route* for blood flow to your heart. A blood vessel from your leg or chest wall is used to create a detour around the blockage in the coronary artery. One or more blocked arteries may be bypassed.

The surgery usually requires several days in hospital, and the recovery time can be weeks, sometimes months.

- *Valve replacement:* On some occasions, it may be necessary to have heart surgery to repair or replace a damaged heart valve.

- *Surgery and devices for heart rhythm problems:* The nerves of the heart can be interrupted by surgery to control or prevent certain types of irregular rhythms. Also, devices such as pacemakers and implantable defibrillators may be permanently attached to the heart to treat abnormal heart rhythms.

Exercising with Heart Disease

Exercise can be both safe and helpful for many people with heart disease, with and without surgery. To make the most of your exercise, you should work closely with your health providers to find the best exercise programme for your needs. Remember that regular, well-chosen exercise is an important part of treatment and rehabilitation. Exercise can lower your risk of developing future problems, reduce the need for hospitalisation, and improve your quality of life.

When Not to Exercise

Some heart conditions limit the kind and amount of exercise you do. You should follow your doctor's advice about exercise and exertion, particularly if you have poor circulation to the heart, called *ischemia*; or if you experience irregular heartbeats or *arrhythmia*; or if your heart is unable to pump enough blood to the rest of your body. If your heart disease is severe, your doctor or cardiologist may want to change your treatment before giving you clearance to exercise. For example, if you have an arrhythmia, they may want to treat you with a medicine that controls your heartbeat. If you have poor circulation to the heart muscle, the doctor may

recommend medications, or bypass surgery, or *balloon angioplasty* to improve blood flow to the heart muscle, before clearing you for conditioning and exercise activities.

Tips for Safe Exercise

If you do not have any restricting conditions or a doctor's warning about the advisability of exercise, then it is safe for you to begin the conditioning exercise programme outlined here. The following, comprises a number of considerations for people with different kinds of heart disease who are about to begin their exercise programme:

- *Strengthening activities, such as isometrics, weightlifting, or rowing, can increase blood pressure and stress your heart:* Remember that *this can be dangerous* if you have high blood pressure or your heart has trouble pumping. However, if you and your doctor think strengthening is important for you, then you will need to pay special attention to how you do it. For example: do *not* hold your breath while you exercise; also remember to breathe out as you exert. One way to make sure you breathe as you exercise is to count out loud, or you can breathe out through pursed lips.

■ *If you have not exercised since your heart disease began; you and your doctor may decide that supervision by experienced professionals will be a good way to start:* Most communities have cardiac rehabilitation programmes or professionally staffed gyms at a local hospital or in a community centre.

■ *Once you are cleared for activity by your doctor, keep the intensity under control:* Keep it well below the level that causes symptoms such as chest pain or severe shortness of breath. If you cannot easily judge when you are staying below your *symptom zone,* you can wear a pulse rate monitor. These are available at medical supply and sporting goods shops and let you check your heart rate at any time. Other ways to monitor the intensity of your exercise are the *talk test* and your *perceived exertion.* For more on this read the information on page 128.

■ *If your heart has a decreased pumping strength you should avoid activities that cause you to strain:* Try safer and more helpful conditioning activities such as light callisthenics, gym exercises, or walking, swimming and stationary cycling.

■ *Exercise while you are lying down:* This is easy when you swim or pedal a special *recumbent* stationary bicycle. Certainly, it can help to improve the efficiency of your heart's pumping action and is less tiring than exercise while standing up.

■ *Always remember that if you develop new or different symptoms you should stop:* Symptoms such as chest pain, shortness of breath, dizziness, or a rapid or irregular heartbeat while at rest or while exercising, should make you stop what you are doing and contact your doctor.

Exercising with Stroke

If you have had a stroke that has affected your arm or leg, you may have had physiotherapy and occupational therapy. You may recognise many of the exercises in this book as the ones you did then. If you are still seeing a physiotherapist or already embarked on a home exercise programme, talk with your physiotherapist about adding some new activities. On the other hand, if you are making your own exercise decisions already, you can use the exercises in this book to continue to improve your flexibility, strength, and endurance. If you have weakness in your arm or leg or have trouble with balance, it is important that you think of safety when you choose which exercises to do. Having another person with you, or sitting instead of standing, and using a table, sturdy chair, or wall rail for support are all ideas for adapting exercises to meet your needs. You can also think about ways for your stronger side can be used to help your weaker side to exercise. A stationary bicycle with toe clips on the pedals will let your stronger leg help both legs exercise. Also, doing arm exercises while holding a cane, walking stick, or towel in both hands will let both your arms move. Remember, even if the arm and leg weakness is permanent, you can still increase your physical activity and general health with exercise.

Exercising with Peripheral Vascular Disease

Exercise for people with leg *claudication*, or *Peripheral Vascular Disease* is generally limited by the leg pain that develops when exercising. The good news is that conditioning exercises can help to improve endurance and reduce the leg pain for most people. Start with short walks or cycling, and continue up to the point when you start to have leg pain. Then, stop and rest or slow down until the discomfort eases, and then start again. At the beginning, repeat this cycle for five to ten minutes, increasing gradually as you become more comfortable. Many people find that they can gradually increase the length of time they can walk comfortably or exercise using this method. A good goal is to be able to keep going for 30 to 60 minutes, which is long enough to get noticeable fitness benefits too. If leg pain continues to prevent you from being physically active, talk to your doctor about other options. Remember, arm exercises won't usually cause leg pain, so be sure to include them as an important part of your overall conditioning programme.

The Outlook

We can do a lot to prevent heart disease and stroke and to help people who suffer from these conditions to live long, full lives. The combination of a healthy lifestyle, the selective use of medications, and cardiac procedures when needed has dramatically lowered the risk of heart attack, stroke, and early death. *You* also have an important job to do. It is up to you to eat well and exercise, manage your stress, and take your medications as prescribed. If you do not do your part, then your health care team will be much less effective. Part of good care and self-management for people with serious heart conditions involves planning for the future and making their personal wishes known regarding end-of-life issues and medical care. These issues are taken up in Chapter 19.

Further Reading

Allen, D. *Bloke with A Stroke*. 2013. Published as an e-Book from Amazon (ISBN 9781301255450).

Burkman, K. *The Stroke Recovery Book: A Guide for Patients and Families* 2nd Edition. Omaha, Nebraska: Addicus Books, 2010.

Casey, A., Benson, H. and O'Neill, B. *Harvard Medical School Guide to Lowering Your Blood Pressure*. New York: McGraw-Hill, 2005.

Freeman, A. E. *Brain Injury and Stroke: A handbook to recovery*. Sydney: Hale and Iremonger, 1998.

Rippe, J. M. *Heart Disease for Dummies*. Hoboke., N.J.: Wiley, 2004.

Taylor, J. B. *My Stroke of Insight: A Brain Scientists Personal Journey*. New York: Viking, 2009.

Other Resources

☐ *British Heart Foundation.* Tel: 0300 330 3311. www.bhf.org.uk.
This organisation has many publications which you can download free or order by telephone.

They include:

- A magazine *Heart Matters* which is published several times a year.

- A large-print Pamphlet on *Blood Pressure.* You can download this free or phone to get a copy.

- A Pamphlet: *Keep your Heart Healthy.*

- A section of the website called *The Women's Room.*

- A DVD on exercise: *Active Heart Healthy Heart.* Obtainable by phoning 0870 600 6566.

☐ *Different Stokes:* This is an organisation for younger stroke survivors. www.differentstrokes.co.uk.

☐ *National Heart Forum:* This site offers information and advice on heart conditions and prevention. Tel: 0207 831 7420. www.heartforum.org.uk.

☐ *National Women's Health Information Center* (This is a USA site). www.womenshealth.gov.

☐ *The National Coalition for Women with Heart Disease; WomenHeart.* www.womenheart.org.

☐ *The Stroke Association.* Tel: 0303 303 3100. www.stroke.org.uk.

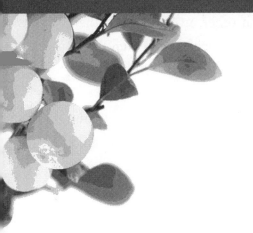

CHAPTER 17

Managing Arthritis and Osteoporosis

*L*ITERALLY, THE WORD *arthritis* means *inflammation of a joint.* However, as the word has come to be used, *arthritis* now commonly refers to virtually any kind of damage to a joint. Although most forms of arthritis cannot be cured, you can learn to the reduce pain, maintain mobility, and use medications to manage symptoms and slow the progression of the disease.

The most common form of arthritis is *osteoarthritis*. This is the arthritis that generally affects us as we age, causing knobby fingers, swollen knees, or back pain. Osteoarthritis is not caused by inflammation, although sometimes it may result in the inflammation of a joint. The cause of osteoarthritis is not precisely known but it involves the wearing away of the cartilage that cushions the ends of bone coupled with a degeneration of the bones, ligaments, and tendons associated with the joint.

Many other kinds of arthritis are due to inflammation. The most common forms are those caused by rheumatic diseases such as rheumatoid arthritis, or by metabolic diseases

277

such as gout, and psoriasis. With these diseases, the lining of the joint becomes inflamed and swollen and secretes extra fluid. As a result, the joint becomes swollen, warm, red, tender, and painful to move. If the symptoms are present for some time, *inflammatory arthritis* can also result in the destruction of cartilage and bone. Such destruction can then lead to deformity. The cause of the inflammation associated with these diseases is not precisely known. However, in the case of gout, it is clearly related to the formation of uric acid crystals in the joint fluid. In the case of rheumatic diseases, they are thought to be an auto-immune reaction: an immune or allergic reaction of the body, against itself.

Most arthritic diseases do not affect the joints alone. Joints are crossed by tendons from nearby muscles that move the joints and by ligaments that stabilise these joints. When the joint lining is inflamed or the joint is swollen or deformed, these tendons, ligaments, and muscles can be affected. They too may become inflamed, swollen, stretched, displaced, thinned out, and even broken. In many places where the tendons or muscles move over each other or over bones, there are lubricated surfaces which ease the movement. These surfaces are called *bursas*. With arthritis, these bursas may also become inflamed or swollen, causing *bursitis*. Thus, arthritis of any kind does not simply affect the joint. It can affect all of the structures in the area around the joint as well.

Consequences of Arthritis

Arthritis results in a number of consequences including the following:

- *The irritation, inflammation, swelling, and joint deformity resulting from arthritis can cause pain.* The pain may be present all the time or only occasionally, as the joint moves. Of all the symptoms of arthritis, pain is the most common.

- *Arthritis can also limit movement.* The limitation may be due to pain, to swelling that prevents normal bending, to deformity of the joint or the tendons, or to weakness in nearby muscles. In addition, arthritis can cause problems in areas distant from the joint. For example, if arthritis affects the joints of one leg, a person's posture can alter during walking or movement. This change places extra burdens on other muscles and

joints, elsewhere. Abnormal posture or extra burdens may therefore create pain on the other side of the body in areas which are distant from the site of the arthritis.

- *Stiffness of joints and muscles may also occur.* This is so particularly after periods of rest such as sleeping and sitting. The stiffness can make it difficult to move. The stiffness may lessen or disappear once you are able to get going. Also it may do so if, for example, you can get heat to the affected joint and muscles using a hot pad or hot shower. For most people, the stiffness lasts only for a short period of time; but for others it can last all day.

- *A common consequence of arthritis is fatigue.* Here again, the precise cause is not known. We know that inflammation itself causes fatigue, but so too does persistent pain, and also the effort of movement when joints and muscles aren't working properly. In addition, it is possible that the fatigue is caused by the worries and fears that often accompany arthritis. Whatever its cause or combination of causes, fatigue is an issue that most arthritis patients must confront.

■ *Depression may also accompany arthritis.* People with arthritis often have trouble doing what they need or want to do. The condition can make them feel helpless, angry, and withdrawn. Understandably, this may lead to depression. Depression can make other symptoms such as pain, fatigue and disability all seem worse. It can reduce an individual's work efficiency and social functioning. It can damage family relationships and undermine the capacity for independent living. This depression is likely to be the *situational* type. This means that it comes from difficulties caused by the arthritis and is not from a mental illness. Often the depression improves when the arthritis improves, but it can also be considerably helped by self-management practices, like those dealt with in Chapter 2; also by managing your pain and depression, which we have featured in Chapter 4, and by the use of antidepressant medication.

Fibromyalgia is a condition that sometimes accompanies arthritis but usually exists alone. Though it is not inflammatory, it creates muscle tenderness and joint pain similar to that of inflammatory arthritis. The cause is not yet known and anti-inflammatory treatment does not usually help. However, much of the self-management therapy which is used by patients with arthritis does seem to be beneficial for people with fibromyalgia.

Overall it is true that although arthritis can have very damaging effects, much can be done to offset or eliminate them. The remainder of this chapter is concerned with appropriate management and with leading you to embrace the helpful self-management techniques described in detail elsewhere in this book.

Prognosis: What Does the Future Hold?

Most arthritic diseases, if left untreated, will have a variety of outcomes for different people. Some people progress more or less steadily, towards increasing disability. Others have experienced disease that has waxed and waned over many years, often, but not always, getting slowly worse. Some individuals might find that the disease or its symptoms disappear spontaneously. Overall, it is the case that with modern treatment, most patients can be helped to reduce the limitations from their arthritis, and for some the progression can be slowed or even stopped.

There is no real cure for any of the forms of arthritis. Nevertheless, for some fortunate people, the arthritis will subside partly or completely on its own. Medical treatment can usually suppress the inflammation and the symptoms but it must often be continued for a long time. Using appropriate self-management techniques can greatly enhance any improvement and prevent or slow the progress of disability. This depends largely on the participation of the person with arthritis and sometimes their family. Therefore, a *prognosis* (a prediction of what the future holds), cannot be very accurate for any individual. It depends partly on medical treatment, partly on the self-management efforts made, and partly on good fortune.

Because there is no cure for arthritis, medical treatment is aimed at preventing or controlling the inflammation, swelling, and pain and improving physical function. The medications commonly used can either help the pain or reduce inflammation and swelling, or do both. When the inflammation is reduced, pain usually declines too, and function increases.

It is important to remember that most people with arthritis can lead normal or nearly normal lives. Proper use of medications and self-management techniques make this possible. So, don't abandon your major life plans just yet! Rather, you should adjust them to accommodate your treatment needs and remember that treatment plans can often be modified to meet your particular needs or wishes.

Common Types of Arthritis and Their Treatment

As we noted earlier, arthritis can be the result of either loss of cartilage or bone in a joint or the result of an inflammation of a joint. Treatment depends on the type of arthritis involved.

Osteoarthritis

Osteoarthritis is a result of degenerative changes in the cartilage and bones in your joints. Cartilage cushions the ends of bones and allows them to move smoothly over one another. Because of degeneration, the bone surfaces become rough and consequently painful when in motion. The roughness may also irritate the joint lining, known as the *synovium*, causing it to produce more than normal amounts of joint fluid. The extra fluid results in swelling. Occasionally, small pieces of damaged cartilage will break off, float in the fluid and catch on a moving surface, thereby increasing the pain. Also, bone endings may grow small spurs, called *osteophytes* and these create, for instance, knobs on fingers and spurs on your heels. Although osteoarthritis can affect any joint, it most commonly affects the hands, knees, hips, shoulders and spine. In general, its presence increases as we get older.

The cause of osteoarthritis is not known, and there is no specific medical treatment to prevent or arrest the degeneration. Treatment is therefore aimed at maintaining joint function and reducing pain.

With osteoarthritis, the saying *use it or lose it* is particularly true. Unless the affected joints are used, they will slowly lose mobility, and the surrounding muscles and tendons will weaken. Fortunately, exercise does not make the osteoarthritis worse and as movement improves with exercise and the surrounding tissues strengthen, the pain will often decline. Thus, exercise is the centrepiece of treatment. Use of exercise is discussed later in this chapter, but you should also consult the advice in Chapters 7 and 8.

Because osteoarthritis damages joint cartilage, an exercise programme should aim at protecting it. Cartilage requires some joint motion and some weight bearing to stay healthy. In much the same way as a sponge soaks up and squeezes out water, joint cartilage soaks up nutrients and fluid and gets rid of waste products by being squeezed when you move the joint. If the joint is not moved regularly, your cartilage will deteriorate.

To help with osteoarthritic pain, the best medications are known as *Non-Steroidal Anti-Inflammatory Drugs* (NSAIDs). When there is no inflammation involved in the arthritis, as is commonly the case, the anti-inflammatory activity of these drugs is not important. The benefit comes instead from their pain-reducing effect, which is similar to that of aspirin. Therefore, aspirin or Paracetamol is usually just as effective as NSAIDs.

Heat to the joint and pain-controlling measures such as relaxation and cognitive distraction can be very helpful, as described in Chapter 5. Heat *before* you exercise can often make the exercise easier. For pain at night in your hands, feet, or knees, you can use gloves, socks, or a sleeve over the knees. These measures can greatly improve your sleep.

When swelling from irritation or mild inflammation is present, then the draining and injection of the joint with a corticosteroid medication can often correct the problem and sometimes do so with lasting benefit.

If the disease progresses to deformity, discomfort, and weakness which makes normal living impossible, then surgical joint replacement is available. The artificial replacement joints commonly function like normal joints and will also permit the recovery of lost strength in your muscles and tendons.

Two additional therapies for osteoarthritis have been used over the last few years. Both are intended to improve damaged cartilage or substitute for it. One is *glucosamine*, taken daily in pill form. The other is *hyaluronan*, injected into the joint as a lubricant. A few years ago the guidance from the *National Institute for Clinical Excellence* (NICE) did not routinely recommend the use of glucosamine. This was because its use was based on studies where the outcomes had not been firmly established. The use of hyaluronic injections was also not routinely recommended. If you want to consider either of these medications you are advised to discuss their use and appropriateness for you, with your doctor or consultant.

Chronic Inflammatory Arthritis

The rheumatic diseases (such as rheumatoid arthritis and lupus erythematosus), psoriasis, and gout are the commonest forms of inflammatory arthritis. Inflammatory arthritis can also occur in association with other inflammatory diseases of the intestines or liver. It may also appear with infections such as Lyme disease (see page 289) or streptococcal and viral illnesses. In these settings, it will sometimes clear with antibiotic treatment or over time, but sometimes it may become long-term.

Please note, that in what follows only generic names have been given and not brand names. You will find some further explanation of these terms in Chapter 14, in the section on *Medications*.

The most commonly used medications for chronic inflammatory arthritis, with the exception of gout, fall into the following categories:

- *Non-Steroidal Anti-Inflammatory Drugs (NSAIDs)*: As noted earlier, these drugs have both pain-reducing and anti-inflammatory effects. They are usually the first drugs used to treat arthritis because they are often helpful and tend to have relatively few severe side-effects. Representatives of this group include *ibuprofen* and *naproxen*. Paracetamol although not an NSAID, is also used to reduce pain, but it has no anti-inflammatory effect. Most of the NSAIDs can damage your stomach and intestines, but this can be minimised by always taking the medications in the middle of a meal. This sounds simple, but many people don't follow this advice consistently.

- A few years ago, three new NSAIDs became available known as *Cox-2 Inhibitors*. There were concerns about their link with heart and blood vessel disease and two were withdrawn and one is still very restricted in its use. Your doctor will discuss with you the issues around prescribing this group of drugs and whether the remaining restricted version is still appropriate for you.

- *Disease-modifying drugs:* The drugs in this category are all anti-inflammatory drugs which are more powerful than the NSAIDs but also potentially more toxic. The term *disease-modifying* implies a slowing of the progression or the reversal of inflammatory arthritis. However, these drugs do not usually result in healing. Members of this group are *gold*, *methotrexate*, *sulfasalazine*, *leflunomide* and *hydroxychloroquine*. These are usually used in inflammatory arthritis if NSAIDs fail. They are not used for osteoarthritis.

    In recent years, evidence has emerged indicating that the earlier use of *disease-modifying*

agents has slowed the progression of the disease. Because the NSAIDs do not achieve such slowing, most patients with rheumatoid arthritis are now receiving treatment with these second-line agents earlier in the course of their disease. Such early benefit from disease-modifying drugs may also be true for other forms of chronic inflammatory arthritis. The use of these medications should be discussed with a doctor who has had special training in treating arthritis and associated diseases, known as a rheumatologist.

- *Corticosteroids:* These are powerful anti-inflammatory drugs that can also suppress immune function. Both effects are helpful with inflammatory arthritis, especially for rheumatic diseases in which the body's immune system appears to play a role in causing the disease. Most corticosteroids in use are synthetic versions of a normal human hormone, *cortisol*, which is present in everybody. Corticosteroids are the most rapid-acting and effective of the anti-arthritic drugs but may cause serious adverse effects when used for long periods of time. *Prednisone* is the most commonly used corticosteroid and is often given with another anti-inflammatory drug in order to get a faster response.

- *Cytotoxic drugs:* These drugs, which were developed to treat cancer, also have anti-inflammatory and immunosuppressive effects. Examples include *ciclosporine*, *cyclophosphamide*, *azathioprine*, *mycophenolate*, and *rituximab*. These drugs can be quite toxic but also very effective. They are usually used only after other drugs have failed to control the problem. They are never used for osteoarthritis.

■ *New biological agents:* A biological material called *Tumour Necrosis Factor* (TNF) plays an important role in dealing with the inflammation of rheumatoid arthritis. Again this medication should be discussed with your doctor or rheumatologist.

For gout: the main treatment goal is to reduce the blood uric acid level by using drugs such as *allopurinol, colchicine, probenecid,* and the newer *febuxostat.* For chronic gout arthritis, most of the drugs and other methods of management for chronic inflammatory arthritis are also used.

For inflammatory arthritis: drugs are frequently used in combination. These combinations are usually based on the individual's response to particular drugs. Thus many combinations are used and sometimes include the biological agents. Although a certain combination may work best for a particular person, recent evidence indicates that no particular combination is clearly superior, in general terms to all the others.

Some years ago, each type of inflammatory arthritis was treated with a particular group of drugs. Nowadays, almost all of the drugs discussed can be used for any type of inflammatory arthritis. The choice of drugs depends on each person's condition and how they respond. Commonly, milder drugs are used first, and more powerful ones follow when these fail. However, as mentioned earlier, stronger drugs are now often used earlier in rheumatoid arthritis in an effort to prevent joint destruction.

General Comments on the Drugs for Arthritis

Here are some issues which you need to consider:

■ *It is almost impossible to predict beforehand whether any of the drugs will be helpful.* Therefore, the treatment of arthritis with drugs is a trial-and-error process. For inflammatory arthritis, only occasionally do drugs, other than corticosteroids provide an immediate benefit. Usually many days or even weeks are necessary before the full effects of the drug are felt.

■ *Problems can be caused by the toxic effects of the drugs.* All drugs can cause harm as well as benefit. Sometimes a particular drug can be very helpful for the arthritis but may also cause so much harm in other respects that it cannot be used.

■ *It is impossible to predict which drugs will be harmful in an individual patient.* With some of the drugs, the toxic effects cannot be recognised by the individual patient. So each patient must be monitored with blood counts, liver function studies, analyses of urine, and other tests.

■ *People starting on any drug treatment for arthritis should make sure they understand the signs and symptoms of potential harm.* They must be alert to symptoms such as rashes, upset stomach, or unusual thoughts, and be quick to notify their doctor if such symptoms appear. Also, you need to discuss with your doctor whether you need to have regular blood or urine tests to monitor for the toxic effects of the prescribed medications.

■ *The unpredictability of benefits and harms from drug therapy creates uncertainty for both the patient and the doctor.* The best way to deal with this uncertainty is to ensure that you understand the treatment plan and know about the alternatives. In addition you should be sure that you have a clear way to communicate with your doctor if the plan is going wrong.

Sometimes, despite drug treatment, your joints may be damaged to the point where they no longer work effectively. Fortunately, modern surgical techniques allow for replacement of many types of joints, and these replacements often function almost as well as natural joints. This is especially true for hips and knees. Modern surgery is efficient, and recovery is usually rapid.

Other Ways to Manage Arthritis

In addition to treatment with drugs or surgery, there are many other management approaches to achieve good results with arthritis.

Using Exercise

The goal of proper management is not just to avoid pain and reduce inflammation; it is to maintain the maximum possible use of the affected joints. This involves maintaining the maximum possible motion of the joint and the greatest strength in the muscles, tendons, and ligaments surrounding it. The key to this goal is exercise, which is an essential part of any good management programme. The exercise you undertake should be regular, consistent, and as vigorous as possible. Exercise will not make your arthritis worse. In fact, failing to exercise can increase arthritis symptoms because of the loss of joint mobility and physical de-conditioning. Although exercise may increase pain temporarily, this is normal during joint and muscle re-conditioning exercise.

Maintaining good posture and the normal motion of joints helps to protect joints from

deterioration, sustains your mobility, and eases pain. The inactivity that results from long time periods spent sitting or lying down can worsen your posture, reduce your joint flexibility, and cause weakness even in the joints not affected by arthritis. Also after inactivity, especially sleeping, stiffness is common. It can be reduced by mild exercise *in bed* before getting up or by a hot bath or shower. For some people, mild exercise before going to bed will reduce stiffness the next morning.

Appropriate exercise programmes are described in Chapters 6, 7, and 8, and there are more specific recommendations for people with arthritis later in this chapter. It is wise to exercise as many joints as possible, including those without arthritis, in order to maintain general physical condition. However, chronic arthritis can affect the bones of the neck. Therefore, in order to prevent nerve damage, it is best to avoid extreme neck movements and strong pressure on the back of the neck or head. Because heat makes exercise easier, it is helpful to exercise when you are warm, for example during or after a bath or, especially for hands and wrists, after washing the dishes.

Using Heat

In addition to improving mobility, heat is also useful to reduce pain in joints and muscles, at least temporarily. When combined with rest, this can be very soothing. Alternatively, some people find that cooling a warm joint with ice is helpful. But, remember that cooling does not increase mobility.

Controlling Your Fatigue

Control of fatigue is important. Rest periods between activities and restful sleep at night are essential for control. Chapter 4 deals with the matter of sleeping better and this may help you. When pain disturbs your sleep at night, different types of beds, such as firm beds, foam beds and air beds, and the use of mild sleep medications can all be a significant help. For some people with arthritis, low doses of anti-depressive medication at bedtime will also effectively control night pain and improve sleep.

Using Assistive Devices

Sometimes, when joint function remains limited, the use of assistive devices can be of benefit. Many types of devices are available including braces, walking sticks, special shoes, grippers, reachers and walkers.

Considering What You Eat

What you eat has little effect on most types of arthritis, particularly osteoarthritis and rheumatoid arthritis. What you eat, however, *is* important for gout, where the consumption of alcohol and eating certain meats can provoke attacks. People with gout should discuss this with their doctor. In rare cases, food allergies can cause attacks of arthritis. There is also some evidence that eating oils from cold-water fish can help people with rheumatoid arthritis; however, the benefit is small. Of course, if you are overweight, then losing weight can reduce the extra burden on joints, especially your hips, knees and feet which bear your weight. People with chronic arthritis should eat balanced, pleasurable meals and maintain a normal weight. Ways in which you can do this are discussed in Chapters 11 and 12.

Combating Depression

It is not surprising that sometimes in the struggle against arthritis, an individual becomes depressed. Usually this is a *situational depression* resulting from the consequences of chronic arthritis and is not a mental illness. It is important to recognise your depression and to seek advice from health professionals. There are many ways to combat depression; the important thing is to know it is present and take steps to control it. Take a look at Chapter 4 for more on this issue.

Most people with arthritis are able to lead productive, satisfying, and independent lives. The most important step in achieving this is to take an active part in managing your own arthritis. All of the components of management mentioned here are the responsibility of the individual involved and must be done with that individual's participation.

Osteoporosis

Osteoporosis is not arthritis, but rather condition that affects the bones and is usually a result of aging. In osteoporosis, bones lose calcium and become more brittle. Then they become more susceptible to fracture.

Normal bone structure is maintained primarily by calcium and vitamin D intake and physical activity. In women, it is also maintained by oestrogen, so after the menopause, when oestrogen production declines, osteoporosis increases. As we age and are less physically active, bone weakening becomes more likely. In addition, the risk of osteoporosis is increased by factors such as smoking and heavy drinking, some endocrine diseases, and by the long-term use of corticosteroids as medications. This last factor is especially important for patients with inflammatory arthritis who must often use corticosteroids for treatment.

Although osteoporosis can cause bone pain, it usually does not cause specific symptoms. Consequently, the diagnosis is made by bone imaging. However, as X-rays can only detect advanced osteoporosis, the imaging is done with a *Dual energy X-ray Absorptiometry* scan (DXA) which measures bone mineral density. Most physicians use the DXA scan for people who are at risk of osteoporosis; the result enables them to establish the diagnosis, determine its severity, and guide the treatment options.

The prevention and treatment of osteoporosis involve the dietary supplements and actions which we have listed in *Advisory Table 17.1*. An appropriate intake of calcium and vitamin D is particularly important, and for more information on calcium and vitamin D you should consult the appropriate section on Healthy Eating in Chapter 11. If the osteoporosis does not respond to these steps or it is severe, there are medications that strengthen bones, primarily oestrogens and bisphosphonates, such as *alendronate*, *ibandronate*, known also as ibandronic acid, and *risedronate*. If you cannot tolerate bisphosphonates, or can't take them for some other medical reason, you may benefit from another class of medicines known as *Selective Oestrogen Receptor Modulators* (SERMs) like *raloxifene*. SERMs produce oestrogen-like effects on bones and reduce the risk of vertebral fractures. They are less effective than bisphosphonates, but they can still be helpful. The use of all these drugs should be discussed thoroughly with your doctor; although they are generally safe, they can have adverse effects.

A mild form of osteoporosis called *osteopenia* can also be diagnosed by DXA scan. This can usually be managed by the supplements and actions which are indicated in *Advisory Table 17.1*. However, medications are unnecessary unless the osteopenia is progressing.

Advisory Table 17.1 **Preventing or Slowing Osteoporosis**

1. *Get enough calcium.* A calcium rich diet is an important part of preventing or managing osteoporosis well. Experts recommended that 1 gram of calcium is eaten every day; foods high in calcium include milk, yoghurt, sardines, cheese, and fortified oatmeal. To check on calcium content read your food labels.

2. *Get enough vitamin D.* Vitamin D is important for bone health and helps the body absorb calcium. You can get vitamin D from some foods such as liver, butter, and the best source being fatty fish such as halibut and mackerel. Vitamin D is made by the skin when exposed to sunlight. You may need to take a supplement so please check with your doctor who will consider your health, age, and lifestyle before prescribing.)

3. *Be physically active.* Get exercise by walking, cycling, or dancing. It is also very important to do strengthening exercises for the shoulders, arms, and upper back.

4. *Avoid lifting heavy objects and high-impact exercise.* Sit up straight, and don't slouch. Good sitting posture puts less pressure on the back. Avoid bending down to touch your toes when standing. This puts unnecessary pressure on your back. If you want to stretch your legs or back, lie on your back and bring your knees up toward your chest.

5. *Maintain a healthy weight.* If you are overweight, losing even a little will help you to reduce pressure on bones.

6. *Don't smoke.* If you do this, then either stop completely or reduce your smoking.

7. *Limit alcohol.* Firmly stick to no more than the recommended number of units a day (see page 234).

8. *Prevent falls.* You can protect yourself from injury in many ways. For example, remove throw rugs, electrical cords and items left on the stairs that may cause you to trip and fall; make sure that your home is well-lit, including staircases and entrances.

9. *Be careful when and where you walk.* Do not walk on ice, polished floors, or other slippery surfaces. Avoid walking in unfamiliar places.

10. *Support your walking.* Use a walking stick, or a walker regularly if your balance is poor. Also install grab bars, especially in the bathroom, to keep you safe at home.

11. *Take care with footwear.* Wear low-heeled shoes with good arch supports and rubber soles.

12. *Keep your eye on the ball.* Check your vision, and get new glasses if you do not see well.

13. *Improve your balance.* Regain and maintain your balance; check out and try out the balance exercises in Chapter 7.

14. *Consider the medication options.* Talk with your doctor about medications if the suggestions here are not adequate.

Exercising with Arthritis or Osteoporosis

Regular exercise is crucial in the management of all types of arthritis and osteoporosis.

Osteoarthritis

Because osteoarthritis begins as primarily a problem with joint cartilage, an exercise programme should include taking care of cartilage. Cartilage requires joint motion and some weight bearing to stay healthy. As noted earlier, just as a sponge soaks up and squeezes out water, joint cartilage soaks up nutrients and fluid and gets rid of waste products by being squeezed when you move the joint. If the joint is not moved regularly, cartilage deteriorates.

Any joint with osteoarthritis should be moved through its full range of motion several times daily to maintain flexibility and cartilage health. Judge your activity level so that pain is not increased. If hips and knees are involved, walking and standing should be limited to two to four hours at a time. This should be followed by at least an hour off your feet to give the cartilage time to decompress.

Using a walking stick on the opposite side to the painful hip or knee will reduce joint stress and often get you through a rough time. Good posture, strong muscles, and good endurance, as well as shoes capable of absorbing the shocks of walking, are important ways to protect cartilage and reduce joint pain.

Knee-strengthening exercises, like exercises 15, 18, and 19 in Chapter 7, performed on a daily basis can help to reduce your knee pain and protect the joint. Being overweight makes knee pain worse, and losing weight will reduce it. Regular exercise is an important part of losing weight and keeping it low.

Chronic Inflammatory Arthritis

Exercise will not damage joints in arthritis and is important for all types of chronic inflammatory arthritis. The purpose of exercise is to maintain joint mobility, strengthen ligaments and tendons around the joint, and maintain or increase the strength of the muscles that move the joint. Gentle flexibility exercises can also help with morning stiffness. When a joint is inflamed, mild exercise in all joint motions is good within the limits defined by pain. When the inflammation is suppressed or eliminated by medication, full regular exercise is desirable. It should be done daily. Some specific types of exercise are described in Chapter 7. They involve all the movements normal to the affected joint and should be done against increasing resistance using weights, elastic bands, compressible balls and spring structures. The object of this is to achieve maximum function for the affected joints, and this Is certainly possible for most people.

Osteoporosis

Regular exercise plays an important part in preventing osteoporosis and strengthening bones which are already showing signs of disease. Endurance and strengthening exercises are the most effective for strengthening bone. Flexibility and back and abdomen strengthening exercises are important for maintaining good posture. Look for the *VIP* exercises and the weight symbol in order to quickly identify strengthening exercises in Chapter 7. You can help yourself with a regular exercise programme that includes some walking and general flexibility and activity geared towards strengthening your shoulders, hips, back, and stomach muscles.

Suggested Further Reading

Anderson, L. *Your Life with Rheumatoid Arthritis: Tools for Managing Treatment, Side Effects and Pain.* Two North Books, 2013. (ISBN 9780991858620)

Backstrom, G. and Rubin, B. *When Muscle Pain Won't Go Away: The Relief Handbook for Fibromyalgia and Chronic Muscle Pain,* 3rd ed. Dallas, Tex.: Taylor, 1998.

Cembrowicz, S. and Allain, T. *Osteoporosis: Answers at Your Fingertips.* London: Class Publishing, 2007.

Foltz-Gray, D. *Alternative Treatments for Arthritis: An A-to-Z Guide.* Atlanta: Arthritis Foundation, 2007.

Jenner, C. *Arthritis: A practical guide to getting on with your life.* Oxford: How to Books Ltd., 2011.

Lorig, K. and Fries, J. *The Arthritis Helpbook,* 6th ed. Reading, Mass.: Perseus, 2006.

Sayce, V. and Fraser, I. *Exercise Beats Arthritis: An Easy-to-Follow Program of Exercise,* 3rd ed. Boulder, Colo.: Bull Publishing, 1998.

Other Resources

☐ *Arthritis Care*: Helpline. Tel: 0808 800 4050; Under 26 Helpline Tel: 0800 800 2000. www.arthritiscare.org.uk.

☐ *Arthritis Research Campaign*: Helpline Tel: 0870 850 5000. www.arc.org.uk.

☐ *The British Pain Society*: The Society has a downloadable pamphlet *Understanding and Managing Pain; information for Patients* (2011). Tel: 0207 269 7840. www.britishpainsociety.org.uk.

☐ *Lupus UK.* Tel: 0170 8731 251. www.lupusuk.org.uk.

☐ NHS has information about Lyme Disease. www.nhs.uk/Conditions/Lyme-disease.

☐ *National Osteoporosis Society.* Tel: 0845 450 0230. www.nos.org.uk.

☐ *National Rheumatoid Arthritis Society*: Tel: 0845 458 3969. www.rheumatoid.org.uk.

☐ *UK Gout Society.* www.ukgoutsociety.org.uk.

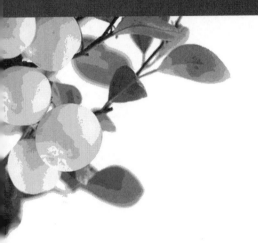

CHAPTER 18

Managing Diabetes

L IVING WELL WITH DIABETES REQUIRES BOTH good medical care and effective self-management. In this chapter we will help you learn about the disease and what you can do to manage it.

What Is Diabetes?

Diabetes is a disease that makes it difficult for the body to turn food into energy. To understand diabetes, it is helpful to know a little about several issues: the digestion process; the function of the pancreas and insulin; and how these relate to diabetes. Take a few moments to study *Figure 18.1* on the next page.

Some of the food we eat, such as sugar, starch, and other carbohydrates, is broken down in the digestion process into a simple sugar called glucose. Glucose is absorbed into the bloodstream from your stomach, causing the level of blood glucose, sometimes

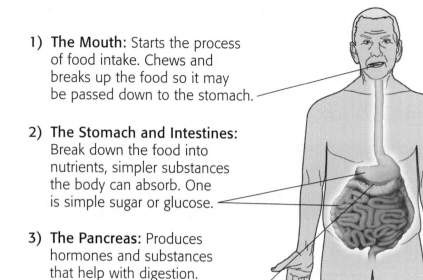

1) **The Mouth:** Starts the process of food intake. Chews and breaks up the food so it may be passed down to the stomach.

2) **The Stomach and Intestines:** Break down the food into nutrients, simpler substances the body can absorb. One is simple sugar or glucose.

3) **The Pancreas:** Produces hormones and substances that help with digestion. One of these hormones is insulin.

4) **Insulin:** Enters the bloodstream. It acts like the key that allows the glucose to enter the cell.

5) **Simple Sugar or Glucose:** Enters the bloodstream, and, with the help of insulin, gives nutrients to the cells, producing energy.

Figure 18.1 **The Digestion Process**

called blood sugar, to rise. The term *blood glucose* is sometimes used interchangeably with the term *blood sugar*. In order to avoid any confusion, only the term *blood glucose* will be used in the rest of this chapter. For the cells of your body to use the glucose as fuel, it needs the help of insulin. Insulin is a hormone produced by the pancreas, a small gland located below and behind your stomach. Insulin helps the blood glucose get from the bloodstream into the cells. Once inside the cells, the glucose is burned to give your body energy.

Glucose in your body can be compared to the petrol in your car; each is a fuel and a source of energy. Petrol alone, however, is not enough to make the car move. We need a key to start the motor, which allows the petrol to be converted into energy. Like the car, our bodies also need a key which will let us use glucose as energy. Insulin is this key; it opens the door for glucose to pass from the bloodstream into the cells, where it produces energy.

For people with diabetes, insulin is not able to carry out this function for one of two reasons:

1. *The pancreas may be producing little or no insulin at all:* This is called *Type 1 diabetes*.

2. *The insulin that is produced cannot be used efficiently by the body:* This second scenario is known as *Type 2 diabetes*.

In both types, the unabsorbed glucose remains in the bloodstream. *Table 18.1* shows the differences between Type 1 and Type 2 diabetes. The significant result is high blood glucose. As a consequence, the excess glucose spills out in the urine when the kidneys filter the blood. This causes two of the symptoms of diabetes: frequent urination and large amounts of glucose in the urine. This is how diabetes got its full name *diabetes mellitus*. The Greek word *diabetes* means *to pass through*, and the Latin word *mellitus* means *sugar* or *honey*.

Table 18.1 **Overview of Type 1 and Type 2 Diabetes**

Characteristics	Type 1 Diabetes (insulin dependent)	Type 2 Diabetes (may or may not need insulin and may need oral medications)
Age	Usually begins before age 20, but can occur in adults.	Usually begins after age 40, but can occur earlier.
Insulin	Little or no insulin is produced by the pancreas.	The pancreas produces insulin, but it may not be enough or it cannot be used by the body.
Onset	Sudden.	Slow.
Gender	Males and females equally affected.	More females are affected.
Heredity	Some hereditary tendency.	Strong hereditary tendency.
Weight	Majority experience weight-loss and are thin.	Majority are overweight.
Ketones	Ketones found in the urine.	Usually there are no ketones in the urine.
Treatment	Insulin, diet, exercise, self-management.	Diet, exercise, self-management, and when necessary, oral medication and/or insulin.

The Cause of Diabetes

The exact cause of diabetes is not known. *Type 1 diabetes*, which requires insulin as medication, usually starts in childhood; it is an auto-immune disease where the body's immune system may damage the pancreatic cells that produce insulin. *Type 2 diabetes* is sometimes called adult-onset diabetes. However, we are seeing more and more young people in their teens and even children developing Type 2 diabetes and this does not seem to be an auto-immune disease. Rather, it tends to run in families and may start as a result of other factors. These include being overweight, lack of exercise, eating and other lifestyle habits or some other illness. It is more common among people who are overweight.

This is because excess body fat does not allow the body to make proper use of insulin. Insulin is still produced, but the body is resistant to it. This resistance prevents the body moving the glucose from the blood and into the cells of the body efficiently. Glucose builds up in the blood because the body cannot use it. Fortunately, we know some ways to prevent this type of diabetes, which we will discuss shortly.

The important difference between the two types of diabetes is that Type 1 requires a daily supplement of insulin, whereas the majority of people with Type 2 may not initially require extra insulin to control the disease. However, if blood glucose levels cannot be well controlled with diet, exercise, and oral medications, supplementary insulin can be tremendously helpful.

Diagnosing Diabetes

Diabetes is usually diagnosed and monitored with blood tests. Monitoring is done by a combination of home testing of blood glucose and laboratory testing of haemoglobin HbA1c. For more information on home testing see page 296. The HbA1c test measures your average blood glucose over the past two to three months. This laboratory test helps you understand how well you are able to keep your diabetes under control. In 2011 the system for expressing the results of HbA1c was changed in the UK. It was previously given as a percentage but is now given as millimoles of HbA1c per mol of haemoglobin. For example, 6% is now expressed as 42 mmol/mol, as you can see from *Table 18.2*.

The HbA1c test is also the test the doctor uses to monitor your diabetes and to judge how well your treatment programme is working to control your diabetes. For most people with diabetes, the usual aim is to keep the HbA1c at 48 mmol/mol as evidence shows this can reduce the risk of developing diabetic complications, such as nerve damage, eye disease, kidney disease and heart disease. Some doctors recommend a slightly higher goal for certain patients, especially those aged over 65 and with other health conditions.

Table 18.2 **Measuring HbA1c Blood Glucose Levels**

(%)	(mmol/mol)
6.0	42
6.5	48
7.0	53
7.5	58
8.0	64
9.0	75

Complications from Diabetes

High blood glucose over months and years can lead to serious complications. For most people, the higher the blood glucose level, the higher the chance of complications.

Although extremely high blood glucose levels can cause loss of consciousness and even death, most complications are related to damage done to blood vessels and nerves throughout the body. This can lead to complications such as: heart disease and stroke, kidney damage, loss of vision, pain and loss of feeling in the feet, and the slow healing of infections and wounds.

Fortunately, you can greatly reduce, or delay such outcomes through healthy eating, exercise, weight management, blood pressure and

Some of the Symptoms of Diabetes

Some people with diabetes have no symptoms, while others may have some or all of the following:

- Extreme tiredness
- Extreme thirst
- Frequent urination, especially at night
- Blurry vision or a change in vision
- Increased hunger

- Unintentional weight loss
- Sores or cuts that heal slowly.
- Numbness or tingling in the feet.
- Frequent infections of skin, gums, bladder, or vagina (yeast infections).

cholesterol control, taking certain medications, and giving up smoking.

Prevention

Type 2 diabetes is a growing epidemic. Like most long-term conditions, diabetes does not happen overnight. Instead it happens slowly over time. There are many people who have a condition known as *pre-diabetes*. This means that their blood glucose levels are higher than normal but not high enough to be diagnosed as diabetes. Pre-diabetes is an early warning sign. But the good news is that maintaining a healthy weight and being physically active can often reverse pre-diabetes and delay or prevent the development of the disease.

Some of the risk factors for diabetes, such as having a brother, sister, or parent with it, cannot be changed. But most of the risks can be reduced by healthy eating, regular exercise and weight control. Sometimes just losing five or ten pounds can stop or slow the development of diabetes.

If you feel that you are at risk of diabetes, talk with your doctor or health care team as soon as possible. Knowing early about diabetes can help you prevent complications. It's worse to have diabetes and not know it.

Self-Management of Diabetes

Successful diabetes management includes maintaining blood glucose in a safe range, detecting early problems, and taking action to prevent complications. This involves working closely with your doctor and health care team and practising effective self-management. Self-management will include all of the following:

- Monitoring your blood glucose level.

- Observing symptoms and knowing what to do about them.

- Following a healthy eating plan.

- Engaging in regular physical activity.

- Managing your stress and emotions.

- Dealing with infections and other illnesses and coping with those days when you are ill.

- Using prescribed medications in a safe and effective way.

- Getting the necessary tests, examinations, and immunisations.

Blood Glucose Monitoring

Management of diabetes is aimed at keeping blood glucose within a safe range. The only way to tell if blood glucose is in this range is to monitor it. Monitoring is *not* a treatment. It is a tool that you can use to find out how you are doing and make any needed day-to-day changes in diet and exercise, as well as changes in your medications, as recommended by your health care team.

There are two ways to monitor blood glucose levels:

1. *Using an HbA1c Glucose Test:* This test was explained earlier in the chapter as a test ordered by your GP and done in a laboratory. It shows your average blood glucose

levels over two or three months. See *Table 18.2* on page 294. The key word here is *average* and like all averages it could be the result of lots of small variations or much larger swings in either direction. For this reason *the test is not useful for making day-to-day adjustments of insulin treatment* but it is a good guide as to whether your treatment is working overall.

2. *Employing home-based blood glucose monitoring:* The daily home glucose monitoring test is designed to provide information about daily adjustments required in your insulin treatment. It consists of a series of blood glucose tests you can do at home using a *small drop of blood, glucose strips,* and a *home glucose meter.* The meter is about the size of a mobile phone and can be taken with you anywhere. The meter is easy to use. You can check your blood glucose at home, at work, or anywhere else. Your diabetes specialist nurse or doctor will instruct you on how to monitor your blood glucose and what equipment you will need. In this way you will ensure accurate results. It is especially helpful to have the doctor or specialist diabetes nurse, observe your technique and give you feedback.

Because blood glucose levels change, often throughout the day and night, you will want to learn how your eating, exercise, medications, stress level, illness, and infections all affect your blood glucose. Monitoring can help with this. Checking your own blood glucose gives you and your doctor more flexibility in making decisions about how to control your blood glucose levels. Checking like this may also help you to evaluate

the situation and take action if your blood glucose is too high or too low. For more information on this take a look at page 308.

How often should I monitor?

How often you check your blood glucose will depend on how you and your health care team are going to use the information. Remember, monitoring is not a treatment. It is used to give you information so that you can make fine adjustments. You may want to monitor several times a day or perhaps once a week. If you are using insulin more than once a day or are using an insulin pump, you should monitor at least three times per day. The truth is that you should monitor anytime you want to know how you are doing with your self-management plan. There are a few times when it is especially important to monitor, including, for example:

- When you start a new medication.

- When you change the dose of medication which you take.

- Any time when you think you might have low or high blood glucose.

- Days when you are feeling ill.

The important thing to remember about monitoring is that the information is *for you.*

Blood glucose targets

The goal for people with diabetes is to keep their blood glucose within a normal range and this does change throughout the day. So when you monitor your own blood glucose, it is important to know what your targets are. Talk with your doctor about your personal targets. the blood glucose targets are as indicated in *Table 18.3.*

Table 18.3 **Target Blood Glucose Levels Recommended by NICE**

Target level by type	Before meals	2 hours after meals
Non-diabetic	4.0 to 5.9 mmol/l	under 7.8 mmol/l
Type 2 diabetes	4 to 7 mmol/l	under 8.5 mmol/l
Type 1 diabetes	4-7 mmol/l	Under 9 mmol/l

Some points to note

If you are not sure how to set up or operate your *Blood Glucose Meter*, ask your GP surgery. You will usually get the advice from the practice nurse or specialist diabetes nurse, or from the diabetes clinic.

You can find further information about this on the *Diabetes UK* website, or from your health care team or diabetes nurse.

In any case, remember that your doctor may recommend slightly different targets for *you*, as an individual.

We suggest that you conduct an experiment. On two days, one a weekday and one a weekend day, monitor your blood glucose five times: first thing in the morning before eating; before a meal; two hours after a meal; before exercising; and finally after exercising. We know that this is a lot of finger lancets, but you only have to do this once, and you will learn a lot. You can plot your blood glucose on the charts we have produced in *Table 18.4* on page 298.

If there are things about these numbers you don't understand or if you want help to work out what these numbers mean, talk to your doctor or diabetes specialist nurse.

Also, you should keep in mind that blood sugar glucose naturally rises and falls during the course of the day. It is usually lowest in the morning when you wake up and highest an hour or two after you eat. Look at *Table 18.3* to check the target ranges. Do not be concerned if your blood glucose fluctuates within this target range and remember your doctor may have set personal targets for you.

What is important is that your blood glucose should be about the same on each day in relation to the same activities, for example, an hour or two after meals or after exercising.

Checking Your Ketones

If your blood glucose tends to be high, you may also be instructed by your doctor or diabetes specialist nurse on how to check your urine at home for ketones. Ketones are the acids remaining when the body burns up its own fat. The body starts to burn up its own fat when there is insufficient insulin to help fuel the body's cells. Ketones are therefore more common in people with Type 1 diabetes than with Type 2. If *ketoacidosis*, a condition in which the ketones are too high, occurs then this will require medical treatment.

If you have been managing your diabetes well, by eating properly, exercising, and taking your medication, and yet your early morning reading is almost always too high, then you should discuss this with your doctor. You may go to bed with your blood glucose in the target range, and then find that the levels jump up in the morning. This is known as the *dawn effect* or *dawn phenomenon*. Your blood glucose level may therefore rise a few hours before getting up in the morning in response to the release of hormones and extra glucose from the liver. To prevent or correct high blood glucose levels in the

Table 18.4 **Your Blood Glucose Profile**

Use the following table to plot your blood glucose profile.
Then ask yourself the questions which follow it.

My Daily Glucose Results

Day 1

When tested	Time of day	Blood glucose level (mmol/l)
First thing in the morning (before eating or taking medicine)		
Before a meal		
2 hours after lunch or dinner		
Before exercising		
After exercising		

Day 2

When tested	Time of day	Blood glucose level (mmol/l)
First thing in the morning (before eating or taking medicine)		
Before a meal		
2 hours after lunch or dinner		
Before exercising		
After exercising		

Questions to Ask Yourself

- Was your blood glucose within the recommended range?

- Are any of your figures under or over your recommended target?

- Do you notice any daily pattern in your results?

- Were there times during the day that your glucose was lower than the target range?

- Were there times during the day that your glucose was higher than the target range?

- Can you think of any reasons why your blood glucose acted as it did?

morning, your doctor may, based on the results of blood testing throughout the night, recommend: not eating carbohydrates close to bedtime; or adjusting your dosage of medication or insulin; or switching to a different medication.

Observing Symptoms and Taking Action

Although it is important to know how you feel when your blood glucose is very low or high, this is not a reliable way to manage your diabetes:

- *Firstly*, this is because many people do not have symptoms until their blood glucose is already very high or very low. Indeed, some people are unaware of any symptoms they may have during periods of high or low blood glucose. This makes it very difficult to stay within a sensible blood glucose range.

- *Secondly*, many of the symptoms are the same for both high and low blood glucose. Without knowing the actual level, it is difficult to know what to do. The only way for you to know about your blood glucose on a day-to-day basis is to monitor it.

Maintaining a Safe Blood Glucose Level

The goal of diabetes management is to keep blood glucose in the target range. Sometimes your blood glucose may rise too high which is *hyperglycaemia*, or it may fall too low which is called *hypoglycaemia*. The causes of hyperglycaemia and hypoglycaemia include the following:

- You are taking too little, or too much, medication or insulin.

- You are not eating properly, maybe by eating at irregular hours or missing or skipping meals.

- You are having too little or too much food, especially carbohydrates.

- You may be drinking too much alcohol.

- You may have increased, or decreased, your level of physical activity.

- You are suffering in some way, perhaps from an illness, infection, or surgery.

- You are under stress emotionally.

It is critically important: that you learn to recognise your specific symptoms; that you take self-care corrective action; and that you know when and how to seek medical assistance. For further guidance take a look now at *Table 18.5*.

We recommend that people with diabetes wear an emergency bracelet or carry an emergency card in their wallet, or that they do both. The emergency card should also contain information about the medications you are taking, your doctor's contact details, and an emergency contact person's name and telephone number. We also recommend that you always carry a *remedy food* such as a boiled sweet or biscuit or any *fast-acting* carbohydrate source with you to quickly manage low blood glucose.

Adopting a Healthy Eating Plan

Healthy eating is the core of diabetes self-management. You are the only one who can manage your blood glucose. The good news is that this is not as hard as it might seem. Small changes in your eating can make important differences in your blood glucose levels and how you feel. Let's start with some reassurance. You do not have to go hungry. You do not need special foods. You can still eat the foods you like. Healthy eating for diabetes is

Table 18.5 **Hyperglycaemia and Hypoglycaemia***

	Hyperglycaemia (blood glucose too high)	Hypoglycaemia (blood glucose too low)
Symptoms	Extreme tiredness. Extreme thirst. Blurred vision or a change in vision. Increased hunger. Increased need to urinate.	Feeling sweaty, shaky, or dizzy. Hard, fast heartbeat. Headache. Confusion or irritability or sudden change in mood. Tingling around your mouth or in your fingers.
What to do if you suspect this condition	If possible, check your blood glucose. If it is above 7.0 mmol/l after fasting or above 11 mmol/l two hours after a meal, take the actions indicated here. If you cannot check your blood glucose and think you have high blood glucose, take the following actions immediately: ♦ Drink water or other sugar-free liquids to prevent dehydration. ♦ If you take insulin, follow your instructions for taking extra insulin. ♦ Check your blood glucose every 4 hours. ♦ Seek immediate medical attention if you develop any of the symptoms described in the next part of this table.	If you feel symptoms of low blood glucose, check your blood glucose immediately. If your blood glucose is below 4 mmol/l or if you are in a place where you cannot test your blood glucose, or still have symptoms of low blood glucose, take the following actions: ♦ Eat a 15g "remedy food" or fast-acting carbohydrate source, for example, 3 glucose tablets, 3 packets of glucose, or 1/2 cup (4 fl. ounces) of fruit juice or a regular soft drink. ♦ Wait 15 minutes, note your symptoms, and, if possible, check your blood glucose again. ♦ After 15 minutes, if the symptoms are not better or your blood glucose level is still glucose is still less than 4 mmol/l eat another remedy food and wait 15 minutes. ♦ If your symptoms are still not better, call the doctor or nurse. Do not wait—it is critical to get immediate medical help. ♦ If your symptoms are better and your next meal is more than one hour away, eat a snack. For example, half a sandwich, some low-fat cheese, a few crackers, or a cup of milk.

300

Table 18.5 **Hyperglycaemia and Hypoglycaemia* (*continued*)**

	Hyperglycaemia (blood glucose too high)	Hypoglycaemia (blood glucose too low)
When to call the doctor or seek immediate medical help	If you feel confused, disoriented, agitated, or weak. If you have symptoms of dehydration, such as extreme thirst, dry mouth, and cracked lips, or have not urinated for eight hours. If you are running a fever, or you are vomiting, or have diarrhoea. If you have a strong, fruity breath, similar to nail polish or acetone. If your breathing is rapid and deep. If your blood glucose level is over 16.6 mmol/l for eight hours, or remains high or much higher than usual. This needs checking with your doctor or diabetes nurse.	If you have slurred speech, poor coordination, or clumsy movements. If you have seizures or a loss of consciousness. If your symptoms are not better after repeating the *what to do* steps. If you have a low blood glucose, of less than 3.3 mmol/l, twice in one day. If your blood glucose is repeatedly lower than usual without an obvious reason.

*Depending on your condition and history, your doctor may provide you with slightly different instructions for managing high or low blood glucoses than the suggestions we make in this table.

You should also note that some people experience symptoms of hypoglycaemia with blood glucose slightly higher than 3.8 mmol/l. This is another reason why it is important for you to check your blood sugar glucose, know your own body and learn how you feel at different levels.

301

healthy eating for your whole family. In Chapter 11 there is information about healthy eating. Here, we will give you the important basics for people with diabetes. If you have diabetes, you need to be more careful than other people about when, how much, and what types of foods you eat. This is because the type of food, the timing of when you eat, and the amount you eat all effect your blood glucose.

All food affects blood glucose. However, carbohydrates are the nutrients that do the most to determine blood glucose levels. Your job is to:

- *Monitor your carbohydrates:* Monitor especially *refined* carbohydrates like sugar. You can do this by learning about the carbohydrate content in different foods.

- *Eat healthy foods:* especially those with fewer carbohydrates.

- *Watch your portion size:* Also know the number of carbohydrates in a portion. All of this is fully discussed in Chapter 11.

- *Choose vegetables, fruits, and whole grains:* These foods give you good nutrients, energy, and fibre, with fewer calories, and with less fat.

- *Limit high-carbohydrate snacks:* Control your consumption of sweets, cakes, biscuits, fizzy drinks, and ice cream. These all raise your blood glucose and add fats and calories without giving you healthy nutrients.

We are not saying you can never have the foods you love. You just need to control your intake of these foods. How much carbohydrate do you need? The actual amount of carbohydrate that your body requires varies depending on your age, weight and activity levels. Some

carbohydrates are better for your overall health than others. This is because they provide vitamins, minerals and fibre. If you eat three meals and two snacks day, limit carbohydrates to about 45–60 grams per meal and 25 grams per snack. It would be useful for you to go back and read some of Chapter 11 on *Healthy Eating*. This will help you to clarify how foods are classified and the purpose each group serves. Remember, that when you are eating, *moderation* is the key to the successful management of blood glucose.

The Glycaemic Index

You may have come across the phrase *Glycaemic Index* in relation to carbohydrates and wondered what it means and what relevance it has for someone with diabetes. Counting carbohydrates is a method we have already discussed as a way of controlling our blood glucose. The Glycaemic Index (GI) is another method which is currently in use and you can apply. GI ranks carbohydrates on a scale from one to 100. Foods with a high Glycaemic Index are those which are rapidly digested and absorbed and therefore will have a marked effect on blood glucose. Foods with a low Glycaemic Index are digested and absorbed slowly and result in a more *gradual* rise in blood glucose levels. Low GI diets have been proven to help improve glucose levels and can also help with weight control. However it is more complicated than at first appears and it is necessary to work out the pros and cons of the GI foods you choose, to get the balance right. For example:

- Some low GI foods, like chocolate pudding, are not healthy choices; and some high GI foods, like watermelon, are healthy.

- The way your foods are cooked, for example boiled, fried or baked, can change their GI.

- The addition of fat will lower the GI of a food.

- The ripeness of both fruit and vegetables can change their GI.

There are many other considerations in getting the balance right if you use the Glycaemic Index. If this is an area you are interested in, it would be beneficial to look at the *Diabetes UK* website and follow the links to the detailed information provided on GI. Also, one small book listed at the end of this chapter provides the nutrition information on hundreds of different foods including their GI.

Planning Meals

When you have diabetes, planning meals may sound complicated. To help you do this, why not try out *The Eatwell Plate* method which we talked about earlier in Chapter 11?

The *Eatwell Plate* (below) is a pictorial summary of the main food groups and their recommended relative proportions for a healthy diet. It is a key method for illustrating the dietary advice recommended by the Department of Health. You can use the *Eatwell Plate* to help you get the balance right. It shows how much of what you eat on a daily basis, should come from each food group.

The plate is divided into five sections of which the first two are the largest:

- *Fruit and vegetables:* Aim for at least five portions of a variety of fruit and vegetables a day. Remember not to include potatoes in this category as they count as starchy foods.

- *Bread, rice, potatoes and pasta and other starchy foods:* Choose whole grain varieties where you can.

- *Milk and dairy products:* These form about a fifth of the plate and include milk, other dairy products and calcium-fortified soya milk.

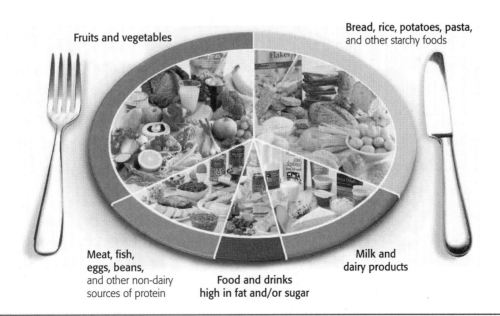

Fruits and vegetables

Bread, rice, potatoes, pasta, and other starchy foods

Meat, fish, eggs, beans, and other non-dairy sources of protein

Food and drinks high in fat and/or sugar

Milk and dairy products

Crown copyright: Department of Health in association with the Welsh Assembly Government, the Scottish Government and the Food Standards Agency in Northern Ireland.

The Eatwell Plate

■ *Non-dairy sources of protein:* This slightly smaller portion is for meat, fish, eggs and other non-dairy sources of protein such as beans and pulses.

■ *Fats and sugars:* The smallest portion on the plate is for foods or drinks which are high in fat or sugar.

Here is one final suggestion. Most people would benefit from eating smaller portions. A portion may be smaller than you think. This does not mean you cannot have more than a portion. It means you need to keep your total grams of carbohydrates per meal down to between 45 and 60. You can learn about portion sizes and the carbohydrate content of common foods by visiting Chapter 11. However, *Table 18.6* may help you.

Getting the balance right

A good way to see if you are achieving the right balance is to think about how many portions of these foods you normally eat and see how this compares to the guidelines provided in *Table 18.6*. Remember, everyone's nutritional needs are different and you may need more or less portions than those suggested.

The number of meals and the time between meals may vary according to your health needs and lifestyle:

■ Many of us eat three regular meals a day every four or five hours, but some people may need to eat smaller meals, more frequently throughout the day, perhaps eating four to six times a day.

■ Be sure not to skip breakfast. This is when your body most needs fuel as you have not eaten for a long time.

■ To learn more about managing your eating, we recommend that you spend some time with a diabetes specialist nurse or a dietician. There are also important programmes run by the NHS which are specifically tailored to learning more, in theory *and* in practice, about diet and nutrition in diabetes. One such programme is called *DAFNE* and another is called *DESMOND*

DAFNE and DESMOND

DAFNE stands for *Dose Adjustment for Normal Eating.* It is a way of managing Type 1 diabetes by providing you with the skills necessary to estimate your carbohydrate intake in each meal and to inject the right amount of insulin. It involves attending a five day course for groups of six to eight participants.

DESMOND stands for *Diabetes Education and Self-Management for On-going and Newly Diagnosed.* It is aimed at recently diagnosed or on-going patients with Type 2 diabetes and is also run in small groups in which a friend or relative can attend with you.

Both programmes are provided by the NHS and are free to participants. These particular programmes are not available in all parts of the UK but each locality will have some similar provision run under a variety of names. Ask your GP or diabetes team where you can access such a course.

Managing Your Physical Activity and Exercise

Regular exercise, along with healthy eating, is a core element of controlling blood glucose levels and improving health for everyone with diabetes. However, if you are taking medication

Table 18.6 **Food Groups and Deciding on the Portions You Eat**

Food groups and what's in a portion	How many portions do you eat in a day?	How many portions should you eat in a day from each group?
Bread, cereals, rice, pasta and potatoes. One portion is equal to: ◆ 2–4 tbsp. cereal. ◆ 1 slice of bread. ◆ Half a small chapatti. ◆ 2–3 crispbreads or crackers. ◆ 2–3 tbsp. rice, pasta, couscous, noodles or mashed potato. ◆ 2 new potatoes or half a baked potato.		**7–14** Include starchy foods at all meals. Choose more slowly absorbed varieties whenever possible.
Fruit and vegetables. One portion is equal to: ◆ A banana or apple. ◆ A slice of melon. ◆ 2 plums. ◆ 3 heaped tbsp. of vegetables. ◆ A handful of grapes. ◆ A cereal bowl of salad. ◆ A small glass of fruit juice or smoothie.		**5 or more** Choose a wide variety of foods from this group, including fresh, frozen, dried and tinned.
Meat, fish, and alternatives. One portion is equal to: ◆ 2–3 oz. (60–85g) of meat, poultry or vegetarian alternative. ◆ 4–5 oz. (120–140g) fish. ◆ 2 eggs. ◆ 2 tbsp. of nuts. ◆ 3 tbsp. of beans, lentils or dhal.		**2–3** Choose the lower fat alternatives whenever possible and eat more beans and pulses.
Milk and dairy foods. One portion is equal to: ◆ 1/3 pint milk. ◆ Small pot of yoghurt. ◆ 2 tbsp. of cottage cheese. ◆ 1½ oz. cheese (40–45g, matchbox size).		**3** Choose lower fat versions of milk and dairy foods.
Fatty and sugary foods. One portion is equal to: ◆ 2 tsp. spread, butter, oil, salad dressing. ◆ Half a sausage. ◆ 1 mini chocolate bar. ◆ 2 tsp. of sugar, jam or honey. ◆ 1 scoop ice cream or 1 tbsp. of cream.		**0–4** Cut down on sugary and fatty foods.

to control the disease, then you should discuss any changes you make in your exercise habits with your doctor, dietician, or diabetes team. A change in activity level often requires some changes in medication and eating schedules.

Exercise is beneficial for people with diabetes in several ways. Mild to moderate aerobic exercise decreases the need for insulin and helps to control blood glucose levels. It does this by increasing the sensitivity of your body cells to insulin and lowering blood glucose levels during and after exercise. This type of regular exercise is also essential for losing weight and reducing cardiovascular risk factors such as high levels of the blood lipids, involved in *cholesterol* and *triglycerides*, and high blood pressure.

The exercise programme recommended for people with diabetes is generally the same as the conditioning programme described in Chapter 7. Mild to moderate exercise (as described in Chapter 8) undertaken for approximately 30 minutes at a time, and performed as part of general conditioning programme, is a safe and effective way to control diabetes and stay healthy. Most people with diabetes should aim for at least 150 minutes a week. If you want to run a marathon, or you simply want to do a lot more exercise, then check with your health care team. You may need to make careful adjustments to your eating, medications, or both of these.

Some additional considerations

When suffering from diabetes you should begin an exercise programme only when your diabetes is well under control. Also, keep in touch with your doctor so that you can make changes in medication and diet if necessary, and co-ordinate your eating, medication, and exercise to avoid low blood glucose. It is often helpful to check your blood glucose levels before and after exercise so that you develop a sense of how your body is responding. If you do not take insulin, plan to be active *within an hour* after eating your meals or snacks so that you can avoid low blood glucose. If you have Type 1 diabetes and your blood glucose is less than 5.5 mmol/l before exercising, then you can eat 15 to 30 grams of carbohydrate before you start exercising *unless you are advised otherwise by your health care team*. Stop exercising right away if you are dizzy, or have shortness of breath, or feel sick, or are in pain. Drink extra fluids before, during, and after your exercise. If you have problems with sensation in your feet or poor circulation, make sure you check them regularly and protect them from blisters and abrasions. It is especially important to inspect your feet and practise good skin and nail hygiene. Don't forget that shoe inserts can be tailored to protect the soles of your feet.

For more information on how to develop and maintain an exercise programme, take a look at Chapter 6.

Managing Stress and Emotions

After learning that you have diabetes or if you develop diabetes-related complications, you may be feeling angry, scared, or depressed. These feelings are normal, understandable, and manageable. In fact, for people with diabetes, stress and emotions such as anger, fear, frustration, and depression can raise blood glucose levels. For this reason, it is important to learn effective ways to deal with your feelings. Hiding or ignoring your feelings is not healthy. You will find lots of tools for dealing with stress and negative emotions in Chapters 4 and 5.

Managing Days When You Are Ill with Infections and Other Illnesses

People with diabetes, like all people, sometimes become ill. When you get an infection, a cold, or the flu, your blood glucose tends to go up. How your body uses food and diabetes medicines will also change. For this reason, it is important to plan for such days and think about what to do and when to seek help. A number of points should be included in your plan, as follows:

Think ahead

■ *Identify a family member or friend who can help you when needed:* This person should know what to do, when to call the doctor, and when to take you to the A&E.

■ *Keep plenty of both sweetened and unsweetened or sugar free liquids close at hand.*

■ *Make sure that you have a thermometer at home:* Make sure you can use it.

■ *Keep your emergency medical information close by you:* This includes your doctor's telephone number and your current list of medications and dosages.

■ *Investigate with your diabetes team the circumstances when you should call them:* Some general guidelines are provided below.

When you are ill

Take your usual dose of insulin or pills: Do this unless you have a special *ill-day plan*, or you are vomiting, or your health care team tells you otherwise.

■ *Test your blood glucose two to four times a day:* If your blood glucose is over 16.6 mmol/l, you should test every three to four hours. Write down the results and times.

■ *Test your urine for ketones:* Do this if you take insulin and your blood glucose is above 16.6 mmol/l. Record whether you have small, moderate, or large amounts.

■ *Watch for symptoms of hypoglycaemia or hyperglycaemia:* Check with *Table 18.5* on pages 300–301.

■ *Track how much fluid you drink:* Try to sip at least eight fluid ounces, which is about half a pint, of fluids every hour while you are awake. This will prevent dehydration. If your blood glucose is over 13.3 mmol/l, use glucose-free drinks such as broth, tea or water. If your blood glucose is low eat or drink half to one pint of a liquid, perhaps fruit juice or a regular soft drink.

■ *Check your temperature:* Do this twice a day and record it.

■ *Keep eating if possible:* Small frequent meals or snacks can help.

■ *Keep in touch with your supporters:* Tell a family member or friend how you are feeling and have this person check in with you frequently.

When to call your health care professional

■ If your blood glucose is less than 3.3 mmol/l two times in one day.

■ If your blood glucose is over 16.6 mmol/l for eight hours or your blood glucoses are much higher than they usually are.

■ If your temperature rises above 101°F or 38.3°C, or if it stays above 100°F or 37.8°C, for more than two days.

■ If you vomit, or have had diarrhoea for more than 24 hours.

- If you are not able to drink liquids, eat food or keep down medications for more than eight hours.

- If you have a small level of ketones in your urine, as indicated on the test strips.

- If you experience deep or troubled breathing, or an extremely dry mouth, or develop a fruity odour to your breath.

- If you have been feeling ill for longer than expected and you are not getting any better.

- If you are not feeling well and are unsure what you should do to care for yourself.

When to seek immediate emergency care

- If your blood glucose is over 27.7 mmol/l.

- If you find moderate to large amounts of ketones in your urine.

  When you call your health care professional, be prepared by having the following information at hand: your type of diabetes, your blood glucose level, if you know it, your temperature, whether you have ketones in your urine, a list of your symptoms and of the medications you are taking, and what you have done so far to treat these symptoms.

Medications: Helping You Control Blood Glucose and Prevent Complications

In addition to healthy eating and exercising, most people with diabetes benefit from medications. These help to keep blood glucose, blood pressure, and cholesterol levels within the target ranges. Although they can be helpful, many people do not like taking medications. For some of us, not taking medications is almost a point of pride. We might want to manage our conditions naturally. It is true that in some cases it is possible to manage without medications. However, most people with diabetes, if they are going to maintain blood glucose control and prevent complications, need to take one or more medications. Medications can help prevent such serious complications as heart attack, stroke, kidney disease, and early death. Unfortunately, you often cannot afford to wait to see what happens without them. It is sensible to take the medications as a risk reduction measure. Once diabetes complications have appeared, they usually cannot be reversed.

Blood glucose medications

Your doctor will recommend medications based on your type of diabetes, how well your blood glucose is controlled, and your other medical conditions.

- *Insulin for Type 1 diabetes:* Insulin is required throughout your life because your body does not produce insulin.

- *Medications for Type 2 diabetes:* There are several types of pills that can be used separately or in combination to help control your blood glucose. Oral or injected insulin is also a safe and effective choice for many people with Type 2 diabetes.

Medications to prevent complications

In addition to using medications to control blood glucose, studies have shown that certain medications can reduce the risk of developing diabetes complications. Because of their protective benefit, these medications are recommended even if your blood pressure and cholesterol are within the target ranges. Depending on your age and medical conditions, common types of preventive medications may include the following:

- *Aspirin:* Low-dose aspirin (75 mg) reduces risk for heart attack and stroke by decreasing the chance of a sudden blockage in an artery. However, patients without known cardiovascular risk need to discuss their individual cases with their health care team rather than taking aspirin as a preventive. Therefore aspirin should only be taken after consultation with your doctor or hospital consultant.

- *ACE inhibitors or ARBs:* These specialised medications to control blood pressure protect your kidneys and reduce the chance of having a heart attack or stroke.

- *Statins:* These decrease inflammation and lower cholesterol, reducing the chance of a heart attack or stroke.

Talk with your doctor if you are not taking these additional preventive medicines to find out whether you should be doing so.

Diabetes medications

Some people with Type 2 diabetes can manage their blood glucose without insulin or other diabetes medications by controlling their exercise, diet, and weight. Sometimes losing only 10 to 15 pounds (4–6 kg) can be enough. As a rule of thumb, a weight loss of 7% will help bring blood glucose into a healthy range. This means losing 14 pounds if you weigh 200 pounds. However, along with diet and exercise, most patients with Type 2 diabetes will need the help of oral medications or insulin to safely control their blood glucose and help prevent complications. These

medications do *not* take the place of healthy eating and regular physical activity.

Using Insulin

Insulin is used to treat everyone with Type 1 diabetes and for many people with Type 2 diabetes. It is used to replace the insulin that is not produced or is inadequately used by the body. Using insulin injections is now one of the safest and most effective ways to control blood glucose and prevent complications. Research now supports using insulin earlier in the treatment of Type 2 diabetes if blood glucose levels are quite high, or if oral medications do not control blood glucose, or if you experience side-effects from oral medications. Some patients are initially fearful of using insulin, but once started, they find that the injections are rather easy and nearly painless. Usually this procedure causes less discomfort than you experience from the finger prick lancet required to check blood glucose! In addition, controlling blood glucose levels is often much easier with the use of insulin. Remember, using insulin is a good thing and likely to be a wise decision when recommended by your doctor.

Types of insulin

There are several types of insulin which are distinguished by how fast and how long they work. It is important that you know the *type* of insulin you are taking, the company that makes it, the dose or number of units you take. In addition, you need to know precisely when to take it, for example before a meal or snack, or soon after taking the first bite of your food. Also make sure that the insulin you are taking has not passed its expiration date. If you feel that you could benefit from learning more about the use of insulin, talk to your doctor or diabetes educator. Look back at the earlier section in this chapter to check on the NHS education courses provided on the use of insulin and diet. Your doctor may also work out a written plan with you for how to adjust your insulin dose on a *sliding scale* based on your own home blood glucose daily measurements. Some patients with diabetes may also benefit from the use of insulin pumps. You will find a more detailed list of resources at the end of this chapter.

Other Medications

If you do need medications, you should know *when* to take them and be aware that you should *never* skip a dose. Most of these drugs are taken once or twice a day, usually just before meals. Check with your doctor before stopping or changing your medicines, even if you don't feel well. When travelling, always keep your medications on your person, not in your luggage.

Other medications, including over-the-counter medications and some natural remedies and dietary supplements, can sometimes interact with diabetes medications. Therefore, it is important that your doctor and pharmacist know *all* the medications you are taking, including prescription and non-prescription drugs and any vitamins, minerals, supplements, herbals, and natural medicines you use.

If you start a new drug and experience side-effects, be sure to tell your health care team straightaway. A simple change in medicine, or in the dosage of the current medicine, can often clear up some side-effects. In *Table 18.7*, we list some of the most common medications used for Type 2 diabetes. If you need more details on any of the medications listed and their characteristics, it is advisable you ask your doctor, pharmacist or diabetes specialist nurse.

Preventing Complications

Diabetes can cause other problems in the body. These can often be delayed and sometimes avoided by maintaining good blood glucose control. Remember that most complications are directly related to inadequate control. The following are the most common complications of diabetes:

- *Heart disease and stroke:* It may surprise you that heart disease and stroke are the biggest killers of people with diabetes. High blood glucose levels can harden and block the arteries. The good news is that there are many things you can do to help reduce these potential problems.

- *Nerve damage:* Diabetes can cause *neuropathy* or damage to the nerves. This results in a burning or tingling sensation, numbness, or severe pain, especially in the feet and hands. Nerve damage can sometimes lead to sexual problems such as erection problems in men and vaginal dryness in women. Nerve damage can also lead to problems with digestion and urination.

Table 18.7 **Some Common Medications Prescribed for Diabetes**

Main groups	How the drug acts	Generic names of medication
Alpha Glucosidase Inhibitor	Slows down the absorption of starchy foods from the intestine thereby reducing after-meal blood glucose peaks.	Acarbose
Prandial Glucose Regulator	Stimulates cells in the pancreas to produce insulin.	Repaglinide Nateglinide
Thiazolidinedione (Glitazones)	Reduces insulin resistance and allows the insulin that the body produces to work more efficiently.	Pioglitazone The European Medicines Agency has advised of a slight risk of bladder cancer and heart problems. Speak to your GP If have any concerns.
Incretin Mimetics	Increases level of a hormone called incretin. Increases insulin when needed and decreases when not needed.	Exanatide
DPP-4 Inhibitors (Gliptins)	Blocks the action of DPP-4, an enzyme which destroys the hormone incretin.	Sitagliptin Vildagliptin Saxagliptin
Biguanides	Slows down the absorption of glucose from the intestine.	Metformin
Sulphonylureas	Stimulates cells in pancreas to produce Insulin.	Glibenclamide Gliclazide Tolbutamide

Note: Many new medications for managing blood glucose are being developed and evaluated each year. It is helpful to discuss with your doctor which medications might be right for you.

- *Kidney damage:* Diabetes can damage the blood vessels in the kidney, especially when the blood pressure is high, causing kidney failure. The first sign may be detected by a test for small amounts of protein in the urine.

- *Vision problems:* Blurred vision can occur when high blood glucose levels temporarily cause the lens in the eye to swell. More serious and permanent damage to the blood vessels in the retina in the back of the eye called *retinopathy*, can lead to poor vision or even blindness.

- *Infections:* Diabetes can decrease immune function and reduce your blood flow, which can lead to slower healing and more frequent infections of the skin, feet, lungs, and other parts of your body.

- *Gum disease:* People with diabetes have a greater risk for gum or *periodontal* disease and infection. So, it is important to discuss your diabetes with your dentist and to get regular dental check-ups.

A Useful Checklist to Manage Complications

Here is a handy checklist to make sure you are doing what's necessary and getting the care required to prevent or delay the complications of diabetes. This may even save your life:

- *Maintain safe blood glucose levels:* The keys to controlling blood glucose levels and preventing complications are a healthy diet, regular exercise, a healthy weight, and necessary medications.

- *Control your blood pressure:* The target blood pressure reading for people with diabetes, is usually 130/80 or less, or as recommended by your doctor. Lower blood pressure means less stress on your heart and blood vessels, eyes, and kidneys. Controlling blood pressure can be as important as controlling blood glucose levels in preventing complications from diabetes.

- *Control your blood cholesterol:* LDL or *bad* cholesterol, rather than total cholesterol, is the measure that is usually monitored for people with diabetes. The target level for people with diabetes is a total cholesterol level of below 4.00 mmol/l. Check with your doctor what is right for you. Remember that taking a statin medication may further reduce the risk of heart attack and stroke even if your cholesterol level is low without the statin.

- *Protect your kidneys:* Along with regular testing, taking an ACE inhibitor or ARB medication can help lower blood pressure as well as protect your kidneys.

- *Get regular check-ups, examinations, and immunisations including the following:*
  - *Have an HbA1c test* at least every six months if your diabetes is well controlled or at three monthly intervals if not well controlled.
  - *Have kidney function test* at least once a year. Recent analysis of diabetes audits suggest that approximately 25% of all diabetes patients are not given this important annual test. So ask your doctor or diabetes team if you think you may not have had the test.
  - *Have cholesterol and lipid tests* at least once a year.
  - *Have eye examinations*, including an inspection of the retina at the back of your eyeball, every one to two years, or as recommended by your doctor. Always report any changes in vision to your doctor. This retinal examination is different from a test by an optometrist, who checks your vision to see if you need glasses or corrective lenses.
  - *Remind a member of your diabetes team to check your feet* at each visit or at least once a year. One way to do this is to always take off your shoes and socks in the examination room.
  - *Have your blood pressure checked at every visit*, or as recommended by your doctor, and keep track of the numbers.
  - *Have a flu jab every year and a pneumonia vaccine at least once.* The latter may need to be repeated after age 65.
  - *Have a dental exam once a year, or as recommended by your diabetes team; floss and brush your teeth at least once a day.*

■ *Check out your feet:* When you have diabetes, your feet need extra care and attention. Diabetes can damage the nerve endings and blood vessels in your feet, making you less likely to notice when your feet are injured. Diabetes also limits your body's ability to fight infection and get blood to areas that need it. If you sustain a minor foot injury, it could become an ulcer or a serious infection. So, take the following precautions:

• *Examine your feet every day.* You should look between the toes and on the tops and bottoms of your feet for cuts, cracks, sores, corns, calluses, blisters, ingrown toenails, extreme dryness, bruises, redness, swelling, or pus.

• *Wash your feet every day.* Use warm, not hot water. Check the water temperature with your wrist or another part of your body and dry thoroughly, especially between the toes. Do not soak your feet.

• *Cut your toenails straight across.* If you can't safely trim your toenails yourself, ask a family member to do it or get some professional help. Also, do not clean under your toenails or remove skin with sharp objects. Many Day Centres have a day or two each month when a professional comes in to cut toenails.

• *If your feet are dry, rub on a mild lotion before going to bed.* Do not put lotion between your toes. Avoid lotions that contain alcohol or other ingredients that end in *-ol*, as these tend to dry out the skin.

• *Wear comfortable shoes and socks and never go barefoot except when bathing or in bed.* Your shoes should support, protect, and

cover your feet. If your feet sweat then use some powder. Before putting on shoes, check inside for rough places or any sharp objects such as tacks or nails inside the sole of the shoe. Break in new shoes gradually. Also avoid socks with tight, elastic tops.

• *Avoid hot spots by not wearing the same shoes two days in a row.* If you have any problems with your feet then change your shoes in the middle of the day.

• *Get a member of your diabetes team or a podiatrist to check your feet at each review.*

• *Always get early treatment for foot problems.* Quite minor irritations can lead to a major problem.

■ Take additional precautionary measures as follows:

• *Be certain to tell your doctor if you are taking aspirin (75mg)* to lessen your risk of heart attacks and stroke.

• *Do not smoke,* or if you do, then take some positive action to stop in future.

• *In general, it is a good idea to avoid alcohol.* For the person with diabetes, alcohol can cause a sudden and drastic drop in blood glucose. It also adds calories that can lead to a weight gain. If you do drink, make sure you have some food with it to avoid a low blood glucose reaction. This can happen if you have alcohol on an empty stomach.

• *Protect your skin.* Don't get sunburned, and keep your skin clean.

• *Wear a MedicAlert necklace or bracelet,* and carry with you a list of all your medications.

◆ *At every visit remind the doctor and nurse that you have diabetes.* This is also important if you are hospitalised or go to A&E.

A reminder – if you are a car driver

Cars can give us a great deal of freedom in our lives. However, when you are diagnosed with diabetes treated with insulin alone or insulin tablets, you must, by law, inform the DVLA as soon as possible after you have been diagnosed. There are other conditions about holding your license, in particular relating to hypoglycaemia. At the end of this chapter we provide contact details for the relevant Section of the DVLA where you can get advice. A revised pamphlet (2013) is available to download called *A Guide to Insulin Treated Diabetes and Driving*.

The Bottom Line: Your Role is Important

Most complications of diabetes can be prevented, delayed, and treated. You have an important role. Let us quickly review what you must do:

- Maintain your blood glucose level within your normal range.

- Be aware of your body and symptoms.

- Report changes early. Time is important.

- Make sure you get regular check-ups, exams, tests, and immunisations.

Table 18.8 is a summary of some of the main tests relating to your diabetes that you may come across or hear about.

To become a good diabetes self-manager, there is certainly a lot to learn. Putting all of this into action is sometimes difficult. So, you should set personal goals to control your diabetes, review them regularly, and revise them as needed. Be sure to talk to your doctor, diabetes team or specialist nurse about your questions, problems, and concerns. Find out about other information and resources in your community. Take a diabetes education programme. Consider joining a diabetes support group either in your community or online. Some additional resources are listed at the end of this chapter.

Table 18.8 **The Main Tests Relating to Your Diabetes**

A list of some tests used for people with diabetes		
Diabetes screening tests	**How the test is done**	**Why the test is done**
C-Peptide Test	After fasting overnight a blood test is taken to find out how much insulin your body produces.	To determine if you have Type 1 or Type 2 diabetes.
Fasting Blood Glucose Test	A blood test is taken to determine blood glucose level after fasting eight hours before a blood test.	To determine, from the results of the blood glucose levels, if you have diabetes or not
Oral Glucose Tolerance Test	After an overnight fast you will be asked to take a glucose drink and your blood glucose Is measured before and after the drink. The test is to find out what stage you may be at in regard to diabetes.	Your test result may be in normal range so you do not have diabetes. Your test shows blood glucose higher than normal but you do not have diabetes. You may have what is called pre-diabetes. Blood glucose high enough to show you do have diabetes.
Self-monitoring Blood Test	Non-fasting blood test done several times or less each day at home using blood glucose meter.	To help you make decisions about your daily diet and adjust your insulin injections.
HbA1c Blood Test	Blood test analysed in the laboratory.	To monitor your average blood glucose control over two to three months.
Urine Test	To test for glucose in the urine using prepared diagnostic strips which are dipped into your urine sample.	Results can be normal or indicate an early sign of pre-diabetes or possible diabetes. Only a doctor can determine the results and what should be done next, if anything.
Ketones Test	Pre-prepared strips are dipped in urine which will show a reaction if ketones are present	Ketones can build up and cause diabetic ketoacidosis. This can lead to coma if not addressed.

Suggested Further Reading

Bierman, J., Valentine, V. and Toohey, B. *Diabetes: The New Type 2: Your Complete Handbook to Living Healthfully with Diabetes Type 2*. New York: Tarcher, 2008.

Chan, W. Counter, *G.I. and G.L.* London: Hamlyn, 2006.
This is a small reference book to hundreds of foods with information on their Glycaemic Index, calories, average portion sizes and nutrition.

Daley, D. *Exercise to Improve Your Health*. London: Cico Books, 2011.
This book has specific exercise suggestions for individual conditions.

Day, J. L. *Living with Diabetes: The Diabetes UK Guide for those treated with Insulin (New Edition)*. Chichester: Wiley Blackwell, 2002.

Keys, A. *Sick Is an Attitude: Living Well with Diabetes*. Create Space: 2013.
The book is written by someone diagnosed with diabetes aged 10 and now in her 60s.

Raymond, M. *The Human Side of Diabetes*. Chicago: Noble Press, 1992.

Schade, D. S., Boyle, P. J. and Burge, M. R. *101 Tips for Staying Healthy with Diabetes and Avoiding Complications*. Alexandria, Va.: American Diabetes Association, 1996.

Walker, R. and Rodgers, J. *Diabetes: A Practical Guide to Managing Your Health*. New York: DK, 2005.

Wright, K. *A Guide to Diabetes*. New Lanark UK: Geddes and Gosset, 2007.

Other Resources

☐ *Blood Pressure Association*: Tel: 0208 722 4994. www.bpassoc.org.uk.

☐ *Diabetes UK*: Helpline: Tel: 0845 120 2960. www.diabetes.org.uk.

☐ *Department of Health*: Follow the links and type in the key words for the topic on which you want information. www.gov.uk/government/organisations/department-of-health.

☐ *DVLA: Driver and Vehicle Licensing Agency*: General Website www.dvla.gov.uk
Important: If you have specific questions or need information regarding diabetes and driving you can telephone 0300 790 6806 or go to www.gov.uk/browse/driving.

☐ *Foods Standards Agency*: Tel: 0207 276 8000. www.food.gov.uk.

☐ *Input*: This is an organisation supporting access to technology for use by people diagnosed with diabetes, in particular insulin pumps. Tel: 0800 228 9977. www.input.me.uk.

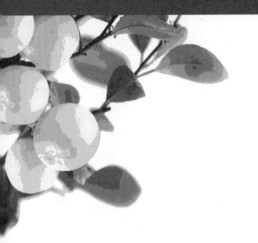

CHAPTER 19

Planning for the Future: Fears and Reality

PEOPLE WITH LONG-TERM CONDITIONS WORRY about what will happen to them should their condition become truly disabling. They fear that at some time in the future they may have problems managing their lives and their health condition. One way people can deal with their fears about the future is to take control and plan for it. They may never need to put their plans into effect, but there is reassurance in knowing that they will be in control, if the events they fear come to pass. We'll examine the most common concerns and offer some suggestions that may be useful to you.

What If I Can't Take Care of Myself Anymore?

Regardless of our state of health, most of us fear becoming helpless and dependent. The fear is even greater among people with potentially disabling health problems. And the fear usually has physical as well as financial, social, and emotional components.

Physical Concerns of Day-to-Day Living

As your health condition changes, you may need to consider changing your living situation. This may involve employing someone to help you in your home or moving to a place where more help is provided. How you make this decision depends on your needs and how they can best be met. Keep in mind that we are talking about physical, social and emotional needs. All these must be considered.

Start by evaluating what you can do for yourself and what Activities of Daily Living (ADLs) will require some kind of help. ADLs are the everyday things such as getting out of bed, bathing, dressing, preparing and eating meals, cleaning the house, shopping, and paying bills. Most people can do all of these things, even though they may have to do them slowly, or with some modification, or with help from gadgets.

However, some people may eventually find one or more of these tasks no longer possible without help. For example, you may still be able to prepare meals but no longer be able to do the shopping. Or, if you have problems with fainting or sudden bouts of unconsciousness, you might need to have somebody around you at all times. You may also find that some things that you enjoyed doing in the past, like gardening, are no longer pleasurable. Sometimes this is because you feel that your garden is now too big. You no longer feel able to manage it on your own or maybe you don't have the energy to do it to the standard you have always maintained.

Using the problem-solving steps discussed in Chapter 2, you can analyse and make a list of what the potential problems might be. Once you have this list, you can solve the problems one at a time. For each problem you can begin by writing down every possible solution you can think of. For example:

I can't go shopping

- Get my daughter, son, other family member, or friend to shop for me.
- Find a local volunteer shopping service.
- Shop at a supermarket that offers a delivery service.
- Ask a neighbour to shop for you.
- Use the Internet more for shopping.
- Get meals on wheels delivered to the door.

I can't manage living on my own any longer

- Employ an around-the-clock carer.
- Move in with a relative.
- Get a Personal Alarm System through an organisation like *Age UK*.
- Move to a residential care home.
- Move into a sheltered housing complex.

When you have listed all your problems and possible solutions, select the one that seems the most workable and acceptable.

The selection will sometimes depends on: your finances; your family; other resources you can call on; and how well the potential solutions address your problem. Sometimes one solution will become the answer for several problems. For instance, if you can't shop and can't be alone, and your household chores are reaching crisis point, then you might consider a sheltered housing complex. This could solve *all* of these problems because most accommodation of this kind will offer meals, regular house cleaning, and help with errands and medical appointments.

Even if you are not of retirement age, many housing organisations will accept younger people. Some facilities for the retired take residents at age 50, or younger if one member of the household has reached the minimum age. If you are a young person, the local centre for people with disabilities or *independent living centre* should be able to direct you to a care facility suitable for you.

Considerations on Levels of Care Offered

When you are looking for a retirement community, consider the levels of care that are being offered. These usually include *independent living,* where you have your own apartment or small house; *assisted living,* where you get some help with dressing, taking medications, and other tasks; and *skilled nursing,* which includes help with all ADLs and some medical care. These options are discussed in more detail later in this chapter.

It may help to discuss your wishes, abilities, and limitations with a trusted friend, relative, or social worker. Sometimes another person can spot things that you might overlook, or would like to ignore. A good self-manager often makes use of a wide range of resources, which is an important step in the problem-solving process laid out in Chapter 2.

Undertake the changes you need to make in your life slowly, one step at a time. You don't need to change your whole life to solve one problem. Remember that you can always change your mind, so don't burn your bridges. If you think that moving out of your own place to another living arrangement, with relatives, or a care home, or elsewhere, is for you. Then be cautious, don't give up your present home until you are settled into your new one and are sure you want to stay.

Options for Day-to-Day Living

There are several options for getting help with your care needs. Of course, these can range from normal daily activities such as shopping, preparing meals, housework, to a more complex situation where your medical needs mean you will require full-time nursing care. Questions you may ask yourself will probably include the following:

> *"If I get some alterations made to my home, like a walk-in-shower, will this solve my problem?"*

> *"If I downsize and move to a smaller more manageable house, will this solve my problems?"*

> *"If I move closer to my family or other relatives, will this provide the help I need?*

> *"If I move into sheltered housing, a residential care home, or a nursing home, will this relieve me of my worry and anxiety about what will happen during an emergency?"*

The next few paragraphs provide a more detailed outline and discussion of these options. In particular, they address the matters you need to consider before you make your final decision and how this will be financed.

At the end of this chapter we provide some useful contact details to enable you to get further advice about whatever decisions you decide to make. It cannot be stressed enough that when you make major changes in your life it is important to look at the long-term planning rather than just at what will solve your immediate problem. There is no point in making big and expensive changes to your home if, in a year's time, you plan to move somewhere else.

Exploring Your Options

Staying in Your Own Home

Many people have worked hard to acquire their own home and they have strong attachments to it and some fond memories. They may also live in a supportive and friendly community. So a decision to move out of their home could be a very emotional one. There are many things you can do to help yourself to continue to live in your own home and retain some independence if it is important and appropriate for you to do so. You have a number of options to consider:

1. Making alterations to your home

Some alterations can make your home safer and more comfortable. These can range from minor matters such as installing hand grips in the bathroom and stair rails, to more substantial changes such as installing a stair lift or a walk-in shower. Some voluntary organisations have schemes where they employ a group of handy men who will come along and do minor alterations at a very small cost. If the alterations are more complicated, Social Services will do an assessment to see what changes would be most appropriate for your needs. This is normally carried out by an occupational therapist.

Funding the changes you want

There are different ways of funding the alterations you may require. You will clearly be expected to buy for yourself very small items, like specialised cutlery for eating your meals. But for larger equipment or alterations an occupational therapist from Social Services will undertake an assessment of your needs. If the proposals will cost less than £1000 they can often be provided free. If, for example, the cost is more than £1000 when installing a downstairs bathroom, then you will have to apply for a *Disabled Facilities Grant* from the Local Authority. The maximum amount currently available is £30,000 in England and £36,000 in Wales. You should take note that, in all we say in this chapter, you may find that the regulations for Scotland, Northern Ireland, and Wales may be different. If this applies to you, then you can get advice either from your Local Authority Housing Department, or Social Services Department, *Age UK,* or the *Citizens Advice Bureau.* The occupational therapist will be able to help you fill in the application form for the Disabled Facilities Grant.

2. Seeking assistance with personal care

You may also need some help with personal care, such as, assistance in getting in and out of bed, bathing, or preparing meals. In these situations you have a range of options. These include home helps to deal with general housework, or home care to assist you with getting dressed or having a bath.

Funding your personal care

The rules governing the cost of this kind of personal help are currently under review by the government. Changes may be made as a result. You should therefore always seek advice at the time when you are thinking of using these services. At the end of this chapter you will find a list of sources from which you can get this sort of advice.

3. Making use of the computer

The use of computers can help in many ways to achieve the objective of staying in your own home. Some people are very computer literate and enjoy using them. Others have never used them at all and are very apprehensive about starting. There are usually local community initiatives where you can learn how to use computers if that is what you would like to do. There is also now a very simple computer with just six keys which has been adapted for ease of use for elderly people and for those who have little confidence. Take a few moments to consider how the computer might help you:

- You can shop online at your local supermarket and have your order delivered direct to your door.

- You can shop for more specialised goods like clothes.

- You can pay your bills on-line.

- You can book and purchase travel tickets.

In fact the resources that become available to you when you are using a computer are vast.

Funding your use of the computer

If you cannot afford to buy your own computer there may be grants available to help you do so.

Ask your Social Services Department or occupational therapist for information about this.

4. Getting involved in the home share scheme

Another option which you may like to consider is to share your home. This is something you need to think carefully about because it is something which involves you living very near to someone you may not know very well. The basis of the *Home Share Scheme* is the exchange of accommodation in return for help in the home. In this scheme, the householder, often an elderly person, with a spare room, offers free or low cost accommodation in exchange for *an agreed level of support*. The support might include shopping, housework, gardening and help with pets. The scheme has a double benefit; *firstly,* it provides housing for someone who may not be able to afford their own home; *secondly,* it enables an elderly person to retain their independence by helping them to continue staying at home. The schemes are usually run by voluntary organisations. *Crossroads* is one such agency.

Funding the home share scheme

The costs related to this scheme are whatever arrangement you and the home sharer feel able to agree on.

5. Installing a personal alarm

If you live alone you may be worried about having a fall or an emergency. One way of addressing the problem might be to use a personal alarm. The *Personal Alarm System* involves you wearing a small pendant or a wrist band into which the alarm system is set. In an emergency you press a small button on your alarm and you are immediately connected to an operator who then arranges the help that you need.

Funding for a personal alarm

The cost of these alarms varies but usually you pay for the system which is a one-off payment of around £100. There are various options to help you pay for this up-front amount. You then pay a weekly amount for the provision of the service. In some cases this weekly amount works out at around £4 inclusive of VAT.

Moving Out of Your Home

There are a range of options to consider when you decide to move out of your home. These include the following:

1. Deciding to downsize

This is one option which you can take whether you own your home or rent it. You may think that it would be easier to manage daily living activities if you lived in a smaller property. Some people worry about managing their garden, whilst others worry about paying basic household bills like heating. Downsizing can certainly resolve some of these issues.

Funding this change

The cost of downsizing will include all the bills related to selling your house and buying another, or if you rent your home privately you will need to consider other factors. For example what does the tenancy agreement with your landlord stipulate? On top of this come the costs of moving yourself and your possessions to your new location.

2. Moving in with a member of your family

This can be an option for some people. Indeed, it can be an ideal solution, but only if you have thought through very carefully all the implications for you *and* your family member. It will be of particular importance that you have discussed all the financial arrangements and the expectations you have of each other.

Funding the move into someone else's home

This will depend on the financial arrangements you discuss with the family into whose home you will be moving.

3. Moving into sheltered housing

This can be an ideal option for people who want to retain their independence, but who need the security of knowing that help is at hand if needed. There are various types of sheltered housing ranging from rented accommodation provided by the Local Authority or by Voluntary Organisations, to housing which is privately owned and run. In the latter situation you can sometimes have the option to buy or rent the property. The advantages of sheltered housing include: the fact that your accommodation is furnished with your own possessions; the presence of a warden on duty full or part-time; and that there are communal facilities where you can meet other residents and socialise. In some cases, sheltered housing will have an optional communal dining room and some even have a leisure centre which in a few places includes a swimming pool!

Funding sheltered accommodation

The cost of this type of accommodation will vary considerably between those run by the local authority, by voluntary organisations and by private providers. It will also depend on whether you decide to buy or rent.

4. Moving into a care home

If you need more help in your daily living than can be provided in Sheltered Housing then moving to a care home can be an option. Care homes are staffed for 24 hours a day and all meals are provided. Some nursing care is also available, but if you need more care than they can offer, then this will not be the right choice. It is important when considering a residential care home, to evaluate the type of residents who are living there to make sure you will fit in. For example, some of these facilities may cater for individuals who are mentally confused. If you are mentally clear, you might not find much companionship there. Equally, if everybody is hard of hearing, you might have trouble finding somebody to talk to! So, it's best to take your time in choosing a care home, go and look round several times and listen to what other people can tell you. It is a major decision to give up your home.

Funding for care home residence

The costs and financial implications are something you will need advice about. The rules about the amount you will be asked to pay are complicated. Currently, in 2013, discussions are under way regarding changes in charges and assessments. At the end of this chapter you will find the names of organisations that can offer you up-to-date guidance about how such matters will affect you.

5. Taking the nursing home option

If you have a medical condition or an illness which requires on-going nursing care, then you will need to find a care home that can provide this. A nurse should be available for 24 hours a day and have appropriate facilities for your care, for example a hoist for lifting you in and out of the bath, perhaps.

Funding for the nursing home

The costs and financial implications of this sort of care are something you will need advice on. The rules about how much you will be asked to pay are complicated and are also currently under review by the government.

I Need Help, but I Don't Want Help: Your Feelings

Let's take some time here to talk about the emotional aspects of needing help.

Every human being emerges from childhood reaching for and cherishing every possible sign of independence. This includes the driver's licence, the first job, your first credit card, the first time you go out and don't have to tell anybody where you are going or when you will be back, and many more. In these and other ways, we demonstrate to ourselves as well as to others that we are *grown up*. We are in charge of our lives and easily able to take care of ourselves without any help from our parents.

When the time comes, we must face the realisation that we can no longer manage completely on our own, it may seem like a return to childhood. It is like letting somebody else take charge of our lives. This can be both painful and embarrassing.

Some people in this situation become extremely depressed and can no longer find any joy in life. Others won't admit they need help, thus placing themselves in possible danger and making life difficult and frustrating for those who would like to help. Conversely, others give up completely and expect other people to take total responsibility for them, demanding attention and services from their children or other family members. If you recognise some of these reactions, you can take steps to help yourself feel better and develop a more positive response.

Making Changes

You should accept the thoughtful idea that we should focus on: *"changing the things I can change, accepting the things I cannot change, and being wise enough to know the difference"*, because this enables us to stay in charge of our own life. You must be able to evaluate your situation accurately and act accordingly. Thus, you must identify the activities that require help from somebody else, like going shopping and cleaning the house, and also celebrate those things that you can still do on your own, perhaps getting dressed, paying bills and writing letters. Another way to look at this is to get help from others for the things you least like to do; giving you the time and energy to do those things you want to do.

All this means *making decisions*. As long as you are making the decisions, you are in charge. It is important to make decisions and take actions while you are still able to do so. Don't let circumstances intervene and make the decision for you. In the end you must be realistic and honest with yourself. You can find more about making decisions on pages 18 and 19.

Getting Help When You Decide to Make Changes

Some people find that talking with a sympathetic listener, either a professional counsellor or a sensible close friend or family member, is both comforting and helpful. An objective listener can often point out alternatives and options you may have overlooked or were not even aware of. These people can provide information, or contribute another point of view or interpret a particular situation in a way that you would not have thought of. This can be an important part of the self-management process.

Nevertheless, be very careful when considering advice from somebody who has something to sell you. There are many people whose solution to your problem just happens to be whatever it is they are selling. This can be health or burial insurance policies, annuities, special and expensive furniture, sunshine cruises, special magazines, or health foods with magical curative properties!

In talking with family members or friends who want to help, be as open and reasonable as you can but, at the same time, try to make them understand that you reserve the right to decide how much and what kind of help you will accept. They will probably be more co-operative and understanding if you say, *"Yes, I do need some help with . . . , but I still want to do . . . myself."* You can find more tips on asking for help in Chapter 9.

You can insist on being consulted. Lay down the ground rules with your helpers early on. Ask to be presented with choices so that *you* can decide what is best for you. You should try to weigh carefully each suggestion made to you and avoid dismissing every suggestion made, out of hand. Your friends will then consider that you are able to make reasonable decisions and will continue to give you the opportunity to do so.

You should be appreciative. Recognise all the goodwill and efforts made by those who want to help. Even though you may sometimes be embarrassed, you will maintain your dignity by accepting the help you need with a good grace. If you are truly convinced that you are being offered help you don't need, then try to decline it with tact and appreciation. For example, you can say, *"I appreciate your offer to have my birthday party at your house, but I'd really like to have it here. I could do with some help, though, maybe with washing-up after the meal?"*

If you reach a point when you feel unable to come to terms with your increasing dependence on others, you should consult a professional counsellor. This should be someone who has experience. Someone who knows the emotional and social issues being faced by people like you, who have disabling health problems. Your local agency providing services to the disabled can refer you to the right kind of counsellor.

In addition, there is an organisation dedicated to serving people with your specific health condition. Organisations such as the *MS Society*, *Parkinson's UK*, *Diabetes UK* and the *British Heart Foundation*, can direct you to support groups and classes to help you in dealing with your condition. You should be able to locate the agency you need through the telephone book or Yellow Pages. Look under the listing for *Social Services and Welfare* organisations. You can also do some research on the Internet.

Gaining Help From Your Family

Rather similar to the fear and embarrassment of becoming physically dependent is the fear of being abandoned by family members who you might expect to provide needed help. Tales abound of being *dumped* in a nursing home by children who never come to visit. These stories haunt many people, who worry that this may happen to them. We need to reach out to family and friends and ask for help when we recognise that we can't go on alone. It sometimes happens that because they expect rejection, people often fail to ask for help. Some people try to hide their need because they think it will cause loved ones to withdraw. Families often complain *"If we'd only known . . ."* when it is revealed to them that a loved one had needs that were left unmet. If it really is the case that you cannot turn to close family or friends because they are unable or unwilling to become involved in your care, then there are agencies dedicated to deal with such situations. Through your local Social Services Department, you should be able to locate a *Case Manager* who will be able to organise the resources in your community to provide the help you need. The *Social Services Department* or *PALS* office in your local hospital can also put you in touch with the right agency.

Grieving: A Normal Reaction to Bad News

When we experience any kind of a loss, even small ones such as losing one's car keys or a letter, or big ones such as losing a life partner or facing a disabling or terminal illness, we go through an emotional process of grieving and coming to terms with the loss.

A person with a long-term, disabling health problem experiences a variety of losses. These include loss of confidence, loss of self-esteem, loss of independence, and the loss of a lifestyle we have known and cherished. Perhaps the most painful of all is the loss of a positive self-image, particularly if your condition has an effect on your appearance, as it often does in the case of rheumatoid arthritis and the residual paralysis following a stroke.

Elizabeth Kübler-Ross has written extensively about this process, and describes the stages of grief in these terms:

- *Shock:* When we feel both a mental and a physical reaction to the initial recognition of the loss.

- *Denial:* When you think, *"No, it can't be true,"* and then proceed for a time to act as if it were not true.

- *Anger:* When we angrily think *"Why me?"* and search for someone or something to blame. This leads to thoughts such as *"if only the doctor had diagnosed it earlier"* or *"if only my job hadn't caused me so much stress."*

- *Bargaining:* When we promise, *"I'll never smoke again,"* or *"I'll follow my treatment regime absolutely to the letter"* or *"I'll go to church every Sunday, if only I can get over this."*

- *Depression:* When awareness sets in and we confront the truth about the situation, and we experience deep feelings of sadness and hopelessness.

- *Acceptance:* When we recognise that we must deal with what has happened and make up our minds to do what we have to do.

We do not pass through these stages in a logical order. We are more likely to vacillate between them. Don't be discouraged if you find yourself angry or depressed again when you thought you had reached acceptance.

I'm Afraid of Death

Fear of death is something most of us begin to experience only when something happens to bring us face-to-face with the possibility of our own death. Losing someone close to us, having an accident that might have been fatal, or learning we have a health condition that may shorten our lives, usually causes us to consider the inevitability of our own eventual death. Many people, even then, try to avoid facing the future because they are afraid to think about it.

Our attitudes about death are shaped by our attitudes about life. This is the product of our culture, our family's influences, perhaps our religion, and certainly our life experiences.

If you are ready to think about your own future, particularly about the near or distant prospect that your life will certainly end at some time, then the ideas that follow will be useful to you. If you are not ready to think about it just yet, put this aside and come back to it later.

As with depression, the most useful way to come to terms with your eventual death is to take positive steps to prepare for it. This means *getting your house in order* by attending to all the necessary details, large and small. If you continue to avoid dealing with these details, you will create problems for yourself and for those involved with your situation. There are a number of components to getting your house in order. Consider the following:

■ *Decide and then convey to others your wishes about how and where you want to be during your last days and hours.* Do you want to be in a hospital or at home? When do you want procedures to prolong your life stopped? At what point do you want to let nature take its course when it is agreed that death is inevitable? Who should be with you? Will it only be the few people who are nearest and dearest to you or all the people you care about and want to see one last time?

■ *Make a will.* Even if your estate is a small one, you may have definite preferences about who should inherit what. If you have a large estate, the tax implications of a proper will may be significant. A will

also ensures that your belongings go where you would like them to go. Without a will, some distant or long-lost relative may end up with your entire estate.

■ *Plan your funeral.* Write down your wishes or actually make arrangements for your funeral and burial. Your grieving family will be very relieved not to have to decide what you would want and how much to spend. Prepaid funeral plans are available, and you can purchase your burial space in the location you approve.

■ *Draw up the documents which will give you control of what happens to you when you can no longer make those decisions for yourself.* There are four documents which you can consider:

  ◆ *Advance Decisions.*

  ◆ *Advance Statements.*

  ◆ *Lasting Power of Attorney (Property).*

  ◆ *Lasting Power of Attorney (Welfare).*

These are discussed later in this chapter. You should also talk over your wishes with your GP, even if he or she doesn't seem interested. Don't forget that your doctor may also have some trouble facing the prospect of losing you. Have a signed written document included in your medical records that indicates your wishes in case you can't communicate them when the time comes.

So What Next?

Be sure that those you want to handle things after your death are aware of all that they need to know about your wishes, your plans and arrangements, and also about the location of necessary documents. You will need to talk to them, or at least prepare a detailed letter of instructions. Give this to someone who can be counted on to deliver it to the right person at the appropriate time. This should be a person close enough to you to know when that time is at hand. You may not want your spouse to have to take on these responsibilities, but your spouse is certainly the best person to keep your letter and know when to give it to your designated agent.

You can keep copies of all your important papers, and information about your financial and personal affairs in a box and in a safe place. This is a handy, concise way of getting everything together that anyone might need to know about. Some of us keep these documents on our computers. If this is the case for you, then make sure the key people can find your passwords and accounts and that for safety reasons it is backed up on your system.

Finish your dealings with the world around you. Mend your relationships. Pay your debts, both financial and personal. Say what needs to be said to those who need to hear it. Do what needs to be done. Forgive yourself. Forgive others.

Talk about your feelings about your death. Most family and close friends are reluctant to initiate such a conversation but will appreciate it if you bring it up. You may find that there is much to say and much to hear from your loved ones. If you find that they are unwilling to listen to you talk about your death and the feelings that you are experiencing, then find someone else who will be comfortable and empathetic in listening to you. Your family and friends may be able to listen to you at a later stage. Remember, those who love you will also go through the grieving process when they have to think about the prospect of losing you.

A large component in the fear of death is fear of the unknown: *"What will it be like?" "Will it be painful?" "What will happen to me after I die?"*

Most people who die of a disease are ready to die when the time comes. Painkillers and the disease process itself will weaken the body and mind, and the awareness of self diminishes without the realisation that this is happening. Most people just *slip away*, with the transition between the state of *living* and that of *no longer living* being scarcely discernible. Reports from people who have been brought back to life after being in a state of clinical death indicate that they experienced a sense of peacefulness and clarity and were not frightened.

A dying person may sometimes feel lonely and abandoned. This is sometimes the result of the fact that many people cannot deal with their own emotions when they are around a person they know to be dying. Because of this they may deliberately avoid contact, or they may engage in superficial chit-chat, broken by long, awkward silences. This is often puzzling and hurtful to those who are dying, who really need companionship and solace from the people they count on.

You can sometimes help by telling your family and friends what you want and need from them. This may be attention, entertainment, comfort, or practical help. Certainly, a person who has something positive to *do* is more able to cope with difficult emotions. So, if you can engage your family and loved ones in specific activities, they will feel needed and be able to relate to you around the activity. This will give you something to talk about, to occupy time, or at least provide some definition of the situation for them and for you.

Palliative Care and Hospice Care

In most parts of the United Kingdom, as well as in many other parts of the world, both *palliative care* and *hospice care* are available. In everyone's life there comes a time when routine medical care is no longer helpful and we need to prepare for death. This preparation means that medical and other care is aimed at making the patient as comfortable as possible and providing the best possible quality of life. This is done by attempting to relieve pain and other distressing symptoms while providing psychological, social and spiritual support. Carers and family also receive the support they need at this time. Some people, because of their condition, may need treatments such as chemotherapy, radiotherapy or other interventions. Palliative care will make these processes more comfortable. Palliative care can take place in a number of locations:

■ *In a hospice*: Hospices can provide individual care more suited to the person in a calm and peaceful atmosphere. There is no charge for hospice care because they are voluntary organisations which raise their own funds. Referral however, must come from your doctor, hospital or district nurse.

■ *In your own home*: Your GP can arrange for community palliative care nurses, like Macmillan nurses, to support you in the best way possible. They are on call 24 hours a day.

■ *In a residential home*: If you are already in a residential home you may find it less distressing to receive any care you need in the home and not go into hospital or a hospice. Some residential homes are accredited by the end of life *Gold Standards Framework*, which means they have specially trained staff and good links with local GPs.

■ *As a day patient in a hospice*: This means you will get the care and support you need without moving away from your own home.

■ *As a day patient in a hospital*: Specialist palliative care teams are available in hospitals; they are sometimes known as the Macmillan Support Team. They can advise hospital staff on the best ways for control pain and recommend the most appropriate options for discharge.

One of the problems with hospice care is that often people wait until the last few days before death to ask for this care. They somehow see asking for hospice care as *giving up*. By refusing hospice care, they often put an unnecessary burden on themselves, their friends, and family. Often, the reverse is also true. Families frequently say they can cope without help. This may be true, but sometimes the patient's life and dying can be improved if the hospice cares for all the medical things and the family and friends are free to give their love and support.

Hospice care can be especially useful in the months before death. Most hospices will only accept people who are expected to die within six months. But, this does not mean that you will be asked to leave if you live longer. It is important to understand that if you, a family member, or a friend is in the end stage of illness, you can make use of your local hospice. It is a wonderful final gift.

Some patients may need support around the time of diagnosis of incurable disease, when a clinical nurse specialist is not available. The focus of palliative care is on patients with a short prognosis. However, it is recognised that there are *grey areas* and members of the team will be happy to discuss these situations where the prognosis is less than a year. Some patients who have progressive terminal disease with a longer prognosis than one year and also have complex needs, can turn to organisations like Macmillan to offer help and advice.

Making Your Wishes Official: Living Wills and Lasting Powers of Attorney

We now have a longer life expectancy than previous generations. So it has become more important and more relevant that we maintain some control over what happens to us in the years ahead. We might feel that some of the strategies which let us take more control suit our needs very well. Others may not be so appropriate and we will neither want nor choose to use them. The options we might want to use come under various headings:

- *A Living Will:* The term *living will* has no legal meaning but it can be used to refer to either an *Advance Decision* or an *Advance Statement.*

- *A Lasting Power of Attorney:* Again this has two types: one known as a *Lasting Power of Attorney (LPA) Property and Affairs* and the other is called a *Lasting Power of Attorney (LPA) Personal Welfare.* These Lasting Powers of Attorney have replaced the old *Enduring Power of Attorney.* The new rules have a much wider application than the old ones.

Most of us find legal documents and phraseology sometimes difficult to get our heads round, so let's examine those mentioned above in more detail. To add some further clarification look at *Figure 19.1* below:

Living Wills

First let's consider an *Advance Decision to Refuse Treatment.* What is this *Advance Decision?* Under normal circumstances you would discuss your

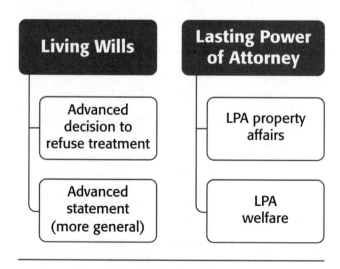

Figure 19.1 **Documents which Assist with Advance Planning**

treatment options with your doctor and reach an agreed decision about your care. There could however be situations when this is not possible: for example if you are unconscious when admitted to hospital or have had a stroke or are suffering from dementia. This situation is one where you are lacking the *mental capacity* to make an informed decision and communicate your wishes. Doctors have a legal and ethical duty to act in your best interests. An exception to this is if you have made an *Advance Decision* to refuse any treatment. If your Advance Decision is valid and applicable to the circumstances, even if your medical professionals feel it is not in your best interests, they are bound to follow your wishes as outlined in your *Advance Decision*. You cannot stipulate what treatment you want, only what treatment you would refuse. This document is legally binding.

You must be over 18 years old and have the mental capacity to make an advanced decision. In other words you must clearly understand the medical implications of your actions, including the fact that they may result in your death. It is clear that an *Advance Decision* is something that you should not make without careful consideration. It is one decision that you should discuss with someone you trust and who understands you. An *Advance Decision* can be cancelled at any time while you have the mental capacity to do so.

An *Advance Decision* cannot be used to stipulate anything illegal such as euthanasia or assisted suicide. It must make clear what type of treatment you wish to refuse – for example, refusing resuscitation in the case of cardiac arrest. Knowing what details to write is sometimes a little complicated. None of us can predict the future or knows the exact circumstances we will find ourselves in. You can get some idea by asking your doctor about the most likely developments for someone with your condition. This may help to guide you in what you want your *Advance Decision* to include. What follows now are some examples of situations you might find yourself in:

- *You have been diagnosed with Alzheimer's disease and other neurological problems that may eventually leave you with little or no mental function:* These are generally not life-threatening, at least not for many years. However, things happen to these patients that can be life-threatening, such as pneumonia and heart attacks. What you need to do is to decide how much treatment you want. For example, do you want antibiotics if you get pneumonia? Do you want to be resuscitated if your heart stops? Do you want a feeding tube if you are unable to feed yourself? Remember, it is your choice as to how you answer each of these questions. You may not want to be resuscitated but may want a feeding tube. If you want aggressive treatment, you may want to use all the means possible to sustain life; alternatively, you may not want any special means to be used to sustain your life. For example, you may want to be fed but may not want to be placed on life-support equipment.

- *You have very bad lung function that will not improve:* Should you become unable to breathe on your own, do you want to be placed in an intensive care unit on a mechanical ventilator? Remember, in this case you will not improve. To say that *you never want ventilation* is very different from saying that *you don't want it if it is used to sustain life when no improvement is likely.* Obviously, mechanical ventilation can be lifesaving in cases such as a severe asthma attack when it is used for a short time until the body can regain its normal function. Here the issue is not whether to use mechanical ventilation *ever* but rather when or under what circumstances you would wish it to be used.

- *You have a heart condition that cannot be improved with surgery:* You are in the cardiac intensive care unit. If your heart stops functioning, do you want to be resuscitated? As with artificial ventilation, the question is not *"Do you ever want to be resuscitated?"* but rather *"Under what conditions do you or do you not want resuscitation?"*

It is vitally important that a copy of your *Advance Decision* is in your hospital *and* in your GP notes. Making your wishes known about how you want to be treated in case of serious or life-threatening illness is one of the most important tasks of self-management. The best way to do this is to prepare an *Advance Decisions* for health care and share this with your family, close friends, and doctor. We have given detailed information on *Advance Decisions* because of the implications. The next section will give you some information on *Advance Statements* which also came under the heading of living wills.

An Advance Statement

An Advance Statement is also used when you are unable to communicate your wishes, but it is a more general statement about how you would like to be looked after. It includes non-medical issues which can include some of the activities of daily living; matters such as your preference for baths or showers or food likes and dislikes. It also takes into account who you would like to be involved when discussions about you need to be made so that you can have your wishes followed even when you are unable to communicate. This can be specified in a *Welfare Lasting Power of Attorney.* The Statement must be considered by those providing your treatment and deciding what is in your best interests but it is not legally binding.

Lasting Powers of Attorney

The earlier *Enduring Power of Attorney* was replaced by a new system called *Lasting Power of Attorney* because the Enduring Power of Attorney could only deal with financial matters. The new Lasting Power of Attorney can deal with both financial affairs and personal welfare. The new system has two separate documents:

1. *Property and Affairs (Lasting Power of Attorney):* This power of attorney allows you to appoint a legally authorised person to make decisions with regard to your property and financial affairs should you become incapable of doing so. It cannot be used until it has been registered with the *Office of the Public Guardian.* It can be registered any time after it has been made. It can also be cancelled at any time using a *Deed of Revocation*, if you have the mental capacity to do so.

2. *Welfare (Lasting Power of Attorney):* This power again allows you to appoint a legally authorised person to make decisions with regard to your personal welfare, including

whether to give consent or to refuse medical treatment, should you become incapable of doing so. This document is also subject to the rules of registration and revocation.

It is very important to note that a *Personal Welfare Power of Attorney* allows the person you have appointed to make decisions on your behalf about the right to refuse treatment. If after making a *Welfare LPA*, you make an *Advance Decision* about your treatment then this will negate the right of your attorney for your *LPA Welfare* to make decisions on refusal of treatment. The crucial element is that you made the *Advance Decision* after you signed the *LPA Welfare*. Any disagreements which arise about the *Advance Decision* are dealt with by the *Court of Protection*.

After reading the information and guidance provided in the last few pages, on different types of living wills and advance decisions, you may feel that the process is both complicated and off putting. If this is true in your case then you will be pleased to learn that there are several organisations that will be able to guide you through, notably *Age UK* who have produced a series of detailed leaflets on every aspect of this subject. Their contact details and references for the leaflets they produce can be found at the end of this chapter. Other organisations that provide similar information are *MIND*, the *Alzheimer's Society* and the *Patients Association*.

Talking about Your Wishes

Now you are ready to talk about your wishes. People frequently don't like to discuss their own death or that of a loved one. Therefore, it is not surprising that when you bring up this subject,

the response is often *"Oh, don't think about that"* or *"That's a long time off"* or *"Don't be so morbid; you're not that sick."* Unfortunately, this is usually enough to end the conversation. Your job, as a good self-manager, is to keep the conversation open. There are several ways to do this. First, plan on how you will have this discussion. Here are some suggestions:

- *Prepare your Advance Decision and then give copies to the appropriate family members or friends.* Ask them to read it and then set a specific time to discuss it. If your family give you one of the avoidance responses, explain that you understand that this is a difficult topic but that it is important to you that you discuss it with them. This is a good time to practise the "I" messages we discussed in Chapter 9, for example, say *"I understand that death is a difficult thing to talk about. However, it is very important to me that we have this discussion."*

- *When you go the hospital, make sure the hospital has a copy of your Advance Decision.* If you cannot bring it, be certain that your agent, your appointed person, knows about giving a copy to the hospital. This is important, as your own doctor may not be in charge of your care in the hospital.

- *There is one thing you should not do.* Do not put your *Advance Decision* in your safe deposit box. This is because no one will be able to get it when it is needed. Incidentally, you do not necessarily need to see a lawyer to draw up an *Advance Decision*. You can do this by yourself or with help from the relevant voluntary agencies.

Now that you have done all the important things, the hard work is over. However, remember that you can change your mind at any time. Also your agent may cease to be available, or your wishes might change. Be sure to keep your documents updated, in particular your *Advance Decision for health care*. Like any legal document, it can be revoked or changed at any time. The decisions you make today are not forever.

Suggested Further Reading

Atkinson, J. M. *Advance Directives in Mental Health: Theory, Practice and Ethics*. London: Jessica Kingsley Publishers, 2007.

Callahan, M. and Kelley, P. *Final Gifts: Understanding the Special Awareness, Needs, and Communications of the Dying*. New York: Bantam Books, 1997.

Carter, R. Lynn, J. and Harrold, J. *Handbook for Mortals: Guidance for People Facing Serious Illness*. Oxford: Oxford University Press, 2001.

Smith, S. W. *End of Life Decisions in Medical Care: Principles and Policies for Regulating the Dying Process*. Cambridge: Cambridge University Press, 2012.

Stolp, H. *When a Loved One Dies: How to Go On After Saying Goodbye*. Hampshire, England: O Books 2005.

Other Resources

☐ *Age UK:* This website has many useful pamphlets which you can download on all the topics covered in this chapter. Tel: 0800 169 6565. www.ageuk.org.uk.

☐ *Alzheimer's Society.* Tel: 0300 222 1122 ask for Factsheet 463. www.alzheimers.org.uk.

☐ *The National Council for Palliative Care:* This is an umbrella organisation for all those involved in palliative, end of life, and hospice care in England, Northern Ireland, and Wales. www.ncpc.org.uk.

☐ *NHS:* This website offers advice and information about the payment charges for residential care where the NHS may make some or all of the contributions. www.nhs.uk/carersdirect/guide/praticalsupport/pages/chargingforresidentialcare.

☐ *The Patients Association.* Tel: 0845 608 4455. www.patients-association.org.uk.

☐ *MIND:* This organisation provides information and support to empower anyone experiencing a mental health problem. Tel: 0300 123 3393. www.mind.org.uk.

Index

Note: Page numbers followed by *b, c, f* and *t* refer to text boxes, charts, figures and tables, respectively.